PROGRESS IN BRAIN RESEARCH

VOLUME 59

IMMUNOLOGY OF NERVOUS SYSTEM INFECTIONS

Recent volumes in PROGRESS IN BRAIN RESEARCH

PROGRESS IN BRAIN RESEARCH

VOLUME 59

IMMUNOLOGY OF NERVOUS SYSTEM INFECTIONS

EDITED BY

P.O. BEHAN, V. TER MEULEN and F. CLIFFORD ROSE

Department of Neurology, Glasgow University, Glasgow, Scotland, U.K.
Institute for Virology and Immunobiology, University of Würzburg, Würzburg, F.R.G.
and
Department of Neurology, Charing Cross Hospital, London, U.K.

Proceedings of the Noble Bodman Symposium on Immunological Aspects of Acute and Chronic Nervous Disorders,
London, U.K., 12-13 November, 1981

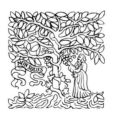

ELSEVIER
AMSTERDAM/NEW YORK/OXFORD
1983

PUBLISHED BY:
ELSEVIER SCIENCE PUBLISHERS B.V.
1 MOLENWERF, P.O. BOX 211
AMSTERDAM, THE NETHERLANDS

SOLE DISTRIBUTORS FROM THE U.S.A. AND CANADA:
ELSEVIER SCIENCE PUBLISHING COMPANY INC.
52 VANDERBILT AVENUE
NEW YORK, NY 10017, U.S.A.

ISBN FOR THE SERIES 0-444-80-104-9
ISBN FOR THE VOLUME 0-444-80-443-9

WITH 117 ILLUSTRATIONS AND 92 TABLES

PRINTED IN BELGIUM

List of Contributors

P. Aasjord, Department of Microbiology and Immunology, The Gade Institute, University of Bergen, Bergen, Norway

A.M. Abdelnoor, Department of Microbiology, Faculty of Medicine, American University of Beirut, Beirut, Lebanon

W. Al Kadiry, Department of Immunopathology, St. Mary's Hospital Medical School, London W2 IPG, U.K.

G. Allsopp, Department of Pathology, Royal College of Surgeons of England, Lincoln's Inn Fields, London WC2A 3PN, U.K.

R.M. Barlow, Moredun Research Institute, Edinburgh EH17 7JH, Scotland, U.K.

P.O. Behan, Department of Neurology, Glasgow University, Glasgow, Scotland, U.K.

W.M.H. Behan, Department of Pathology, Glasgow University, Glasgow, Scotland, U.K.

H. Bernheimer, Neurologisches Institut der Universität Wien, Schwarzspanierstrasse 17, A-1090 Vienna, Austria

E.L. Berrie, Department of Microbiology, University of Bristol, Bristol, U.K.

W.A. Blyth, Department of Microbiology, University of Bristol, Bristol, U.K.

D. Brigden, The Wellcome Research Laboratories, Beckenham, Kent BR3 3BS, U.K.

F. Brown, The Animal Virus Research Institute, Pirbright, Woking, Surrey GU24 ONF, U.K.

M.E. Bruce, ARC and MRC Neuropathogenesis Unit, West Mains Road, Edinburgh EH9 3JQ, Scotland, U.K.

R. Capildeo, Department of Neurology, Charing Cross Hospital, Fulham Palace Road, London W6 8RF, U.K.

M.J. Carter, Institute for Virology and Immunobiology, University of Würzburg, Versbacherstrasse 7, D-8700 Würzburg, F.R.G.

A.K.R. Chaudhuri, Monklands District General Hospital, Airdrie, Lanarkshire, Scotland, U.K.

G.B. Clements, Institute of Virology, Church Street, Glasgow G11 5JR, Scotland, U.K.

A.M. Denman, Connective Tissue Diseases Research Group, Clinical Research Centre, Harrow, Middlesex, U.K.

S.S. Dhib-Jalbut, Department of Medicine, Faculty of Medicine, American University of Beirut, Beirut, Lebanon

M. Egghart, Neurologisches Institut der Universität Wien, Schwarzspanierstrasse 17, A-1090 Vienna, Austria

R.L. Epstein, Department of Neuroscience, Children's Hospital Medical Center and Department of Medicine, Sections of Neurology and Infectious Diseases, Brigham and Women's Hospital, Boston, MA 02115, U.S.A.

M.M. Esiri, Department of Neuropathology, Radcliffe Infirmary, Oxford, U.K.

J.O. Fleming, University of Southern California, School of Medicine, 2025 Zonal Ave, Los Angeles, CA 90033, U.S.A.

A. Fontana, Department of Neuroscience, Children's Hospital Medical Center and Department of Medicine, Sections of Neurology and Infectious Diseases, Brigham and Women's Hospital, Boston, MA 02115, U.S.A.

P. Forsberg, Department of Infectious Diseases, University Hospital, S-581 85 Linköping, Sweden

H. Fraser, ARC and MRC Neuropathogenesis Unit, West Mains Road, Edinburgh, EH9 3JQ, Scotland, U.K.

D.S. Freestone, The Wellcome Research Laboratories, Beckenham, Kent BR3 3BS, U.K.

K. Frese, Institut für Virologie und Veterinär Pathologie, Justus-Liebig Universität Giessen, D-6300 Giessen, F.R.G.

R.S. Fujinami, Scripps Clinic and Research Foundation, Department of Immunopathology, 10666 N. Torrey Pines Road, La Jolla, CA 92037, U.S.A.

R.G. Gold, Department of Immunopathology, St. Mary's Hospital Medical School, London W2 IPG, U.K.

D.E. Griffin, Howard Hughes Medical Institute, Departments of Medicine and Neurology, Baltimore, MD 21205, U.S.A.

F.S. Haddad, Department of Surgery, Faculty of Medicine, American University of Beirut, Beirut, Lebanon

D.A. Harbour, Department of Microbiology, University of Bristol, Bristol, U.K.

S.L. Hauser, Department of Medicine, Section of Neurology, Brigham and Women's Hospital, Boston, MA 02115, U.S.A.

A. Henriksson, Department of Neurology, University Hospital, S-581 85 Linköping, Sweden

T.J. Hill, Department of Microbiology, University of Bristol, Bristol, U.K.

R.L. Hirsch, Department of Neurology, The Johns Hopkins University School of Medicine, Baltimore, MD 21205, U.S.A.

S.J. Illavia, Neurovirology Unit, Department of Neurology, The Rayne Institute, St. Thomas' Hospital, London SE1 7EH, U.K.

R. Jones, Department of Neurology, Charing Cross Hospital, Fulham Palace Road, London W6 8RF, U.K.

S. Kam-Hansen, Department of Neurology, Karolinska Institutet, Huddinge University Hospital, S-141 86 Huddinge, Stockholm, Sweden

K. Kitz, Neurologisches Institut der Universität Wien, Schwarzspanierstrasse 17, A-1090 Vienna, Austria

J.A. Kirby, Department of Biology, University of York, Heslington, York YO1 5DD, U.K.

S.C. Knight, Clinical Research Centre, Watford Road, Harrow, Middlesex HA1 3UJ, U.K.

M. Koga, Institute for Virology and Immunobiology, University of Würzburg, Versbacherstrasse 17, D-8700 Würzburg, F.R.G.

H. Lassmann, Neurologisches Institut der Universität Wien, Schwarzspanierstrasse 17, A-1090 Vienna, Austria

H. Link, Department of Neurology, Karolinska Institutet, Huddinge University Hospital, S-141 86 Huddinge, Stockholm, Sweden

C. Love, Department of Infectious Diseases, Ruchill Hospital, Glasgow, Scotland, U.K.

N.P. Luckman, Department of Neurology, Charing Cross Hospital, Fulham Palace Road, London W6 8RF, U.K.

J. Mertin, Clinical Research Center, Watford Road, Harrow, Middlesex, HA1 3UJ, U.K.

F. Mokhtarian, Department of Neurology, The Johns Hopkins University School of Medicine, Baltimore, MD 21205, U.S.A.

J.F. Mowbray, Department of Immunopathology, St. Mary's Hospital Medical School, London W2 IPG, U.K.

W.H. Murphy, The Department of Microbiology and Immunology, The University of Michigan School of Medicine, Ann Arbor, MI 48109, U.S.A.

O. Narayan, Department of Neurology and Comparative Medicine, Johns Hopkins School of Medicine, Baltimore, MD 21205, U.S.A.

A.A. Nash, Department of Pathology, University of Cambridge, Tennis Court Road, Cambridge, U.K.

J.F. Nawrocki, The Department of Microbiology and Immunology, The University of Michigan School of Medicine, Ann Arbor, MI 48109, U.S.A.

H. Nyland, Department of Neurology, Broegelmann Research Laboratory for Microbiology, The Gade Institute, University of Bergen, Norway

M.B.A. Oldstone, Scripps Clinic and Research Foundation, Department of Immunopathology, 10666 N. Torrey Pines Road, La Jolla, CA 92037, U.S.A.

M.M. Park, Department of Neurology, The Johns Hopkins School of Medicine, Baltimore, MD 21205, U.S.A.

S. Pathak, Neurovirology Unit, Department of Neurology, The Rayne Institute, St. Thomas' Hospital, London SE1 7EH, U.K.

L.R. Pease, The Department of Microbiology and Immunology, The University of Michigan School of Medicine, Ann Arbor, MI 48109, U.S.A.

M.L. Powers, Department of Neuroscience, Children's Hospital Medical Center and Department of Medicine, Sections of Neurology and Infectious Diseases, Brigham and Women's Hospital, Boston, MA 02115, U.S.A.

A. Preece, Department of Neurology, Charing Cross Hospital, Fulham Palace Road, London W6 8RF, U.K.

A.B. Rickinson, Department of Pathology, University of Bristol, The Medical School, Bristol BS8 1TD, U.K.

F. Clifford Rose, Department of Neurology, Charing Cross Hospital, Fulham Palace Road, London W6 8RF, U.K.

R. Rott, Institut für Virologie und Veterinär-Pathologie, Justus-Liebig Universität Giessen, D-6300 Giessen, F.R.G.

M.G. Rumsby, Department of Biology, University of York, Heslington, York YO1 5DD, U.K.

W.C. Russell, Division of Virology, National Institute for Medical Research, Mill Hill, London NW7 1AA, U.K.

L. Saland, Departments of Medicine, Microbiology and Anatomy, University of New Mexico, Albuquerque, NM 87131, U.S.A.

B. Schwerer, Neurologisches Institut der Universität Wien, Schwarzspanierstrasse 17, A-1090 Vienna, Austria

M. Siegert, Kinderklinik der Freien Universität, Berlin, F.R.G.

H. Siemes, Westfälische Landeskinderklinik-Universitätsklinik, Alexandrinenstrasse 5, 4630 Bochum, F.R.G.

A.J. Steck, Department of Neurology, Centre Hospitalier Vaudois, 1011 Lausanne, Switzerland

J.H. Subak-Sharpe, Institute of Virology, Church Street, Glasgow G11 5JR, Scotland, U.K.

A.J. Suckling, Department of Biology, University of York, Heslington, York YO1 5DD, U.K.

H.K. Tamer, Department of Microbiology, Faculty of Medicine, American University of Beirut, Beirut, Lebanon

M. Tardieu, Department of Neuroscience, Children's Hospital Medical Center and Department of Medicine, Sections of Neurology and Infectious Diseases, Brigham and Women's Hospital, Boston, MA 02115, U.S.A.

C. Taylor, Departments of Medicine, Microbiology and Anatomy, University of New Mexico, Albuquerque, NM 87131, U.S.A.

V. Ter Meulen, Institute for Virology and Immunobiology, University of Würzburg, Versbacherstrasse 7, D-8700 Würzburg, F.R.G.

E.J. Thompson, The Institute of Neurology, The National Hospital, Queen Square, London WCIN 3BG, U.K.

A.B. Tullo, Department of Microbiology, University of Bristol, Bristol, U.K.

J.L. Turk, Department of Pathology, Royal College of Surgeons of England, Lincoln's Inn Fields, London WC2A 3PN, U.K.

D.E. Van Epps, Departments of Medicine, Microbiology and Anatomy, University of New Mexico, Albuquerque, NM 87131, U.S.A.

M. Vandevelde, Institute of Comparative Neurology, University of Berne, Berne, Switzerland

J. Veitch, University of Glasgow, Department of Pathology, Western Infirmary, Glasgow G11 6NT, Scotland, U.K.

R.W.H. Walker, The Institute of Neurology, The National Hospital, Queen Square, London WC1N 3BG, U.K.

R. Watanabe, Institute for Virology and Immunobiology, University of Würzburg, Versbacherstrasse 7, D-8700 Würzburg, F.R.G.

H.E. Webb, Neurovirology Unit, Department of Neurology, The Rayne Institute, St. Thomas' Hospital, London SE1 7EH, U.K.

A.D.B Webster, Clinical Research Centre, Harrow, Middlesex, U.K.

H. Wege, Institute for Virology and Immunobiology, University of Würzburg, Versbacherstrasse 7, D-8700 Würzburg, F.R.G.

H.L. Weiner, Department of Neuroscience, Children's Hospital Medical Center, Boston, MA 02115, U.S.A.

L.P. Weiner, University of Southern California, School of Medicine, 2025 Zonal Ave, Los Angeles, CA 90033, U.S.A.

K. Whaley, University of Glasgow, Department of Pathology, Glasgow G11 6NT, Scotland, U.K.

R.C. Williams, Jr., Departments of Medicine, Microbiology and Anatomy, University of New Mexico, Albuquerque, NM 87131, U.S.A.

Preface

One of the most important questions in neurology is that of the differing contributions of infection and immunity to the production of disease. The central nature of this question becomes obvious when it is realized how little we understand of the mechanisms by which infection initiates acute or chronic disorders of the central nervous system. It has become clear, however, that in some of these illnesses, the main damage to the tissues is brought about by diverse immunological effects. Knowledge of the precise role of immune factors, and how they may be related to viruses and other agents, is essential for the development of rational modes of therapy. This work brings together a variety of specialists from neurology, immunology, virology and the veterinary sciences, in an attempt to answer the questions raised. The relationship between infection and immunology in the nervous system is discussed fully. The work will appeal to clinicians and laboratory workers who wish to know more of this rapidly developing area, and will be of use to both established investigators and newcomers to the field.

Acknowledgements

We are grateful to the trustees of the Andrew Noble and Lee Bodman Fund for their financial assistance, and to the Medical Society of London for their hospitality in holding the Symposium at Lettsom House.

Contents

xiv

Immunology of Nervous System Infections, Progress in Brain Research, Vol. 59, edited by P.O. Behan, V. ter Meulen and F. Clifford Rose
© *1983 Elsevier Science Publishers B.V.*

A Molecular Approach to the Diagnosis of Virus Infections

F. BROWN

The Animal Virus Research Institute, Pirbright, Woking, Surrey GU24 ONF (U.K.)

INTRODUCTION

Virus diseases are traditionally diagnosed by serological methods and diagnostic laboratories possess large collections of antisera and antigens which have been prepared over many years as new aetiologic agents have been recognized. Many different serological methods have been developed, and with the introduction of reagents labeled with either radioactivity, enzymes or fluorescent chemicals, their sensitivity is now very high. For example, as little as 1 ng/ml of a virus or virus protein can be detected by both radioimmune assay (RIA) or enzyme-linked immunosorbent assay (ELISA). The use of labeled reagents also means that viruses and virus antigens can often be identified in situ without extracting them from the infected tissues.

While conventional serology has played, still plays and will continue to play, a very important role in diagnosis, the specificity of the reactions is limited by the number of antigenic sites which may be present on a virus. Thus conventional serology places Coxsackie B5 virus of man and swine vesicular disease virus (which cause different diseases in the two species) in the same group and does not readily differentiate between them, although competition RIA or ELISA tests will do this.

The advent of monoclonal antibodies has provided a new dimension in serology since each antibody reacts with only one antigenic site. The pioneering work of Gerhard, Koprowski and their colleagues (see review by Koprowski et al., 1980) with influenza and rabies viruses provides excellent examples of the great potential of these reagents for the refined analysis of closely related virus strains, and there is no doubt that there will be considerable activity in this area of virology during the next few years.

The increasing information that is becoming available on the physical and chemical properties of viruses and the rapid advances made in the methods used for the examination of nucleic acids and proteins provide alternative techniques whereby the identity of viruses can be determined with great precision. The purpose of this article is to outline these methods and provide some examples of their application. Most of the examples in this chapter are taken from the field of veterinary medicine where one is faced not only with a wide spectrum of diseases but also with a wide variety of animal species. The methods described, however, are equally applicable to the study of viruses isolated from man and are being applied increasingly in medical and public health laboratories.

While the methods have been used principally for the identification of viruses in acute infections, some of them have obvious application to the study of neurological disorders caused by viruses. In the last decade several chronic degenerative disease states of the CNS have been shown to be associated with specific viruses and these findings have given rise to the concept that viruses may be involved in a wide variety of such diseases. This has stimulated much work on the application of physico-chemical methods for the detection of viruses in these conditions. The method of in situ nucleic acid hybridization in particular has been singled out for its applicability to the examination of these diseases. While it is still too early to know whether this method will find widespread application, it is probably the most sensitive virus detection method available. Evidence of virus infection may be found by hybridization even when it cannot be obtained by the most sophisticated serological techniques (Kohne et al., 1981).

PROPERTIES OF VIRUS PARTICLES

Those virologists interested in the classification and taxonomy of viruses recognized more than 30 years ago that the properties of the virus particles themselves would be of more relevance in their identification than the description of the diseases they caused. This is accepted now with hardly any dissent. More recently, the veritable explosion in our knowledge of the chemistry of viruses has provided a framework of more than 50 virus families within which most of the known viruses can be fitted. This classification work has been a valuable contribution to virology and has obvious value in characterizing new viruses.

Early attempts at virus classification included a cryptogram, proposed by Wildy and his colleagues (Gibbs et al., 1966) which included 6 physicochemical properties which they considered to be the most important at that time. These were: (1) the nature of the nucleic acid, i.e. DNA or RNA; (2) its strandedness i.e. single or double; (3) the molecular weight of the nucleic acid; (4) the percentage of the nucleic acid in the virus particle; (5) the symmetry of the virus particle; and (6) the symmetry of the nucleocapsid. Although our knowledge has increased greatly since that time, probably the most important additional properties which can contribute to classification are morphology, the presence or absence of a lipid coat and, for the RNA viruses, the number of segments in the genome. DNA viruses do not have segmented genomes.

Morphology

The advent of the electron microscope and the discovery of negative staining added a completely new dimension to virology and paved the way to an understanding of virus structure. The dissection of virus particles into subunits, some of them biologically active, has given us an insight into the organization of virus particles which would otherwise have been unobtainable. Additional information can also be obtained by combining electron microscopy with serology (Fig. 1).

Effect of lipid solvents

The differential effect of lipid solvents and mild detergents on virus particles has for many years provided a very powerful tool for characterizing viruses. The group which is labile in lipid solvents contains an outer membrane consisting of lipoprotein, derived from the host cell. Removal of the membrane and outer coat with lipid solvents renders the virus non-infections. Naked virus particles are unaffected by lipid solvents.

VIRUS   VIRUS+IgM

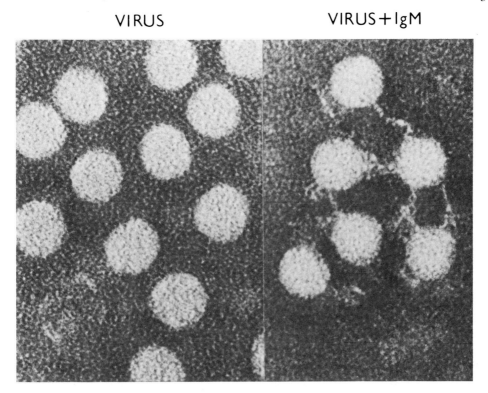

VIRUS+IgG

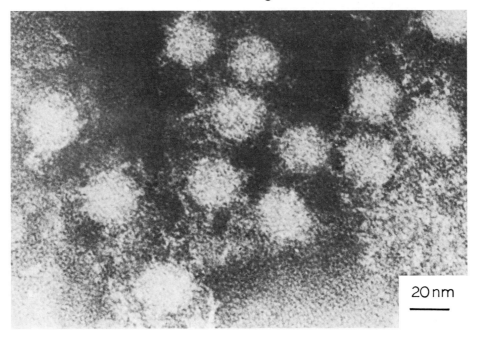

20 nm

Fig. 1. Immune complexing of foot-and-mouth disease virus with the type specific IgM and IgG.

4

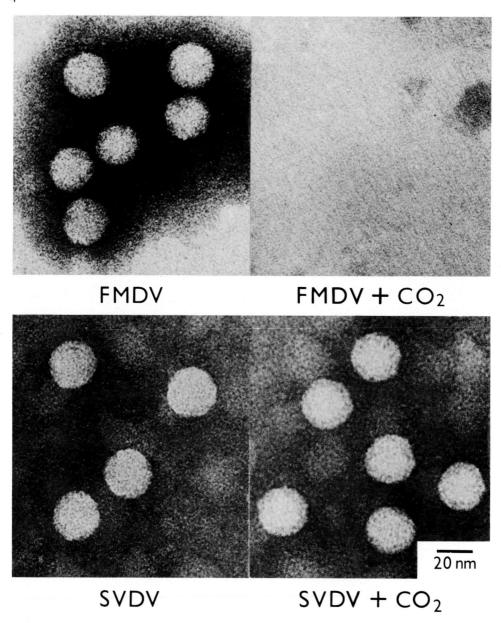

FMDV   FMDV + CO₂

SVDV   SVDV + CO₂

Fig. 2. Effect of carbon dioxide on the morphology of the acid-labile foot-and-mouth disease virus and acid-stable swine vesicular disease virus.

Other properties

The effect of pH has proved to be very useful in the differentiation of the picornaviruses. Members of this family of viruses contain one molecule of ssRNA, molecule weight 2.5×10^6 and 60 copies of each of 4 proteins. Three of the proteins have molecular weights of approximately 25×10^3 and one has a molecular weight of approximately 10×10^3. All the picornaviruses look alike in the electron microscope, but enteroviruses (e.g. poliovirus) can be distinguished from, for example, foot-and-mouth disease virus, by their much greater stability below pH 7. Enteroviruses are stable, even at pH 3, whereas foot-and-mouth disease virus disintegrates below pH 7. This difference in stability proved to be extremely valuable in showing that a virus causing a foot-and-mouth disease-like illness in pigs belonged to the acid-stable enterovirus group (Fig. 2, Nardelli et al., 1968).

Measuring virus density in caesium chloride is also of diagnostic value within the picornavirus family. Thus the enteroviruses (polio, Coxsackie, ECHO) and cardioviruses (encephalomyocarditis, Maus Elberfeld, Mengo) have a density of 1.34 g/ml, whereas the human rhinoviruses and foot-and-mouth disease viruses have densities of 1.40 and 1.43 g/ml respectively (Table I). The density can be correlated with the stability of the virus below pH 7: those with the higher density are more porous, allowing the caesium ions to penetrate the particles to react with the RNA, and the RNA-protein and protein–protein bonds are more easily broken.

TABLE I

BUOYANT DENSITY OF THE DIFFERENT GENERA OF PICORNAVIRUSES AND THE BASE COMPOSITION OF THEIR RNAs

Genus	Buoyant density in CsCl (g/ml)	Base composition (%)			
		Adenylic acid	Cytidylic acid	Guanylic acid	Uridylic acid
Entero	1.34	29	23	24	24
Cardio	1.34	26	25	24	25
Human rhino	1.40	34	20	19	27
Aphtho (foot-and-mouth disease)	1.43	26	28	24	22
Equine rhino	1.45	26	24	23	27

PROPERTIES OF THE VIRUS NUCLEIC ACID

The advances made during the last 3 decades in improving methods for extracting nucleic acids from tissues and subsequently analyzing them have been applied to the study of many viruses. Even the most fundamental property of nucleic acids, the sequence of their bases, has been determined for a few viruses, e.g. poliovirus RNA (Kitamura et al., 1981; Racaniello and Baltimore, 1981) and many more will become available within the next few years. It is not envisaged, however, that this degree of sophistication will be required for the identification of viruses because many other properties, requiring much less effort, are available for this purpose.

IN RNA VIRUSES

RNA viruses contain either single-stranded or double-stranded RNA and the genome can occur as one molecule or in segments. In viruses containing segmented genomes the number of segments can vary from two single-stranded species (e.g. Nodamura virus which is found in mosquitoes) to 11 double-stranded species (rotaviruses which are important causal agents of diarrhoea in young animals and children). The RNAs have been analyzed by several different methods.

Rate of sedimentation and mobility of RNA in polyacrylamide gels

These two properties are related in that the RNAs with the greater sedimentation coefficients travel more slowly through polyacrylamide gels. In recent years, polyacrylamide gel electrophoresis has been used increasingly because of its greater resolving power and it provides a valuable diagnostic tool, particularly for the viruses with segmented genomes. For example, the influenza virus genome occurs as 8 pieces of single-stranded RNA and the mobility of the different segments can be used to distinguish between isolates. Although there are potential pitfalls which must be considered, such as a change in mobility which may reflect only minor differences in nucleotide sequence, this type of analysis is extremely valuable for the rapid comparison of isolates (Palese and Schulman, 1976). A similar approach has been made in studying the epidemiology of the rota and bluetongue viruses which contain segmented double-stranded RNA genomes (Kalica et al., 1978; Gorman, 1979).

Base composition

This measures the proportion of each of the nucleotides, adenylic, cytidylic, guanylic and uridylic acid and is useful in providing basic information on individual viruses. It has allowed the subdivision of the picornaviruses into 4 genera, the enteroviruses, cardioviruses, rhinoviruses and aphthoviruses, each having a different base composition (Table I, Newman et al., 1973). It has also allowed the so-called equine rhinoviruses to be clearly differentiated from the rhinoviruses infecting man and correlates observations regarding their widely differing densities in caesium chloride.

Base sequence homology

A much more stringent comparison of the nucleic acids of different virus isolates can be made by estimating the extent of their homology. Thus the different serotypes of poliovirus, which have the same base composition, have sequences which are about 50% homologous. A similar degree of hybridization has been found between the different serotypes of foot-and-mouth disease virus. Different isolates belonging to the same serotype exhibit approximately 70–80% homology.

This type of test proved extremely valuable in establishing that a virus with the same morphology as the caliciviruses (Fig. 3), which was found in aborting sea lions, is more closely related to vesicular exanthema virus than to feline calicivirus. The sea lion virus could not be established as belonging to either the feline or swine virus group by serological methods. Moreover, the base composition of all 3 viruses is similar, but by the use of hybridization methods it was found that the sea lion virus was closely related to vesicular exanthema virus and could be regarded as another serotype of that group of viruses (Burroughs et al., 1979). Subsequent work has shown that there are at least 10 serotypes of the sea lion virus, the multiplicity of serotypes being similar to that found with the vesicular exanthema virus group.

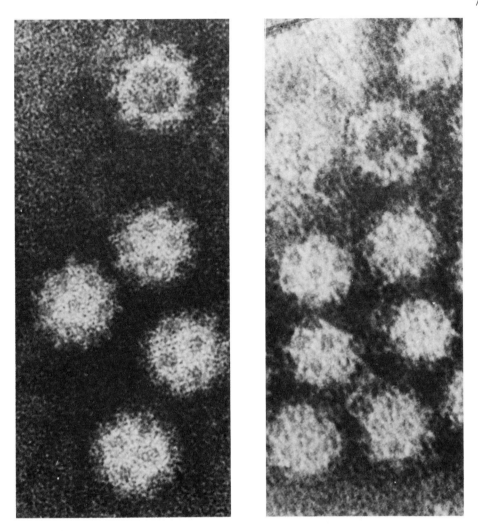

Fig. 3. Electron micrographs of vesicular exanthema virus and feline calicivirus showing their indistinguishable morphology.

Fingerprinting of ribonuclease T1 oligonucleotides

In this method, which has added a new dimension to the identification of RNA viruses, the RNA is cut at guanylic acid residues with the enzyme and the resulting mixture of oligonucleotides is separated in two dimensions, one separation depending on the charge of the oligonucleotides and the second on their size (de Wachter and Fiers, 1972). Each RNA gives its own distinctive pattern and even closely related strains of a particular virus can be distinguished by this method. Its value in epidemiological studies was clearly demonstrated in recent outbreaks of foot-and-mouth disease in the United Kingdom, when it was possible to relate them unequivocally to similar outbreaks in France (King et al., 1981, Fig. 4).

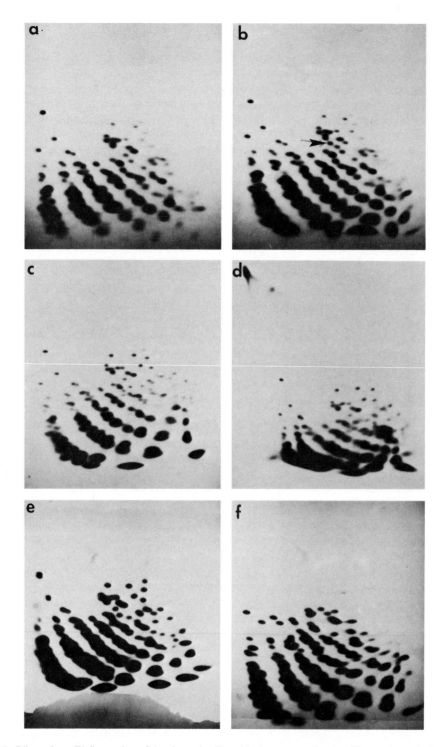

Fig. 4. Ribonuclease T1 fingerprints of the viruses implicated in the recent outbreaks of foot-and-mouth disease in France and the U.K.. The maps in a (Brittany), b (Jersey), d (Lausanne), and e (Isle of Wight) are indistinguishable apart from one spot (shown arrowed) in the Jersey map. The map in c of a mixture of a and d has no extra spots, providing evidence that the maps (and hence the RNAs) are indistinguishable. The map in panel f of a foot-and-mouth disease virus isolated in Austria in 1981 is included to show the difference between the maps of the related viruses and a virus unconnected with the outbreak.

IN DNA VIRUSES

The genome in DNA viruses is either single- or double-stranded, but no DNA virus with a segmented genome has been described so far. As with the RNA viruses, homology tests have been valuable for determining relationships between viruses. In addition, the density of the virus DNA can be correlated with its content of deoxyguanylic and deoxycytidylic acids (GC content), thus allowing a rapid method for its identification.

By far the most important method for the rapid analysis of DNA molecules, however, has come from the use of restriction enzymes. These enzymes cleave double-stranded DNA molecules at specific nucleotide sequences so that a relatively small number of fragments are then separated according to their size by gel electrophoresis. By using enzymes with different specificities it is possible to construct maps so that a very precise comparison of different DNAs can be made. This method has been applied to studies of pox viruses (Esposito et al., 1978) and herpes viruses (Buchman et al., 1978) and will no doubt be applied to many other groups.

VIRUS PROTEINS

Proteins can be analyzed by a variety of methods and these have been applied widely to virus proteins during the last decade. Separation of the proteins according to their size by polyacrylamide gel electrophoresis is one of the most frequently used techniques in biochemical virology and the original paper (Shapiro et al., 1967) is one of the most frequently quoted. It is interesting that the proteins of different isolates of the same virus often give different patterns of separation. We provided an example of this with different isolates of Coxsackie B5 and swine vesicular disease viruses (Harris and Brown, 1975). The method can also be applied to an examination of the virus-specific proteins in the infected cell and this approach has been used by Bedson and his colleagues in a study of pox viruses (Harper et al., 1979).

Virus structural and induced proteins can also be examined by iso-electric focusing in polyacrylamide gels. This separation method depends on the difference in charge of the proteins and has been used, for example, to distinguish between closely related strains of foot-and-mouth disease virus in the recent outbreaks in France and the United Kingdom (King et al., 1981).

A more precise identification of virus proteins can be achieved by examining the products obtained by hydrolysis with various proteolytic enzymes. Trypsin has been the enzyme most frequently used for this purpose. Cleavage occurs at arginine and lysine residues and the products of hydrolysis, which are different for each protein, can be separated by a combination of electrophoresis and chromatography or by ion exchange chromatography.

CONCLUSIONS

The biochemical study of viruses has had an important spin-off in diagnostic virology. Unlike serological methods, which only measure antigenic sites, biochemical analyses provide a picture of the entire genome. By using the methods described in this paper a much more precise identification of viruses can be achieved. The term 'fingerprinting', which has been applied to both ribonuclease T1 mapping of RNAs and tryptic peptide analysis of proteins is an apt one. Such have been the advances in biochemical technology that even these methods, with their apparently high degree of resolution, can be performed quickly and simply. Their use has, in general, been restricted to problems where large amounts of virus were available for analysis, but their application to the study of more difficult questions such as the identification of those agents causing unresolved or chronic infections is already in progress and should provide valuable information within the next few years.

ACKNOWLEDGEMENTS

I wish to thank Miss Joan Crick for valuable discussion, Mrs. P. Thomas for considerable help with the preparation of the manuscript and Mr. C.J. Smale for the micrographs.

REFERENCES

Buchman, T.G., Roizman, B., Adams, G. and Stover, B.H. (1978) Restriction endonuclease fingerprinting of herpes simplex DNA: a novel epidemiological tool applied to a nosocomial outbreak. *J. infect. Dis.*, 138: 488–498.

Burroughs, N., Doel, T. and Brown, F. (1979) Relationship of San Miguel sea lion virus to other members of the calicivirus group. *Intervirology*, 10: 51–59.

De Wachter, R. and Fiers, W. (1972) Preparative two-dimensional polyacrylamide gel electrophoresis of ^{32}P-labeled RNA. *Analyt. Biochem.*, 49: 184–197.

Esposito, J.J., Obijeski, J.F. and Nakano, J.H. (1978) Orthopoxvirus DNA: strain differentiation by electrophoresis of restriction endonuclease fragmented virus DNA. *Virology*, 89: 53–66.

Gibbs, A.J., Harrison, B.D., Watson, D.H. and Wildy, P. (1966) What's in a virus name? *Nature (Lond.)*, 209: 450–454.

Gorman, B.M. (1979) Variation in orbiviruses. *J. gen. Virol.*, 44: 1–15.

Harper, L., Bedson, H.S. and Buchan, A. (1979) Identification of orthopoxviruses by polyacrylamide gel electrophoresis of intracellular polypeptides. 1. Four major groupings. *Virology*, 93: 435–444.

Harris, T.J.R. and Brown, F. (1975) Correlation of polypeptide composition with antigenic variation in the swine vesicular disease and Coxsackie B5 viruses. *Nature (Lond.)*, 258: 758–760.

Kalica, A.R., Sereno, M.M., Wyatt, R.G., Mebus, C.A., Chanock, R.M. and Kapikian, A.Z. (1978) Comparison of human and animal rotavirus strains by gel electrophoresis of viral RNA. *Virology*, 87: 247–255.

King, A.M.Q., Underwood, B.O., McCahon, D., Newman, J.W.I. and Brown, F. (1981) Biochemical identification of viruses causing the 1981 outbreaks of foot-and-mouth disease in the United Kingdom. *Nature (Lond.)*, 293: 479–480.

Kitamura, N., Semler, B.L., Rothberg, P.G., Larsen, G.R., Adler, C.J., Dorner, A.J., Emini, E.A., Hanecak, R., Lee, J.J., van der Werf, S., Anderson, C.W. and Wimmer, E. (1981) Primary structure, gene organization and polypeptide expression of poliovirus RNA. *Nature (Lond.)*, 291: 547–553.

Kohne, D.E., Gibbs, C.J., White, L., Tracy, S.M., Meinke, W. and Smith, R.A. (1981) Virus detection by nucleic acid hybridisation: examination of normal and ALS tissues in the presence of poliovirus. *J. gen. Virol.*, 56: 223–233.

Koprowski, H., Gerhard, W. and Croce, C.M. (1980) Study of genetic variability of viruses through the use of monoclonal antibodies. In B.N. Fields, R. Jaenisch and C.F. Fox (Eds.), *Animal Virus Genetics*, I.C.N.–U.C.L.A., Symposia on Molecular and Cellular Biology, Vol. 18.

Nardelli, L., Lodetti, E., Gualandi, G.L., Burrows, R., Goodridge, D., Brown, F. and Cartwright, B. (1968) A foot-and-mouth disease syndrome in pigs caused by an enterovirus. *Nature (Lond.)*, 219: 1275-1276.

Newman, J.F.E., Rowlands, D.J. and Brown, F. (1973) A physico-chemical subgrouping of the mammalian picornaviruses. *J. gen. Virol.*, 18: 171-180.

Palese, P. and Schulman, J.L. (1976) RNA pattern of 'swine' influenza virus isolated from man is similar to those of other swine influenza viruses. *Nature (Lond.)*, 263: 528-530.

Racaniello, V.R. and Baltimore, D. (1981) Molecular cloning of poliovirus cDNA and determination of the complete nucleotide sequence of the viral genome. *Proc. nat. Acad. Sci. U.S.A.*, 78: 4887-4891.

Shapiro, A., Vinuela, E. and Maizel, J.V. (1967) Molecular weight estimation of polypeptide chains by electrophoresis in SDS-polyacrylamide gels. *Biochem. Biophys. Res. Commun.*, 28: 815-820.

Immunology of Nervous System Infections, Progress in Brain Research, Vol. 59, edited by P.O. Behan, V. ter Meulen and F. Clifford Rose
© *1983 Elsevier Science Publishers B.V.*

Immune Responses to Acute Alphavirus Infection of the Central Nervous System: Sindbis Virus Encephalitis in Mice

DIANE E. GRIFFIN [1], FOROOZAN MOKHTARIAN [2], MAHIN M. PARK [2] and ROBERT L. HIRSCH [2]

[1] *Howard Hughes Medical Institute, Departments of Medicine and Neurology, and* [2] *Department of Neurology, The Johns Hopkins University School of Medicine, Baltimore, MD 21205 (U.S.A.)*

INTRODUCTION

Togaviruses are responsible for a large proportion of epidemic viral encephalitis and alphaviruses are particularly associated with mosquito-borne epidemics in the New World (Shope, 1980). The morbidity and mortality from these infections occur during the acute phase of the illness. Permanent neurologic damage may occur, but there is no evidence of persistent infection and the disease is monophasic without progressive deterioration. For this reason, the interactions which occur between viral replication, immune responses and nonspecific defenses during the early weeks of infection are most important in determining the outcome from the encephalitis.

We have been studying an animal model of acute alphavirus encephalitis in order to examine these interactions more thoroughly. Sindbis virus is the Old World counterpart of Western equine encephalitis, being found in Africa, Australia and South-Eastern Asia where, in humans, it is a cause of fever without encephalitis (Chamberlain, 1980). In mice, this virus causes an acute encephalitis after intracerebral inoculation and an acute myositis with subsequent encephalitis after peripheral inoculation (Johnson et al., 1972). The outcome of this encephalitis is dependent on the strain of virus (Griffin and Johnson, 1977) and the age of the animal (Taylor et al., 1955; Griffin, 1976). Intracerebral infection of weanling mice with a non-neuro-adapted strain of virus produces a predictable, non-fatal encephalitis. This model, therefore, allows the study of the immune responses during the recovery phase, as well as the acute phases, of this central nervous system (CNS) infection.

METHODS AND MATERIALS

Virus

Sindbis virus, strain AR339 (ATCC) is grown in baby hamster kidney (BHK-21) cells and assayed by plaque formation in BHK-21 cells. For use in in vitro assays, the virus is purified on sucrose gradients (Hirsch and Griffin, 1979) and contains 10^{10} pfu (1 mg of protein)/ml.

Animal manipulations

Three- to five-week-old BALB/c mice (Charles River, Wilmington, MA) or athymic *nu/nu* mice bred on BALB/c background (Sprague–Dawley, Madison, WI) were used. Intracerebral inoculations used 1000 plaque-forming units (pfu) Sindbis virus in 0.03 ml and subcutaneous inoculations used 10^5 pfu in 0.03 ml into each of the 4 footpads.

Some mice were immunosuppressed by thymectomy at 3 weeks of age combined with lethal irradiation (732 rads) at 4 weeks of age (Park et al., 1981). Immediately after irradiation mice were reconstituted with 10^7 bone marrow cells (AT × B), with or without $6 × 10^7$ spleen and lymph node cells (AT × BT) from normal donors. Sensitized T cells were obtained from donor mice 6 days after subcutaneous infection (AT × TRs).

Mice treated with reserpine received 5 mg/kg intraperitoneally on days 2 and 4 after infection.

Animals were bled by severing the axillary artery. Cerebrospinal fluid (CSF) was obtained by puncturing the cisternal space with a micropipette and aspirating the fluid (Griffin, 1981a).

Cell preparations

Lymph node cells were taken from the popliteal, brachial and axillary lymph nodes of subcutaneously inoculated mice. Meningeal exudate cells were obtained by removing the skull in Hanks balanced salt solution and gently scraping the meninges (Morishima and Hayashi, 1978). Populations of certain lymphoid cells were depleted using anti-Thy-1.2 (New England Nuclear, Boston, MA), anti-mouse IgG (Miles Laboratories, Elkhart, IN), or arsanilate-conjugated anti-Lyt-1 and Lyt-2 (Becton Dickenson, Sunnyvale, CA) plus complement (Mokhtarian et al., 1982). Adherent cells were obtained by plating cells in RPMI containing 20 % fetal calf serum (FCS) onto plastic tissue culture dishes for 1–2 h at 37° C. Non-adherent cells were obtained by passing LNC over a G10 column (Mokhtarian et al., 1982).

Chemotaxis assays

Lymph node cells were cultured at a density of $5 × 10^6$ cells/ml in RPMI-1640 (GIBCO, Grand Island, NY) containing 50 μg/ml gentamicin and 10 % FCS. For stimulation with virus, 5 μg ($5 × 10^7$ pfu) purified virus was added to $5 × 10^6$ cells, and supernatant fluids were harvested at 72 h. This fluid was tested for chemotactic activity using blind-well chambers (Neuroprobe, Bethesda, MD), 5 μm polycarbonate filters (Nucleopore, Pleasonton, CA) (Boetcher and Meltzer, 1975) and peritoneal exudate cells induced 1 week before with 100 μg concanavalin A (Meltzer et al., 1975). Chemotactic chambers were incubated for 3 h, the filters were wiped, removed, stained with Diff-Quick and the migrated cells counted. All assays were done in triplicate and 10–20 high-power fields were counted.

Antibody and protein assays

Antibody was measured either by 50 % plaque reduction (Griffin, 1976) or by a solid-phase radioimmunoassay (Griffin, 1981a). Albumin was measured by radial immunodiffusion and IgG, IgM and IgA were measured by solid-phase radioimmunoassay (Griffin, 1981a).

Measurement of inflammation

Central nervous system inflammation was measured by the accumulation of ^{125}IUDR-labeled cells in the brain (Anders et al., 1979), counting the numbers of cells in the CSF or meninges, and/or by grading the inflammation in formalin-fixed, paraffin-embedded brains which had been sectioned at 4 levels and stained with hemotoxylin and eosin (Hirsch and Griffin, 1979).

RESULTS AND DISCUSSION

Intracerebral inoculation of unadapted Sindbis virus into 4-week-old BALB/c mice results in a nonfatal encephalitis characterized by rapid virus growth, a neutralizing antibody response which is first IgM, followed rapidly by IgG, and infiltration of the brain with mononuclear cells (McFarland et al., 1972; Griffin and Johnson, 1977). Virus growth in the brain is maximal on day 2 and is completely cleared 7–8 days after infection (Fig. 1).

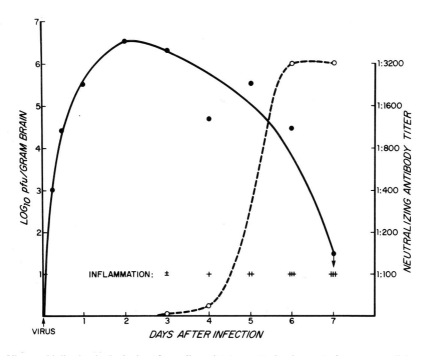

Fig. 1. Virus multiplication in the brains of weanling mice (●——●), development of serum neutralizing antibody (o----o) and inflammation after intracerebral inoculation with Sindbis virus. (From Griffin, 1975. Reprinted with permission from Academic Press.)

Cellular response

The local immune response of this acute viral infection of the CNS consists of both cellular and humoral components. The cellular immune response results in a mononuclear inflammatory reaction found focally in the brain parenchyma, especially around blood vessels, in the meninges, and in the CSF beginning approximately 3 days after infection by the intracerebral route (Table I). Inflammation is maximal in the CSF on days 3 and 4, in the meninges on day 6 and in the brain on day 8. For Sindbis (Johnson, 1971), as well as other togavirus infections (Doherty, 1973; Kitamura, 1975; Blinzinger et al., 1978), the inflammatory cells are primarily monocytes, with a minority of the cells being lymphocytes, and resemble the cell types found in the classical delayed type hypersensitivity (DTH) response (Waksman, 1976).

14

TABLE I

INFLAMMATORY RESPONSE IN THE CSF, MENINGES AND BRAINS OF MICE INFECTED INTRACEREBRALLY WITH SINDBIS VIRUS

Cells	Days after infection				
	Day 0	Day 2	Day 4	Day 6	Day 8
CSF (per mm^3)	50	1000	3150	2500	1300
Meninges	10^5	10^5	10^6	$10^{6.4}$	$10^{5.9}$
Brain	−	±	+	++	+++

Previous studies, using passive transfer of lymphoid cells into cyclophosphamide-immuno-suppressed mice have shown that the induction of this response is immunologically specific (McFarland et al., 1972). It therefore seemed likely that T-lymphocytes were responsible for the specificity of the response and amplified it by attracting other mononuclear cells from the blood. To determine whether virus-sensitized T-lymphocytes respond with proliferation and/or lymphokine production upon re-exposure to the virus, lymph node cells were cultured in vitro. Mice were injected subcutaneously with Sindbis virus or diluent, and cells from the draining lymph nodes were taken at various times after infection and cultured with and without added virus. In one experiment, the cells were tested for lymphoproliferation of tritiated thymidine (Griffin and Johnson, 1973), and in another, the supernatant fluids were tested for the presence of mononuclear chemotactic activity (Mokhtarian et al., 1982) (Fig. 2). The

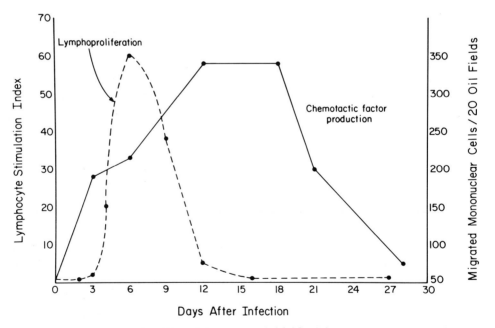

Fig. 2. In vitro responses of lymph node cells draining an area of Sindbis virus infection. Mice were infected subcutaneously with 10^5 pfu Sindbis virus on day 0. Lymphoproliferation was measured by the incorporation of [^{3}H]thymidine (Griffin and Johnson, 1973) and the mononuclear chemotactic factor produced was measured by the induction of cell migration through a polycarbonate filter (Mokhtarian et al., 1982).

sensitized cells, but not the control cells, responded both by proliferating and producing a factor chemotactic for mononuclear cells. These responses were dose-dependent and specific for the virus inoculated (Griffin and Johnson, 1973; Mokhtarian et al., 1982). Although both tests measured T-cell responses to antigenic challenge, the time-courses were different. Maximal lymphoproliferation occurred before maximal lymphokine production and was terminated earlier. This is consistent with other observations reporting a dissociation of lymphoproliferation and lymphokine production (Bloom et al., 1972; Rocklin, 1973) which may reflect two cell populations or two different responses of the same population.

TABLE II

THE EFFECT OF CELL DEPLETION ON THE IN VITRO PRODUCTION OF CHEMOTACTIC FACTOR IN RESPONSE TO SINDBIS VIRUS

Cells	Monocytes/hpf
Unfractionated LNC	196 ± 4
Antiserum treatment	
anti-Thy-1.2	83 ± 13
anti-IgG	161 ± 29
anti-Lyt-1	92 ± 15
anti-Lyt-2	185 ± 37
Adherence	
non-adherent	84 ± 21
adherent	75 ± 6

The cell responsible for the production of chemotactic factor was investigated by selectively depleting certain populations of lymph node cells, using adherence properties and antisera to surface antigens (Table II). In vitro production of this lymphokine in response to antigen, required both T-lymphocytes bearing the Lyt1 antigen and adherent cells. The need for adherent cells is consistent with the known accessory cell requirement of T-cells for lymphokine production (Wahl et al., 1975). It therefore seems likely that during the first few days after CNS infection with Sindbis virus, T-lymphocytes are sensitized in the peripheral lymphoid tissue, then leave this tissue and circulate to the site of antigen replication where they stop and are stimulated to release lymphokines locally. At least one of these lymphokines attracts circulating blood monocytes to enter the site of infection, thus expanding the cellular infiltration.

The development of immune responses within the CNS is undoubtedly influenced by the presence of the blood–brain barrier. This barrier is localized anatomically to the tight junctions which connect the capillary endothelial cells, arachnoid cells, and choroid plexus epithelial cells (Reese and Karnovsky, 1967; Brightman and Reese, 1969; Brightman et al., 1970; Davson, 1972). Tight junctions are also found between endothelial cells in the capillaries supplying the epidermis and, in the mouse, it has been shown that monocytes cannot, of their own accord, participate in the DTH response unless entry of monocytes into the tissue is facilitated. This is accomplished through tissue mast cells. In the mouse, these cells are numerous in skin sites where a DTH response can be elicited (footpads) but lacking in unresponsive areas (flank skin). Mast cells, in response to a lymphokine, produced locally by sensitized T-cells, release serotonin which increases the permeability of the capillary tight junctions, thus allowing the influx of monocytes from the blood in response to the chemotactic factor lymphokine. If serotonin release is prevented (reserpine), or its pharmacologic action is blocked (cyproheptadine), monocyte accumulation does not occur in the area of antigenic stimulation (Gershon et al., 1975; Askenase, 1977; Askenase et al., 1980).

To determine whether there is a similar requirement for mast cells and serotonin release within the CNS in order to facilitate monocyte entry into the inflammatory reaction of viral encephalitis, infected mice were treated with reserpine. This drug depletes mast cells of vasoactive amines by blocking the transport system of the storage granules, allowing intracellular degradation by monoamine oxidase (Shore, 1962). The inflammatory response in the CSF, meninges and brain parenchyma were compared on days 4 and 6 for untreated infected mice and infected mice treated with reserpine (Table III). The inflammatory response is diminished in all compartments in the reserpine-treated mice suggesting that the release of vasoactive amines may also be important for full expression of the inflammatory response in the rodent CNS.

TABLE III

EFFECT OF RESERPINE (R) ON DEVELOPMENT OF THE INFLAMMATORY RESPONSE TO SINDBIS VIRUS (SV) ENCEPHALITIS

Location	Inflammation			
	Day 4		Day 6	
	SV	SV + R	SV	SV + R
CSF (cells/mm^3)	3150	375	2500	850
Brain — ^{125}IUDR (cpm/brain)	350	105	200	85
— histology	+	±	+++	+

To determine whether inflammation is necessary for recovery from viral encephalitis, experiments were done using genetically (athymic *nu/nu*) and experimentally (adult thymectomized, irradiated, bone marrow-reconstituted) T-cell-deficient mice. Athymic nude mice developed only a minimal inflammatory response but survived the infection and cleared virus from the brain at the same time as normal BALB/c mice (Hirsch and Griffin, 1979). Likewise, thymectomized, irradiated mice reconstituted only with normal bone marrow cells (AT × B) had no detectable inflammation, survived the infection and cleared virus at the same time as mice receiving a source of T-normal cells in addition (AT × B,T) (Park et al., 1981, Fig. 3). T-cell-deficient mice of both types produced only IgM neutralizing antibody, but this, in addition to natural defense mechanisms, may have contributed to their recovery. If only sensitized T-cells are transferred (AT × Ts) the antibody response is minimal, but inflammation is present and virus is cleared earlier (day 10 rather than day 14) (Fig. 4). If both bone marrow cells and sensitized T-cells are transferred (AT × BTs), the antibody, inflammation and virus clearance resemble that of the normal mouse (Figs. 1 and 4). Therefore, although the mononuclear inflammatory response may contribute to clearance of Sindbis virus from the brain, it is not necessary.

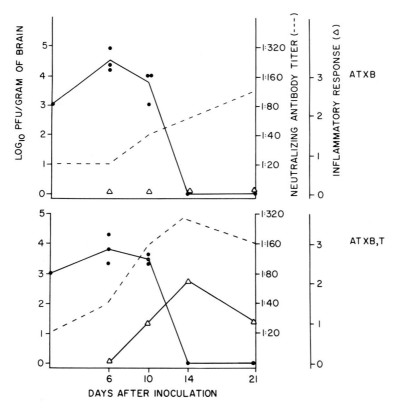

Fig. 3. Virus clearance (●———●), antibody response (------) and inflammation (△———△) after intracerebral Sindbis virus infection of adult thymectomized, lethally irradiated mice reconstituted with normal bone marrow cells (AT × B) or with normal bone marrow cells and normal spleen and lymph node cells (AT × BT).

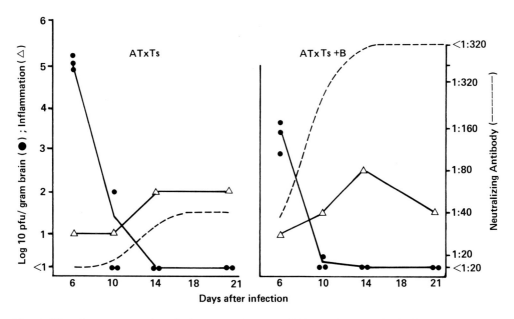

Fig. 4. Virus clearance (●———●), antibody response (------) and inflammation (△———△) after intracerebral Sindbis virus infection of adult thymectomized, lethally irradiated mice reconstituted with Sindbis virus-sensitized lymph node cells (AT × Ts) or sensitized lymph node cells plus normal bone marrow cells (AT × Ts + B).

18

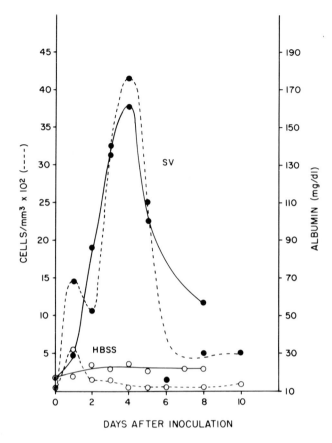

Fig. 5. Changes in the amounts of albumin (●——●) and in the number of leukocytes (o---o) present in the cerebrospinal fluid of weanling mice after intracerebral inoculation of 1000 pfu Sindbis virus.

Antibody response

The antibody response to Sindbis virus encephalitis is both systemic (Figs. 1, 3 and 4) and local (Griffin, 1981a). To examine the local humoral immune response, CSF was sampled at frequent intervals after infection. The cells were counted and the fluid assayed for albumin as a measure of total serum proteins (Fig. 5), for IgM, IgG and IgA, and for antibody to Sindbis virus. There was an initial (days 3–5) increase in all serum proteins in the CSF which coincided with the pleocytosis and was indicative of generalized blood–brain barrier dysfunction (Fig. 5). Immunoglobulins were present in the CSF proportionately to their representation in serum. Similar disruption of blood–CSF barrier function is found in other fatal (Doherty and Zinkernagel, 1974; Griffin, 1981b) and nonfatal (Griffin et al., 1979) viral encephalitides and may contribute in some instances to a fatal outcome (Doherty and Zinkernagel, 1974).

The albumin concentration and cell numbers normalized over the next several days and the immunoglobulin concentrations also fell (Griffin, 1981a), but again began to rise about 8 days after infection (Table IV). All immunoglobulin classes, including IgM and IgA, increased in the CSF but the proportionate rises were most dramatic for IgG1, IgM and IgA. Furthermore, specific antiviral antibody in the CSF was associated with IgA as well as IgG (Griffin, 1981a).

TABLE IV

CSF IMMUNOGLOBULIN CONCENTRATIONS DURING RECOVERY FROM SINDBIS VIRUS ENCEPHALITIS

Immunoglobulin	Immunoglobulin concentrations ($\mu g/ml$)				
	Day 0	Day 4	Day 8	Day 15	Day 30
IgG1	0.7	17.4	24.3	12.6	6.5
IgG2A	0.39	0.8	1.35	1.28	0.47
IgG2B	1.25	4.5	6.2	7.4	5.2
IgG3	0.54	0.78	1.07	0.87	1.24
IgM	0.13	0.29	5.6	2.7	0.55
IgA	0.18	1.03	6.9	8.4	1.8

Studies using iodinated proteins to track the entry of proteins from the CSF into serum demonstrated transudation only during the early (days 3–4) inflammatory phase and not later during the recovery phase when CSF immunoglobulins were most increased. Serum immunoglobulin levels did not change significantly during the period of study. Mice examined 4 months after infection still had increased levels of IgG and IgA in the CSF (Griffin, 1981a). Therefore, the phase of recovery from infection is marked by a local antibody response which does not reflect the isotype composition of antibodies present in the serum, and is not due to transudation of proteins from the serum.

SUMMARY

Sindbis virus is an alphavirus which produces an acute nonfatal encephalitis in mice. The local immune responses to this virus are both cellular and humoral. The cellular response is characterized by an infiltration of mononuclear cells into the CSF, the meninges, and the brain parenchyma. This inflammatory response is initiated by sensitized T-lymphocytes which are stimulated, by exposure to viral antigen, to produce a lymphokine which is chemotactic for mononuclear cells. These T-cells may also produce a lymphokine which stimulates mast cells to release vasoactive amines which facilitate monocyte entry from the blood. Inflammation is not necessary for clearance of virus from the brain. Humoral immune responses are initially systemic and, in the CNS, reflect transudation of serum antibody. During recovery, there is local production of antiviral IgA as well as IgG.

ACKNOWLEDGEMENTS

This work was supported in part by a grant from the National Multiple Sclerosis Society and Research Grants NS-15721 and NS-07000 from the National Institutes of Health.

REFERENCES

Anders, E.M., Miller, J.F.A.P. and Gamble, J. (1979) A radioisotopic technique for measuring the mononuclear inflammatory response in Sindbis virus-induced encephalitis of mice. *J. immunol. Meth*, 29: 167–171.

Askenase, P.W. (1977) Role of basophils, mast cells and vasoamines in hypersensitivity reactions with a delayed time course. *Progr. Allergy,* 23: 199–320.

20

Askenase, P.W., Bursztajn, S., Gershon, M.D. and Gershon, R.K. (1980) T cell-dependent mast cell degranulation and release of serotonin in murine delayed-type hypersensitivity. *J. exp. Med.*, 152: 1358–1374.

Blinzinger, K., Herrlinger, H., Luh, S. and Anzil, A.P. (1978) Ultrastructural cytochemical demonstration of peroxidase-positive monocyte granules: an additional method for studying the origin of mononuclear cells in encephalitic lesions. *Acta Neuropathol.*, 43: 55–61.

Bloom, B.R., Gaffney, J. and Jimenez, L. (1972) Dissociation of MIF production and cell proliferation. *J. Immunol.*, 109: 1395–1398.

Boetcher, D.A. and Meltzer, M.S. (1975) Mouse mononuclear cell chemotaxis: description of system. *J. nat. Cancer Inst.*, 54: 795–799.

Brightman, M.W. and Reese, T.S. (1969) Junctions between intimately apposed cell membranes in the vertebrate brain. *J. Cell. Biol.*, 40: 648–677.

Brightman, M.W., Klatzo, I., Olsson, Y. and Reese, T.S. (1970) The blood–brain barrier to proteins under normal and pathological conditions. *J. neurol. Sci.*, 10: 215–239.

Chamberlain, R.W. (1980) Epidemiology of arthropod-borne togaviruses: the role of arthropods as hosts and vectors and of vertebrate hosts in natural transmission cycles. In R.W. Schlesinger (Ed.), *The Togaviruses: Biology, Structure, Replication*, Academic Press, New York, pp. 175–227.

Davson, H. (1972) The blood–brain barrier. In G.H. Bourne (Ed.), *The Structure and Function of Nervous Tissue, Vol. IV*, Academic Press, New York, pp. 321–405.

Doherty, P.C. (1973) Quantitative studies of the inflammatory process in fatal viral meningoencephalitis. *Amer. J. Pathol.*, 73: 607–621.

Doherty, P.C. and Zinkernagel, R.M. (1974) T-cell-mediated immunopathology in viral infections. *Transplant Rev.*, 19: 89–120.

Gershon, R.K., Askenase, P.W. and Gershon, M.D. (1975) Requirement for vasoactive amines for production of delayed-type hypersensitivity skin reactions. *J. exp. Med.*, 142: 732–747.

Griffin, D. (1975) Immune response-pathogenicity of viral infection. In C. Koprowski and H. Koprowski (Eds.), *Viruses and Immunity: Toward Understanding Viral Immunology and Immunopathology*, Academic Press, New York, pp. 67–82.

Griffin, D.E. (1976) Role of the immune response in age-dependent resistance of mice to encephalitis due to Sindbis virus. *J. infect. Dis.*, 133: 456–464.

Griffin, D.E. (1981a) Immunoglobulins in the cerebrospinal fluid: changes during acute viral encephalitis in mice. *J. Immunol.*, 126: 27–31.

Griffin, D.E. (1981b) CSF changes during acute encephalomyocarditis virus meningoencephalitis in mice. *Ann. Neurol.*, 10: 55–57.

Griffin, D.E. and Johnson, R.T. (1973) Cellular immune response to viral infection: in vitro studies of lymphocytes from mice infected with Sindbis virus. *Cell. Immunol.*, 9: 426–434.

Griffin, D.E. and Johnson, R.T. (1977) Role of the immune response in recovery from Sindbis virus encephalitis in mice. *J. Immunol.*, 118: 1070–1075.

Griffin, D.E., Narayan, O., Bukowski, J., Adams, R.J. and Cohen, S. (1979) The cerebrospinal fluid in visna, a slow viral disease of sheep, *Ann. Neurol.*, 4: 212–218.

Hirsch, R.L. and Griffin, D.E. (1979) The pathogenesis of Sindbis virus infection in athymic nude mice. *J. Immunol.*, 123: 1215–1218.

Johnson, R.T. (1971) Inflammatory response to viral infection. In Immunological Disorders of the Nervous System, *Res. Pub. Assoc. Res. Nerv. Ment. Dis.*, 69: 305–312.

Johnson, R.T., McFarland, H.F. and Levy, S.E. (1972) Age-dependent resistance to viral encephalitis: studies of infections due to Sindbis virus in mice. *J. infect. Dis.*, 125: 257–262.

Kitamura, T. (1975) Hematogenous cells in experimental Japanese encephalitis. *Acta Neuropathol.*, 32: 341–353.

McFarland, H.F., Griffin, D.E. and Johnson, R.T. (1972) Specificity of the inflammatory response in viral encephalitis. I. Adoptive immunization of immunosuppressed mice infected with Sindbis virus. *J. exp. Med.*, 136: 216–226.

Meltzer, M.S., Jones, E.E. and Boetcher, D.A. (1975) Increased chemotactic responses of macrophages from BCG-infected mice. *Cell. Immunol.*, 17: 268–276.

Mokhtarian, F., Griffin, D.E. and Hirsch, R.L. (1982) Production of mononuclear chemotactic factors during Sindbis virus infection of mice. *Infect. Immun.*, 35: 965–973.

Morishima, T. and Hayashi, K. (1978) Meningeal exudate cells in vaccinia meningitis of mice: role of local T cells. *Infect. Immun.*, 20: 752–759.

Park, M.M., Griffin, D.E. and Johnson, R.T. (1981) Analysis of the role of immune responses in recovery from acute Sindbis virus encephalitis: studies in adult thymectomized lethally irradiated mice. *Infect. Immun.*, 34: 306–309.

Reese, T.S. and Karnovsky, M.J. (1967) Fine structural localization of a blood–brain barrier to exogenous peroxidase. *J. Cell. Biol.*, 34: 207–217.

Rocklin, R.E. (1973) Production of migration inhibitory factor by non-dividing lymphocytes. *J. Immunol.*, 110: 674–678.

Shope, R.E. (1980) Medical significance of togaviruses: an overview of diseases caused by togaviruses in man and in domestic and wild vertebrate animals. In R.W. Schlesinger (Ed.), *The Togaviruses*, Academic Press, pp. 47–82.

Shore, P.A. (1962) Release of serotonin and catecholamines by drugs. *Pharmacol. Rev.*, 14: 531–550.

Taylor, R.M., Hurlbut, H.S., Work, T.H., Kingsbury, J.R. and Frothingham, T.E. (1955) Sindbis virus: a newly recognized arthropod-transmitted virus. *Amer. J. Trop. Med. Hyg.*, 4: 844–846.

Wahl, S.M., Wilton, S.M., Rosenstreich, R. and Oppenheim, J.J. (1975) The role of macrophages in the production of lymphokines by T and B lymphocytes. *J. Immunol.,* 114: 1296–1301.

Waksman, B.H. (1976) Immunoglobulins and lymphokines as mediators of inflammatory cell mobilization on target cell killing. *Cell. Immunol.*, 27: 309–315.

Immunology of Nervous System Infections, Progress in Brain Research, Vol. 59, edited by P.O. Behan, V. ter Meulen and F. Clifford Rose

Viral Interactions with Receptors in the Central Nervous System and on Lymphocytes

HOWARD L. WEINER, MARC TARDIEU, ROCHELLE L. EPSTEIN, ADRIANO FONTANA and M. LINDA POWERS

Department of Neuroscience, Children's Hospital Medical Center and Department of Medicine, Sections of Neurology and Infectious Diseases, Brigham and Women's Hospital, Boston, MA 02115 (U.S.A.)

INTRODUCTION

It has been observed clinically for some time that viruses cause different diseases based on their tissue tropism; for example, poliovirus to anterior horn cells in the spinal cord, rhinoviruses to tissues of the upper respiratory tract, and Coxsackie B viruses to cardiac muscle (Meager and Hughes, 1977; Tardieu et al., 1982). It is probable that a major determinant of tissue tropism involves the recognition of a portion of the susceptible host-cell membrane by the virus and that this cell surface structure serves as a viral-receptor. Furthermore, the specific interaction of a viral particle with the host cell membrane is most probably determined by a specific protein or structure on the outer surface of the virus itself. To study these issues of viral-receptor interactions, we have used reovirus as a model system, both in the central nervous system (CNS) and in the immune system.

Reoviruses are double-stranded RNA (dsRNA) viruses whose genome consists of 10 segments which are named according to size classes; 3 large segments (L1, L2, L3), 3 medium segments (M1, M2, M3), and 4 small segments (S1, S2, S3, S4). The dsRNA is surrounded by a double capsid shell (Joklik, 1974). The outer capsid consists of 3 polypeptides, $\sigma 1$, $\sigma 3$, and $\mu 1C$ which are derived from genome segments S1, S4, and M2, respectively (Mustoe et al., 1978; McCrae and Joklik, 1978). Using recombinant clones derived from crosses between reovirus types 1 and 3 and consisting of genome segments derived from both parents, we have previously shown that the hemagglutinin of reovirus is the $\sigma 1$ outer capsid polypeptide encoded by the S1 genome segment (Weiner et al., 1978). As described below, we have used the natural biologic polymorphism of reovirus types 1 and 3 in the study of reovirus interactions both in vivo and in vitro with the central nervous system and the immune system.

IN VIVO INTERACTIONS OF REOVIRUS WITH THE CENTRAL NERVOUS SYSTEM

When reovirus type 3 is injected into newborn mice, all animals die of a necrotizing encephalitis that consists histologically of prominent neuronal damage with sparing of ependymal cells. Inoculation of newborn animals with reovirus type 1 causes a non-lethal infection of the brain with the histological pattern in many animals consisting of ependymal cell necrosis and hydrocephalus. There is no damage seen to neuronal cells. These observations suggested that the differing tropism of the two serotypes of reovirus, type 3 for neurons and type 1 for ependymal cells, might be a major determinant of viral virulence. To study this question, recombinant viral clones were injected into animals. After a variety of experiments using a large number of clones which contained various mixtures of genes from one parental serotype or the other, it became clear that one genome segment was the primary determinant of the pattern of histologic damage and virulence. This genome segment was the S1 gene, the gene encoding the viral hemagglutinin (Weiner et al., 1977). Two single-segment recombinant clones were then generated which conclusively established the role of the viral hemagglutinin in these patterns of virulence and tropism, and these clones have subsequently been used for a variety of studies of viral receptor interactions (Weiner et al., 1980a).

Clone 3.HA1 contains 9 genes from type 3 and one gene, the S1 gene (which encodes the viral hemagglutinin) from type 1. Clone 1.HA3 is the reciprocal clone. When clone 3.HA1 is injected into newborn animals, it behaves identically to parental type 1, even though it has 9 genes from the type 3 virus. Thus, both type 1 and clone 3.HA1 cause a non-lethal infection of ependymal cells, leading to hydrocephalus in most animals. There is no damage to neuronal cells. Similarly, clone 1.HA3 causes a pattern of virulence identical to the parental type 3, namely, a necrotizing encephalitis with damage to neuronal cells, which causes death in all animals but no damage to ependymal cells. Not only are patterns of virulence and histologic changes in the central nervous system linked to the viral hemagglutinin, but viral growth patterns are linked as well. Thus, type 3 and clone 1.HA3 grow to titers of between 10^9 and 10^{10} plaque-forming units (pfu) per ml in the brains of newborn animals, whereas type 1 and clone 3.HA1 only grow to titers of 10^7 pfu (Weiner et al., 1980a).

These in vivo studies suggest that the interaction of the σ1 outer capsid polypeptide with a specific structure on the surface of either the neuron or ependymal cell determines tissue tropism and ultimate pattern of virulence of the viral serotypes. Of note is that the σ1 outer capsid polypeptide comprises a small portion of the outer capsid, representing only between 1 and 2% of the viral protein coat.

CENTRAL NERVOUS SYSTEM IN VITRO INTERACTIONS

In order to test the hypothesis that viral binding to the cell surface was a major determinant of tissue damage, in vitro studies were performed. The first set of experiments were performed with isolated ependymal cells. Single cell suspensions of viable ependymal cells were prepared from the central nervous system of adult mice by the technique described by Manthorpe et al. (1977). In this technique, viable ciliated ependymal cells can be prepared following stripping of the ependymal cell surface and preparation of cells on a BSA gradient as modified by Tardieu and Weiner (1982). Following this, 500,000 ependymal cells were incubated with $40\,\mu$l of cesium chloride-purified reovirus type 1 or 3 at titers of 5×10^9 pfu (plaque-forming units)/ml. The particle-to-plaque-forming ratio of reovirus is 100:1. Thus, 5×10^9 pfu/ml is approximately 5×10^{11} viral particles. After incubation of cells for 20 min at 4°C and washing, the presence of viral binding to the ependymal cell surface was demonstrated using an indirect immunofluorescence technique with rabbit anti-reovirus antibody and then FITC-conjugated goat anti-rabbit immunoglobulin. In these experiments, bright ring fluorescence was seen surrounding ciliated ependymal cells when incubated with reovirus type 1, while no staining was seen with reovirus type 3. Maximal staining was observed between titers of 10^9–10^{11} pfu, and minimal staining was seen between titers of 10^7 and 10^8 pfu.

In order to demonstrate that viral binding was indeed a property of the viral hemagglutinin, recombinant clones were then tested. Clone 3.HA1 bound to ependymal cells in an identical fashion as reovirus type 1, while clone 1.HA3 did not. These results demonstrate that in vitro binding and specificity of reovirus for ependymal cells mimic in vivo patterns of CNS damage.

Identical patterns of binding were found for reovirus binding to ependymal cells of newborn animals compared to adult animals. These latter experiments suggest that the age-dependent hydrocephalus observed in animals is probably not due to the presence or absence of viral receptors on the ependymal cell surface.

Hydrocephalus following reovirus type 1 infection has been reported for mice, rats, hamsters, and primates. In order to determine if similar in vitro tropism for reovirus type 1 existed in humans, we prepared viable ciliated ependymal cells from the brain of a 6-month-old child obtained 8 h postmortem. The same specificity of viral binding was observed with human as with murine ependymal cells. Reovirus type 1 bound to 90% of the ciliated cells, while reovirus type 3 bound only to 18%. Control staining obtained when human ependymal cells were incubated with antiviral antibody and FITC-Garig alone was 12%.

Although reovirus rarely causes illness in humans, a group of viruses exists which causes disease in humans and which has been reported to have specific tropism for ependymal cells. These and other viruses were tested for binding to isolated murine ependymal cells in an effort to determine the specificity of ependymal cell binding for a panel of viruses. Herpes virus type 1, parainfluenza type 3, measles, and mumps bound to ependymal cells, while herpes virus type 2 and poliovirus type 1 did not. Of note is that the percentage of cells staining with the various viruses was dependent on the titer of the particular viral stock, and was remarkably similar to the percentages obtained with the various titers of reovirus type 1. These results suggest that, irrespective of the virus, a similar minimal number of viral particles was required to demonstrate staining. The structure on ependymal cells to which these viruses bind remains to be identified. These receptors could be shared by different viruses or be specific for each of them. Little is known about the different antigens present on the surface of ependymal cells. We have found histocompatibility antigens to be present on ependymal cells and are developing a panel of monoclonal antibodies against these cells (Tardieu and Weiner, 1982; Tardieu et al., 1982). We have not found Fc receptors or Thy 1.2 on the ependymal cell surface.

The binding of reovirus type 3 to neuronal cells has also been studied. In preliminary experiments using primary cortical cultures of both mouse and rat neurons, we have been able to demonstrate the binding of reovirus type 3 (and not type 1) to neurons in culture. Using recombinant clones, binding was seen with 1.HA3 and not 3.HA1. Thus, it appears that the reciprocal in vitro specificity of binding of reovirus type 3 to neurons (and not of type 1) can be studied.

INTERACTION OF REOVIRUS WITH LYMPHOCYTES

Viral receptors have been demonstrated on lymphocytes, and in some instances the biological consequences of the specific interaction of a virus with the lymphocyte membrane have been demonstrated (Greaves, 1976). Using a similar approach to that used with ependymal cells, we studied the binding characteristics of reovirus serotypes to both human and murine lymphocytes (Weiner et al., 1980b). It was found that reovirus type 3, but not reovirus type 1, bound to the surface of a subpopulation of both murine and human lymphocytes. These studies were performed by incubating lymphocytes with purified viral particles, labeling attached virus with FITC-labeled antiviral antibody, and analyzing binding characteristics on a fluorescence-activated cell sorter. Maximal staining of lymphocytes varied between 34% and 45% positive cells per 100,000 cells counted on the cell sorter. An identical range for positive cells was obtained when cells were counted visually under the fluorescence microscope. To determine the viral gene product responsible for interaction of reovirus type 3 with murine splenic lymphocytes, recombinant clones were tested, and it was found that the viral hemagglutinin determined these binding characteristics. Thus, clone 1.HA3 bound to murine and human lymphocytes, while clone 3.HA1 did not. Different lymphocyte subpopulations were then tested for their binding characteristics. These experiments showed binding of virus to both T-cells and B-cells in both mouse and man. Specifically, 55% of murine splenic B-cells bound virus, while 26% of murine splenic T-cells bound virus. In addition, 21% of murine lymph node cells bound reovirus type 3. In humans, 27% of peripheral blood T-cells bound reovirus type 3, whereas binding was seen in 56% of peripheral blood B-cells. Similar numbers were obtained when human splenic B- and T-cells were studied. These binding characteristics were further shown using ^{125}I-labeled virus, which demonstrated pronounced binding of type 3 to the lymphocyte with minimal binding of type 1. Furthermore, in these studies, we were able to competitively inhibit the binding of ^{125}I-labeled type 3 virus with unlabeled type 3, but not with unlabeled type 1. Of note, however, is that using radiolabeled virus, some binding of type 1 to the lymphocyte surface was observed.

To study further the interaction of reovirus type 3 with the lymphocyte surface, capping studies were performed (Epstein et al., 1981). Using purified reovirus type 3 particles as a ligand, followed by FITC-labeled antiviral antibody, we were able to demonstrate viral-induced capping of the reovirus receptor on both B- and T-cells. Kinetic studies and inhibition experiments using cytochalasin B and colchicine demonstrated that reovirus-induced capping of the viral receptor on both B- and T-cells shows characteristics identical to the capping of immunoglobulin on B cells by anti-immunoglobulin reagents.

In order to determine whether there was a functional concomitant to the presence of reovirus receptors on lymphocytes, functional studies were undertaken (Fontana and Weiner, 1980). It was found that reovirus type 3, but not type 1, inhibited the in vitro proliferative response of murine splenic lymphocytes to concanavalin A (ConA). By analyzing recombinant clones we were able to demonstrate that this effect was a property of the viral hemagglutinin. In addition, we found that reovirus type 3, but not type 1, generated suppressor T cells in vitro capable of suppressing ConA proliferation and that this property was also secondary to the viral hemagglutinin. These effects were observed whether ultra-violet-inactivated or live virus was used. Furthermore, reovirus type 3 inhibition of the proliferative response of murine splenic lymphocytes to ConA was blocked by anti-reovirus type 3 antibody, but not by anti-reovirus type 1 antibody. Antiviral antibody had no effect on the ability of reovirus type 3-induced suppressor cells to inhibit ConA proliferation. These results demonstrate that suppressor cells were indeed generated and that suppression was not secondary to the carry-over of virus. Repeated attempts to demonstrate a mitogenic effect of reovirus type 3 have not been successful.

In addition, results from our laboratory using affinity plating techniques demonstrate that reovirus type 3 binds specifically to the Ly 2,3 subset of murine lymphocytes and to the T8 subset of human lymphocytes (Epstein et al., 1982). These subsets represent the suppressor/cytotoxic cell, and it may be that the generation of suppressor cells that we have demonstrated with reovirus is secondary to the presence of a receptor for the virus on this particular subset of cells.

SUMMARY

The approach we have taken has utilized a biologically relevant model for the study of viral-receptor interactions both in the nervous system and the immune system. Further work is in progress to identify the receptor(s) to which reovirus types 1 and 3 bind on the cell surface. One approach we have taken involves the generation of anti-idiotype antibodies directed against the hemagglutinin of type 3 which may serve as a probe for the structure to which the virus binds. (Nepom et al. 1982). The investigation of viral receptor interactions has important implications for determining specificity of viral injury and explaining possible mechanisms of autoimmunity. Moreover, the varying natural specificities of viruses may make them powerful biologic probes for the study of cell surface receptors.

ACKNOWLEDGEMENTS

Supported by Grant NSAI16998 from the NIH.

REFERENCES

Epstein, R., Powers, M.L. and Weiner, H.L. (1981) Interaction of reovirus with cell surface receptors. III. Reovirus type 3 induces capping of viral receptors on murine. *J. Immunol.,* 127: 1800–1803.

Epstein, R.L., Powers, M.L., Finberg, R. and Weiner, H.L. (1982) T-Lymphocyte receptors for the hemagglutinin of reovirus type 3 are expressed predominantly on murine Lyt 2,3+ and human T8+ cells. *Fed. Proc.,* 41: 568 (abstr.).

Fontana, A. and Weiner, H.L. (1980) Interaction of reovirus with cell surface receptors. II. Generation of suppressor T cells by the hemagglutinin of reovirus type 3. *J. Immunol.,* 125: 2660–2664.

Greaves, M.F. (1976) Virus "receptors" on lymphocytes. *Scand. J. Immunol.,* Suppl 5, 5: 113–120.

Joklik, W.K. (1974) Reproduction of reoviridae. *Comp. Virol.,* 2: 297–298.

Meager, A. and Hughes, R.C. (1977) Virus receptors. In P. Cuatrecasas and M.F. Greaves (Eds.), *Receptors and Recognition,* John Wiley, New York, pp. 143–195.

McCrae, M.A. and Joklik, W.K. (1978) The nature of the polypeptide encoded by each of the 10 double-stranded RNA segments of reovirus type 3. *Virology,* 89: 578–593.

Manthorpe, C.M., Wilkin, G.P. and Wilson, J.E. (1977) Purification of viable ciliated cuboidal ependymal cells from rat brain. *Brain Res.,* 134: 407–411.

Mustoe, T.A., Ramig, R.F., Sharpe, A.H. and Fields, B.N. (1978) Genetics of reovirus: identification of the dsRNA segments encoding the polypeptides of the mu and sigma size classes. *Virology,* 89:594–604.

Nepom, J.T., Weiner, H.L., Dichter, M.A., Tardieu, M., Spriggs, D.R., Gramm, C.F., Powers, M.L., Fields, B.N. and Greene, M.I., (1982) Identification of a hemagglutinin-specific idiotype associated with reovirus recognition shared by lymphoid and neural cells. *J. exp. Med.,* 155: 155–167.

Tardieu, M. and Weiner, H.L. (1982) Viral receptors on isolated murine and human ependymal cells. *Science,* 215: 419–421.

Tardieu, M., Noseworthy, J.H., Perry, L., Greene, M.I. and Weiner, H.L. (1982) Generation of a monoclonal antibody which binds selectively to murine ependymal cells. *Brain Res.,* in press.

Weiner, H.L., Drayna, D., Averill, D.R. and Fields, B.N. (1977) Molecular basis of reovirus virulence: role of the S1 gene. *Proc. nat. Acad. Sci. U.S.A.,* 74: 5744–5748.

Weiner, H.L., Ramig, R.F., Mustoe, T.A. and Fields, B.N. (1978) Identification of the gene coding for the hemagglutinin of reovirus. *Virology,* 86: 581–584.

Weiner, H.L., Powers, M.L. and Fields, B.N. (1980a) Absolute linkage of virulence and central nervous system cell tropism of reoviruses to viral hemagglutinin. *J. infect. Dis.,* 141: 609–616.

Weiner, H.L., Ault, K.A. and Fields, B.N. (1980b) Interaction of reovirus with cell surface receptors. I. Murine and human lymphocytes have a receptor for the hemagglutinin of reovirus type 3. *J. Immunol.,* 124: 2143–2148.

Immunology of Nervous System Infections, Progress in Brain Research, Vol. 59, edited by P.O. Behan, V. ter Meulen and F. Clifford Rose

Humoral and Cellular Immunity in Patients with Acute Aseptic Meningitis

HANS LINK[1], SLAVENKA KAM-HANSEN[1], PIA FORSBERG[2] and ANNEMARIE HENRIKSSON[3]

[1]*Department of Neurology, Karolinska Institutet, Huddinge University Hospital, S-141 86 Huddinge, Stockholm, and* [2]*Department of Infectious Diseases and* [3]*Department of Neurology, University Hospital, S-581 85 Linköping (Sweden)*

INTRODUCTION

A number of chronic central nervous system (CNS) diseases of unknown etiology, the most common and notable among them being multiple sclerosis, are characterized by an immune response within the CNS cerebrospinal fluid (CSF) compartment, which is reflected by abnormalities in humoral as well as cell-mediated immune variables in the CSF, while the corresponding variables in peripheral blood are frequently normal. In multiple sclerosis, this local immune response is characterized by inter alia mononuclear pleocytosis, elevated concentrations of IgG, IgA and IgM, oligoclonal IgG with γ_1 heavy chain and κ light chain predominance, which is exaggerated compared to normal, production of antibodies directed against various viral, bacterial and auto-antigens, low or absent proliferation of CSF lymphocytes on stimulation in vitro with the mitogens phytohaemagglutinin, concanavalin A and pokeweed mitogen, and low numbers of so-called active T-cells (for reviews see Kam-Hansen, 1980; Laurenzi, 1981; Roström, 1981).

Acute aseptic meningitis (AM) is mostly a self-limiting, self-healing disease of acute onset and short duration. The etiology can often be established, and the pathogenesis is comparatively well worked out. Definition of the immune reactions seen in CSF, in comparison to those in peripheral blood, in patients with AM should expand our understanding of a compartmentalized immune response, and increase the possibility of elucidating the immune mechanisms involved in the pathogenesis of diseases like multiple sclerosis.

This chapter summarizes our knowledge of the spread of virus in the CNS, and includes data collected mainly from our laboratory over the last few years regarding the humoral and cell-mediated immune responses in AM.

SPREAD OF VIRUS IN CNS

Acute RNA virus infections of the human nervous system are common. Effective immunization procedures have practically eliminated poliomyelitis and rabies, and will probably conquer measles, mumps and rubella. Many of the other RNA infections produce only mild and often clinically insignificant infections of the nervous system, frequently yielding non-specific clinical manifestations. They are difficult to diagnose and almost certainly under-reported.

The DNA agents, herpes simplex virus (HSV) serving as a prototype, are responsible for a significant percentage of all virus infections which involve the human nervous system. The clinical features of HSV meningoencephalitis vary from mild symptoms, where the diagnosis is often overlooked, to severe meningoencephalitis of acute or subacute onset with headache, fever, confusion, meningismus and various focal neurological symptoms including convulsions. The course may be progressively downhill to death, or it may be arrested at any point and followed by gradual improvement, depending on the extent of the structural injury to the brain. This disease is due to the infection of neurons and glia as a result of viremia, although rapid spread also occurs in the ventricular CSF, involving ependymal surfaces as well as the leptomeninges. After infection of susceptible cells, HSV redirects its metabolic activity to produce new virus.

Once complete herpes simplex virions have been synthesized in the host cell, they may cause an acute lytic infection that destroys the cell and liberates the virus. After that, the virus may spread either by the extracellular route (type I spread) or from cell to cell (type II spread) (Notkins, 1974), the latter being particularly important in the nervous system (Johnson and Mims, 1968). Type I spread is readily prevented by extracellular antiviral antibody, but arrest of type II spread requires that the virus-infected cells are destroyed. This process is dependent on sensitized lymphocytes elaborating mediators capable of performing these functions (Shore et al., 1974). Before the infected cells are destroyed, however, the virus may be transmitted to contiguous cells, and therefore the infection is not stopped. Sensitized leukocytes have been shown to inhibit in vitro cell-to-cell spread of HSV experimentally and to convert type II spread to type I spread (Notkins, 1974). This results from the actions of soluble mediators, particularly interferon and lymphotoxin, which are released from these leukocytes. Together they seem to abort viral replication by acting on uninfected cells and interrupting type II spread of virus. Once this occurs, infection can usually be eliminated by the action of antibody and complement, followed by phagocytosis. The latter effect is another function mediated in part by the sensitized lymphocytes which are antibody producers. The obvious conclusion from these observations is that recovery from HSV infection is primarily host-dependent, and anything that interferes with this, particularly an agent that suppresses T-cell function, is potentially detrimental.

The precise etiologic diagnosis is difficult to establish for most viral infections of the nervous system at the time that the patient is symptomatic because: (1) the causative agent is rarely recoverable from the blood or CSF; (2) the demonstration of significant serum antibody changes requires examination of paired serum samples taken at an interval of about 14 days and the exclusion of large numbers of potential viral agents, so that in clinical practice this procedure is less useful in identifying a newly acquired infection; (3) a CSF picture of moderate pleocytosis, slight blood–brain barrier damage, normal glucose concentrations, elevated immunoglobulin concentrations and oligoclonal bands, is not diagnostic for the specific etiologic agent in question.

EVIDENCE FOR SYNTHESIS OF IMMUNOGLOBULINS AND COMPLEMENT WITHIN THE CNS

On calculation of the relative concentrations of IgM, IgA and IgG in CSF, i.e. expressed as percent of the total protein concentration of CSF, we described elevated values in 9%, 27%

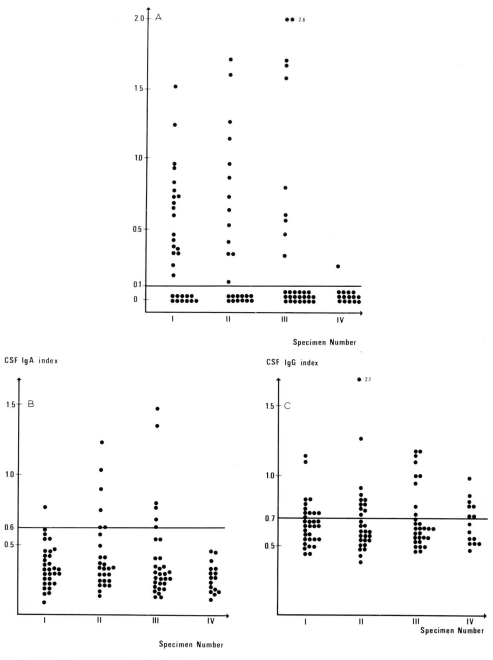

Fig. 1. Values of CSF IgM index (A), CSF IgA index (B) and CSF IgG index (C) in 38 patients with acute aseptic meningitis at different times after onset of symptoms: on the day of admission (specimen I); about 5 days later (specimen II); 1–2 months later (specimen III); more than 3 months after admission (specimen IV). The interval between onset of meningitis symptoms and admission was 0–5 days (mean 2 days). Lines represent upper reference levels in our laboratory, being 0.1 for CSF IgM index, 0.6 for CSF IgA index and 0.7 for CSF IgG index. (Modified from Frydén et al. (1978b).)

and 36%, respectively, of 39 patients with various CNS infections which were mostly of viral etiology (Link and Müller, 1971). An extended study of immunoglobulin levels was done in our laboratory by Frydén et al. (1978b) on two or more CSF and serum specimens obtained over the course of disease from 19 patients with mumps meningitis and 19 with AM of other viral etiology. The CSF values for IgM, IgA and IgG were calculated in the form of CSF immunoglobulin indices, which take into account the concentration in serum of the corresponding immunoglobulin, as well as the influence of the blood–brain barrier, by the inclusion of the CSF/serum albumin ratio (Tibbling et al., 1977). In this way, evidence was obtained of intrathecal synthesis of IgM in 63%, IgA in 26% and IgG in 55% of the patients where upper reference values of 0.1, 0.6 and 0.7, respectively, were applied for the corresponding CSF immunoglobulin indices (Fig. 1). Elevated values were most frequently registered during the acute stage of AM, but when examined more than 3 months after onset of AM, no less than 7 out of 15 patients had elevated CSF IgG index and one out of 15 had elevated CSF IgM index in the presence of normal CSF cell counts. The occurrence of elevated CSF immunoglobulin indices had no influence on the prognosis of AM.

Determination of the concentrations of the complement factors C_3 and C_4, and calculations of their CSF/serum ratios in relation to the patient's CSF/serum albumin ratios revealed elevated C_3 and C_4 values in CSF in about 20% of patients during the acute stage of mumps meningitis (Frydén et al., 1978b). This abnormality may also be interpreted as reflecting intrathecal synthesis.

OLIGOCLONAL REACTION

The occurrence of oligoclonal bands on electrophoresis or isoelectric focusing of CSF in about one of 3 patients with AM is well known (Laterre et al., 1970; Link and Müller, 1971). Among 19 patients with mumps meningitis, 7 had oligoclonal bands in CSF (Frydén et al., 1978b). The oligoclonal bands had disappeared one year after the onset of symptoms in one of these patients. In two of them, the oligoclonal bands remained when the last lumbar puncture was carried out one year after onset, and in two patients oligoclonal bands were detected in all CSF samples obtained over 2.5 years after onset, even though the course of AM in these patients also was completely uneventful. The persistence for one year of oligoclonal bands in CSF obtained from children with mumps meningitis has also been described (Vandvik et al., 1978). These observations indicate that the possible occurrence of oligoclonal bands in CSF for one or more years after ordinary AM has to be kept in mind when separation of CSF IgG by electrophoresis or isoelectric focusing for the demonstration of oligoclonal bands is used as a diagnostic tool, e.g. in multiple sclerosis.

The 7 mumps meningitis patients with oligoclonal bands in the group of 19 mentioned above had an elevated CSF IgG index (Table I). However, 5 of the 12 patients with mumps meningitis and normal findings on agarose electrophoresis of CSF also displayed an elevated CSF IgG index. This observation might indicate intrathecal production of polyclonal IgG in AM (vide infra).

Determination of the κ/λ light chain ratio of CSF in relation to the corresponding ratio in serum is an alternative method for demonstration of an oligoclonal reaction in CSF (Link and Zettervall, 1970). In patients with AM, both abnormally low and abnormally high CSF κ/λ ratios have been found, reflecting intrathecal synthesis either predominantly of IgG λ, or IgG κ, respectively (Link and Müller, 1971; Frydén et al., 1978b).

TABLE I

RELATION BETWEEN OLIGOCLONAL BANDS DEMONSTRABLE BY AGAROSE ELECTROPHORESIS OF CSF, AND OTHER LABORATORY VARIABLES IN 19 PATIENTS WITH ACUTE MUMPS MENINGITIS

(Modified from Frydén et al., 1978b.)

Laboratory abnormality	Oligoclonal bands in CSF	
	Present (n = 7)	Absent (n = 12)
CSF IgG index > 0.7	7	5
CSF IgA index > 0.6	2	2
CSF IgM index > 0.1	6	7
Abnormal CSF κ/λ ratio	3	3
Mumps virus antibody synthesis within the CNS	4	3

Immunofixation with monospecific antisera after separation of CSF and serum by agarose electrophoresis was carried out in 10 patients with AM; this revealed free λ light chains migrating as bands in two patients, and oligoclonal IgM bands, in addition to oligoclonal IgG bands in two patients (Frydén and Link, 1979). These observations indicate that the oligoclonal reaction within the CNS-CSF compartment in viral CNS diseases is not restricted to IgG production, but may also include synthesis of oligoclonal immunoglobulins belonging to other classes, as well as the excessive production of free light chains. These abnormalities are not specific for any inflammatory CNS disease. They may occur in acute AM of well-defined etiology, as well as in multiple sclerosis.

INTRATHECAL ANTIBODY PRODUCTION

Using 3 different conventional serological methods, intrathecal production of mumps antibodies was detected in only 7 of 19 patients with mumps meningitis (Frydén et al., 1978b). Four of these 7 patients had oligoclonal bands in CSF. Three additional patients had oligoclonal bands in CSF but no serological evidence of intrathecal mumps antibody synthesis (Table I).

Studies in HSV encephalitis and meningitis carried out by Sköldenberg et al. (1981) have confirmed the superiority of micromethods, in this case a solid-phase radioimmunoassay (RIA), for the demonstration of virus specific intrathecal antibody response. Evidence of intrathecal production of HSV RIA IgM, IgA and/or IgG antibodies was regularly obtained within 10 days after the onset of symptoms in all 11 patients with HSV encephalitis. In two patients with repeated CSF and serum examinations, evidence of intrathecal synthesis of HSV RIA IgG antibodies was obtained on days 6 and 7, respectively, when oligoclonal IgG bands were still not demonstrable by agarose electrophoresis. These observations underline the diagnostic potential in viral CNS infections of the recently developed, highly sensitive tests for class-specific antibody determinations carried out on CSF and serum specimens which have been obtained simultaneously. Calculation of the CSF/serum antibody ratio in relation to the CSF/serum albumin ratio (CSF antibody index) should yield reliable information about the presence of intrathecal synthesis of the antibody in question.

34

We have recently examined 24 adult patients with mumps meningitis regarding intrathecal production of antibodies against mumps and other viruses (Link et al., 1981). CSF and serum were separated by polyacrylamide gel isoelectric focusing (PAG IF) followed by immuno-fixation with viral antigen and subsequent autoradiography. Bands of mumps antibodies on the CSF autoradiograms without counterparts in the corresponding serum autoradiograms (Fig. 2) were found in 10 patients, while one patient had distinctly fainter bands in serum than CSF. Both these findings were considered to represent evidence of intrathecal mumps antibody production. In 11 of the 24 patients, only an extrathecal specific antibody response was demonstrable, characterized by mumps antibody bands which were stronger or about equally strong on the serum autoradiograms compared to the corresponding CSF autoradiograms. In the two remaining patients, no mumps antibody response was detectable with the present technique, neither inside nor outside the CNS. Vandvik et al. (1983) have reported higher frequencies of intrathecal mumps antibody synthesis, but their patients with mumps meningitis were children, and the mumps antigen preparation used was different from ours.

Five of our 24 patients with mumps meningitis had oligoclonal IgG bands in CSF demon-strated by PAG IF. All oligoclonal IgG bands in 3 of these patients and some of the bands in the remaining two were found to contain mumps antibodies. Fig. 2 shows the patterns on the autoradiograms after immunofixation with mumps virus, compared to the pattern on PAG IF of

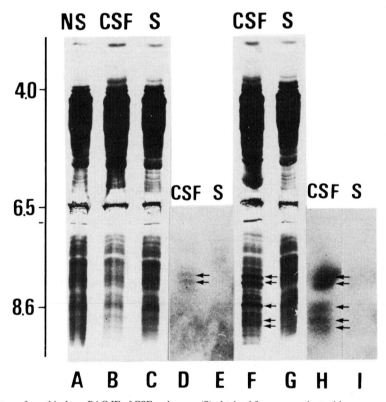

Fig. 2. Patterns from thin-layer PAG IF of CSF and serum (S) obtained from one patient with mumps meningitis on day 3 (B, C) and 43 (F, G) after onset, and the corresponding autoradiograms after immunofixation with mumps virus (D, E and H, I, respectively). Arrows on autoradiograms denote visible bands corresponding to intrathecally synthesized mumps antibodies. These bands had their counterparts in some of the oligoclonal CSF Ig bands. Normal serum (NS) was run as a control (A). Values on the ordinate refer to pH.

CSF and serum taken from one of the patients in the acute phase of mumps meningitis and during convalescence. It is apparent that oligoclonal CSF IgG bands containing mumps antibodies appeared during the observation time in this patient.

Bands of mumps antibodies detected on the CSF autoradiograms from 8 of our 24 patients with mumps meningitis could be traced to polyclonal IgG separated by PAG IF (Table III). Explanations for this phenomenon may be: (1) intrathecal synthesis of polyclonal mumps antibodies; (2) co-migration of oligoclonal IgG in polyclonal IgG zones appearing on PAG IF; (3) artefact due to the separation procedure used. Even though the two last-mentioned alternatives have not been ruled out, the occurrence of elevated CSF IgG index and/or serological evidence for mumps antibody synthesis within the CNS in the absence of oligo-clonal bands in CSF (Table I) favour the first explanation. Indirect evidence for intrathecal production of polyclonal IgG (Laurenzi et al., 1980) with virus antibody activity (Roström et al., 1981) has previously been presented in patients with multiple sclerosis.

In the group of 24 patients with mumps meningitis, only one displayed local production of antibodies to other viruses (measles and HSV) which could then be traced to polyclonal CSF IgG (Tables II and III). On the other hand, local production of mumps antibodies is not specific for mumps meningitis, but can also be demonstrated in other inflammatory CNS diseases, especially in multiple sclerosis, where locally synthesized viral antibodies of various specifi-cities can be traced to oligoclonal as well as polyclonal CSF IgG (Roström et al., 1981). Similar observations have been reported in patients with acute cerebrovascular disease who have been selected on the basis of the presence of oligoclonal IgG bands in CSF (Tables II and III) (Roström et al., 1981). The main difference between the specific local immune response, as it occurs in mumps meningitis, and the non-specific as in multiple sclerosis or cerebrova-scular disease, is that the majority of oligoclonal IgG bands found in mumps meningitis contain mumps antibodies which can be absorbed almost completely with a concentrated suspension of mumps virus, while locally synthesized viral antibodies, e.g. in multiple sclerosis, represent only a minor fraction of the total CSF IgG (Vandvik et al., 1976; Roström et al., 1981). Release of structural brain components as a consequence of brain damage have been proposed to induce polyclonal B-cell activation, leading to the non-specific intrathecal immune response detectable in patients with multiple sclerosis or cerebrovascular disease (Roström et al., 1981). AM, on the other hand, is a benign disease where severe parenchymal brain damage is rare and this is probably the reason why intrathecal "by-stander" antibody production is uncommon in this disease.

TABLE II

INTRATHECAL SYNTHESIS OF VIRAL ANTIBODIES DETECTED BY ANTIGEN IMMUNOFIXATION AND AUTORADIOGRAPHY, AND OCCURRENCE IN PATIENTS WITH MUMPS MENINGITIS, MULTIPLE SCLEROSIS (MS) AND CEREBROVASCULAR DISEASE (CVD)

The patients with CVD were selected on the basis of the demonstration of oligoclonal IgG bands in CSF. n.d., not determined.

Type of local viral antibody production	Mumps meningitis (n = 24)	MS (n = 25)	CVD (n = 9)
Mumps	46%	12%	0
Measles	4%	76%	67%
Herpes simplex type 1	4%	36%	56%
Rubella	0	12%	0
Varicella	n.d.	2 of 10	22%
Cytomegalovirus	n.d.	0 of 10	0
Oligoclonal IgG in CSF	21%	96%	100%

TABLE III

RELATION BETWEEN AUTORADIOGRAPHY FINDINGS OF INTRATHECALLY PRODUCED VIRAL ANTIBODY, AND POLYACRYLAMIDE GEL ISOELECTRIC FOCUSING PATTERNS OF CSF IgG IN PATIENTS WITH MUMPS MENINGITIS, MULTIPLE SCLEROSIS AND CEREBROVASCULAR DISEASE

The patients with cerebrovascular disease were selected on the basis of the demonstration of oligoclonal IgG bands in CSF. n.d., not determined.

Type of local viral antibody production seen on autoradiography	Intrathecally produced antibodies in relation to CSF IgG patterns								
	Mumps meningitis (n = 24)			Multiple sclerosis (n = 25)			Cerebrovascular disease (n = 9)		
	Oligoclonal (n = 5)	Polyclonal	Total number of patients with intrathecal antibody production	Oligoclonal (n = 24)	Polyclonal	Total number of patients with intrathecal antibody production	Oligoclonal (n = 9)	Polyclonal	Total number of patients with intrathecal antibody production
Mumps	5	8	11*	3	2	3*	0	0	0
Measles	0	1	1	17	11	19*	6	3	6*
Herpes simplex type 1	0	1	1	7	3	9*	5	3	5*
Rubella	0	0	0	2	2	3*	0	0	0
Varicella	n.d.			n.d.			1	2	2*
Cytomegalovirus	n.d.			n.d.			0	0	0

* There were patients who had antibodies which could be traced to oligoclonal as well as polyclonal IgG.

TABLE IV

PLAQUE FORMING CELLS (PFC) IN PERIPHERAL BLOOD AND CSF IN PATIENTS WITH ASEPTIC MENINGITIS (AM) DURING THE ACUTE PHASE (GROUP I) AND CONVALESCENCE (GROUP II)

Diagnosis and numbers of subjects			PFC per 20×10^3 lymphocytes							
			IgG		IgA		IgM		IgG + IgA + IgM	
			Blood	CSF	Blood	CSF	Blood	CSF	Blood	CSF
AM Group I (n = 20)	Absolute numbers	Range	0–319	0–716	7–295	0–596	4–104	0–326	21–516	4–1508
		Median	31	15.5	82.5	28.5	17.5	9	129	74
		Mean	79.5	86.4	118.2	104.3	33.8	56.9	231.5	214.3
	Percentage	Range	0–1.6	0–3.6	0.04–1.48	0–3.0	0.02–0.52	0–1.63	0.11–2.6	0.02–7.54
		Median	0.16	0.08	0.41	0.14	0.09	0.05	0.65	0.37
		Mean	0.4	0.43	0.6	0.52	0.17	0.28	1.16	1.07
AM Group II (n = 15)	Absolute numbers	Range	0–26	0–11	8–220	0–186	0–28	0	18–236	0–86
		Median	8	3	27	6	3	0	34	9
		Mean	9.2	4.7	54.6	30.4	7.3	0	75.4	18.2
	Percentage	Range	0–0.13	0–0.01	0.04–1.1	0–0.93	0–0.14	0	0.09–1.18	0–0.43
		Median	0.04	0.02	0.14	0.03	0.02	0	0.17	0.05
		Mean	0.05	0.02	0.27	0.15	0.04	0	0.38	0.09
Healthy individuals (n éY 27)	Absolute numbers	Range	0–20		4–42		0–7		8–68	
		Median	7		12		0		21	
		Mean	7.0		13.3		2.7		23.2	
	Percentage	Range	0–0.1		0.02–0.21		0–0.4		0.04–0.34	
		Median	0.04		0.06		0		0.11	
		Mean	0.04		0.07		0.01		0.12	

IMMUNOGLOBULIN-PRODUCING CELLS IN PERIPHERAL BLOOD AND CSF

The adoption of the hemolysis-in-gel plaque-forming cell (pfc) assay (Jerne and Nordin, 1963) to study single cell immunoglobulin production and secretion, and the application of this technique to human lymphocytes, has suggested new possibilities for in vitro study of a function of cells belonging to B cell lineage in humans.

We have modified the protein-A plaque assay of Gronowicz et al. (1976) for 20×10^3 cells, thereby allowing the immunoglobulin-producing cells in CSF to be counted (Henriksson et al., 1981). Only 3 of 11 patients with AM examined 2–10 days after onset of symptoms had increased numbers of IgM-, IgA- as well as IgG-producing cells in CSF than in peripheral blood, while among patients with multiple sclerosis, 10 out of 11 had higher numbers of IgG-producing cells, 5 had more IgM-producing cells, and 3 had more IgA-producing cells in CSF than in peripheral blood. The patients with AM had higher numbers of IgM-, IgA-, IgG- and IgM + IgA + IgG-producing cells in blood when compared with healthy individuals. These data indicate that even though an intrathecal immune reaction, as reflected by high numbers of immunoglobulin-producing cells, occurred in at least 7 of the 11 patients with AM, an intense immune response outside the CNS was also the rule in this disease.

We have recently extended this study in AM to include 20 patients who were examined during the acute phase (days 1–10; group I) with 15 of the 20 being studied also during convalescence (days 19–38; group II) (Forsberg and Kam-Hansen, manuscript in preparation). Table IV gives the range, median and mean values of immunoglobulin-producing cells in peripheral blood and CSF as absolute numbers and percentages among the patients with AM, and in peripheral blood only in a group of 27 healthy individuals.

The patients in group I, compared to those in group II, had significantly higher numbers of IgG- and IgM-producing cells in peripheral blood as well as in CSF, while no such difference was observed for IgA-producing cells. Even though a predominance of immunoglobulin-producing cells was again observed in peripheral blood, the reverse, i.e. higher CSF values was found in about 25% of the patients in group I for each class of immunoglobulin-producing cells. In group II (15 patients), predominance of immunoglobulin-producing cells in CSF was rare or absent. IgA-producing cells dominated in peripheral blood in both groups of AM patients, as in healthy controls (Table V). In the CSF, about equal numbers of AM patients had mostly IgG- and IgA-producing cells, while in two patients IgM-producing cells predominated. In this respect, the patients with AM differed from those with multiple sclerosis, since IgG-producing cells predominated in the CSF from 27 out of 37 patients, and IgM-producing cells in 7 of the remaining (Table V) (Henriksson et al., manuscript in preparation).

TABLE V

DISTRIBUTION OF DOMINATING CLASS-SPECIFICITY OF Ig-PRODUCING CELLS IN PERIPHERAL BLOOD (PB) AND CSF IN PATIENTS WITH ASEPTIC MENINGITIS (AM) DURING THE ACUTE PHASE (GROUP I) AND CONVALESCENCE (GROUP II), PATIENTS WITH MS, AND HEALTHY CONTROLS

Ig class	AM group I (n = 20)		AM group II (n = 15)		Healthy controls (n = 27)	MS (n = 37)	
	PB	CSF	PB	CSF	PB	PB	CSF
IgG	3	8	1	6	2	2	27
IgA	15	9	12	8	24	34	2
IgM	2	2	1	0	0	1	7
IgG = IgA	0	0	1	0	1	0	1
IgG = IgM	0	1	0	0	0	0	0

A positive correlation was demonstrated in patient group I between the numbers of each of the 3 classes of immunoglobulin-producing cells in the CSF, and the corresponding CSF immunoglobulin indices. No such correlations were found in group II. Several of the patients in both groups, however, had elevated numbers of immunoglobulin-producing cells in CSF in the presence of normal values of the corresponding CSF immunoglobulin index, most probably because the latter is a less sensitive indicator of intrathecal immunoglobulin production than is the counting of immunoglobulin-producing cells. This observation is also corroborated by the finding that a few patients belonging to the convalescent group (group II) had normal white cell counts per μl of CSF, while at the same time considerable proportions of the CSF cells were still active immunoglobulin producers.

Conclusions from these studies are:

(1) As expected, there is an obvious decrease of cells producing different classes of immunoglobulins in both peripheral blood and CSF over the course of AM. This feature seems to parallel the previously described decrease of the concentrations of free immunoglobulins.

(2) The dominating immunoglobulin class-specificity of immunoglobulin-producing cells in peripheral blood in AM is IgA, just as in healthy individuals, while in the CSF compartment the predominance of IgA-producing cells is hardly obvious in relation to the predominance of IgG-producing cells (Table V).

(3) This study strengthens the hypothesis that elevated CSF immunoglobulin index means that some of the CSF immunoglobulins are produced intrathecally in AM, even though the picture is confused by the well-known passage of immunoglobulins from serum through a damaged blood–brain barrier in this disease. The CSF immunoglobulin index corrects for this blood–brain barrier damage by the inclusion of the CSF/serum albumin ratio (Tibbling et al., 1977).

(4) On the other hand, this study also shows that enumeration of immunoglobulin-producing cells in CSF is a much more sensitive indicator of the immune status intrathecally, since, for example, free IgG is the sum of IgG produced over the last month, because the half-life of IgG is about 25 days (6 days for IgA and 5 days for IgM) (Hood et al., 1978).

Finally, it must be stated that future development of techniques enabling analysis not only of class-specific immunoglobulins, but also of specific antibodies on the single cell level in AM and other inflammatory CNS diseases, will have a profound impact on our understanding of the pathogenesis of such disorders.

B- AND T-LYMPHOCYTES AND ACTIVE T-CELLS IN PERIPHERAL BLOOD AND CSF

Results from our laboratory (Frydén, 1977), show that patients with AM have significantly higher T- and lower B-lymphocyte values in CSF than in blood. Similar findings have been reported in multiple sclerosis despite the chronicity of this disease (Kam-Hansen et al., 1978).

When AM patients were divided into 3 groups depending on the stage of the disease (days 1–4, 5–10 and > 20 days after onset of symptoms), those examined on days 1–4 did not show any difference for T-cell distribution in CSF compared to that in peripheral blood, but significantly higher T-cell values were registered in CSF than peripheral blood in the two groups examined during the later AM stages (Frydén et al., 1980).

In experimental viral infections of the CNS in mice, T-lymphocytes are necessary for recovery (Hapel, 1975). The significantly higher mean T-lymphocyte values in the CSF than in

40

the blood of AM patients may be interpreted in the same way, and this T-lymphocyte predominance may obviously last for longer periods of time than clinical symptoms of AM.

A subpopulation of T-cells which has been claimed to reflect cell-mediated immuno-competence more properly than total T-cells in, inter alia, viral diseases, are called "active" T-cells. These are characterized by their ability to form temperature-stable (at 37°C) rosettes with sheep red blood cells. In patients examined over the course of AM (days 1–4, 5–10 and > 20 days after onset of symptoms), higher proportions of active T-cells were measured in CSF than in peripheral blood in all 3 phases of disease (Frydén et al., 1980). However, percentages of active T-cells in the CSF decreased significantly from phase II to phase III, although they were stationary in peripheral blood, possibly reflecting the normalization of intrathecal immune processes reflected by this group of T-cells (cytotoxic cells?), and occurring slightly after clinical improvement.

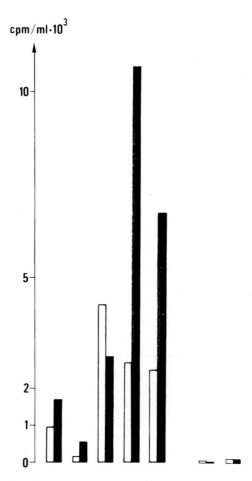

Fig. 3. Effect of mumps virus on peripheral blood lymphocytes (unfilled bars) and CSF lymphocytes (filled bars) from 5 patients with mumps meningitis and two patients with aseptic meningitis due to other causes. The results are expressed as mean net counts/min (cpm)/ml/culture × 10^3.

LYMPHOCYTE RESPONSE TO MITOGENS AND SPECIFIC ANTIGEN IN MUMPS MENINGITIS

An indicator of immuno-competence is the in vitro proliferative response of lymphocytes to stimulation with mitogens. In our study of 15 patients with AM, peripheral blood lymphocytes (PBL) and CSF lymphocytes were stimulated with phytohaemagglutinin (PHA), concanavalin A (ConA), and pokeweed mitogen (PWM), and their responses were measured by the incorporation of radiolabeled thymidine into cellular DNA. The PBL responded more strongly than CSF lymphocytes on exposure to all 3 mitogens, but the CSF lymphocytes were always capable of proliferation. No predominance of either PHA population or ConA population of lymphocytes could be registered among PBL or CSF lymphocytes. The latter appeared to be much more sensitive to small changes of culture conditions than PBL (Frydén and Link, 1978).

The next step was to study the proliferative response on in vitro exposure to mumps virus, of PBL and CSF lymphocytes from patients with mumps meningitis, and from patients with AM of other etiology. In 4 out of 5 patients with mumps meningitis, the CSF lymphocyte proliferation was higher than that obtained with the corresponding numbers of PBL (Fig. 3). The control virus in this study was Newcastle disease virus, and the proliferative responses after stimulation with this virus were at background level. These results indicate the expansion of clones of specifically sensitized lymphocytes inside the diseased organ (Frydén et al., 1978a).

MLC RESPONSE OF CSF LYMPHOCYTES COMPARED WITH THAT OF AUTOLOGOUS PERIPHERAL BLOOD LYMPHOCYTES

The importance of the complex relation between the major histocompatibility complex (MHC) of the host and the virus infecting the host is well established, although far from completely clarified. The ability of lymphocytes, in this case T-cells, to respond on exposure to mononuclear cells with foreign MHC antigens on their surfaces, in so-called mixed lymphocyte culture (MLC), has been shown to be one of the fundamental immune reactions. In healthy humans, positive correlation has been found between MLC responses and mitogenic polyclonal T-cell activation, in spite of the different mechanisms involved (Nanra and Boettcher, 1980).

Recently, MLC has been applied in our laboratory to CSF lymphocytes and PBL from patients with AM (Kam-Hansen et al., 1982). In 8 patients with acute AM, the CSF lymphocytes were regularly MLC reactive, and in 3 of them, more so than the corresponding PBL (Fig. 4). All 7 patients with subacute or chronic AM also responded in the MLC on one or more occasions (Fig. 4), which might be due to different stages of the disease as well as to different sources of stimulator cells. Two of the 3 patients with chronic AM had higher responses of CSF lymphocytes than of PBL, and the same was the case in one of the 4 patients with subacute AM. No statistically significant difference was scored between CSF lymphocyte and PBL responses. The stimulator cells in 11 of the patients with AM (4 acute, 5 subacute and 2 chronic) consisted of PBL from patients with multiple sclerosis. Compared to other sources of stimulator cells (patients with AM and healthy subjects), no differences in MLC responses were found.

42

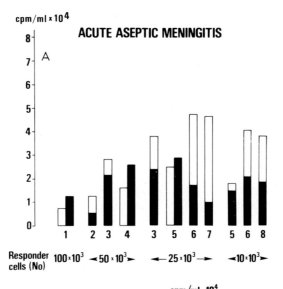

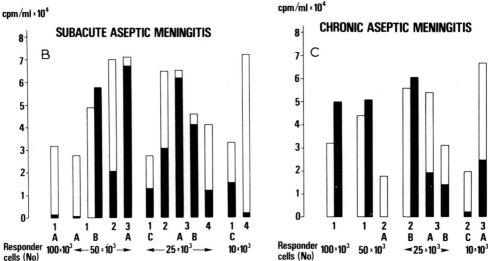

Fig. 4. Mixed lymphocyte culture responses of peripheral blood lymphocytes (unfilled bars) and CSF lymphocytes (filled bars) in patients with acute (A), subacute (B), and chronic aseptic (C) meningitis. Arabic numerals in the figure correspond to the number of the individual patient, while A, B and C underneath these numbers denote different specimens from the same subject obtained at different occasions. The results are peak values, expressed as mean net counts/min (cpm)/ml/culture $\times 10^4$.

In one acute AM patient, 25×10^3 autologous irradiated CSF lymphocytes were used as stimulator cells for both 10×10^3 PBL and 10×10^3 CSF lymphocytes, covering days 3–7 of culture. The maximal response of PBL was 16,472 cpm/ml and that of CSF lymphocytes 640 cpm/ml. When autologous PBL were used as stimulators, the highest PBL response was 4408 cpm/ml and the highest CSF lymphocyte response was 2118 cpm/ml. The fact that autologous CSF cells are better stimulators than autologous PBL may be explained by the possible alteration of MHC antigen of CSF cells by virus or by the selection of clones in CSF which are highly auto-antigenic. This localized MLC response needs further studying, but this is, however, difficult to perform with the current technique available for CSF lymphocytes.

In the patients with AM, no consistent MLC patterns were noticed in relation to clinical or CSF findings, the latter consisting of the degree of pleocytosis or blood–brain barrier damage, CSF IgM, IgA and IgG indices, and IgG synthesis rate within the CNS per 24 h. Comparing MLC responses of PBL in patients with AM, multiple sclerosis, and healthy controls, no significant differences were registered. Nor was this the case when comparing MLC responses of CSF lymphocytes in AM and multiple sclerosis. Even when the highest MLC background values were considered, no significant differences were found when PBL and CSF lymphocyte background values in AM were compared to those in multiple sclerosis. A similar result was obtained when the background values of PBL were compared in AM, multiple sclerosis and healthy controls. MLR backgrounds of CSF lymphocytes showed higher responses in AM than in multiple sclerosis ($P < 0.05$), perhaps as a reflection of the acuteness of AM.

The results of mostly well-reacting CSF lymphocytes in MLC, as well as our previous observation regarding responses of CSF lymphocytes from patients with AM on stimulation with the mitogens PHA, ConA and PWM, show that a majority of individuals suffering from a benign viral CNS disease like AM most probably have immuno-competent lymphocytes intrathecally, as judged by these basic immune tests.

SUMMARY

Acute aseptic meningitis (AM) is a self-limiting, benign disease where the etiology can often be established and the pathogenesis is relatively well worked out. Host-dependent factors, including sensitized lymphocytes and antiviral antibodies, are probably responsible for inhibition of viral spread and elimination of the infection. Abnormalities in the form of increased immunoglobulin concentrations and oligoclonal bands, have previously been described in CSF from patients with AM, and resemble those seen in chronic inflammatory CNS diseases, the most important of them being multiple sclerosis, where the etiology is unknown. Careful dissection of the humoral and cell-mediated immune reactions within the CNS as reflected in CSF, compared to peripheral blood, in patients with AM, will most likely give us fundamental information about the localized immune response in the CNS–CSF, and improve our ability to interpret and utilize new data about immune reactions, e.g. in multiple sclerosis. The following results have emerged over the last years from studies performed on patients with AM.

Humoral immunity

The majority of the patients have elevated CSF indices for IgM, IgA and/or IgG, and some have elevated CSF/serum ratios of the complement factors C_3 and C_4, most probably secondary to intrathecal production. Separation of CSF by electrophoresis or isoelectric focusing revealed oligoclonal bands which most frequently consisted of IgG but sometimes of IgM or even of free λ light chains in about one-third of patients. An elevated CSF IgG index may persist for months after the onset of symptoms, and oligoclonal bands may be detected in CSF for at least 2.5 years after uneventful AM. Intrathecal production of mumps antibodies can be demonstrated in about half of adult patients with mumps meningitis, using immunofixution with mumps virus and subsequent autoradiography. The majority of oligoclonal IgG bands occurring in such patients contain locally synthesized mumps antibodies. Such antibodies can, however, also be traced to polyclonal IgG in some of the patients.

In contrast to the specific intrathecal immune response occurring in AM, the intrathecal viral antibody response that may occur in patients with multiple sclerosis or cerebrovascular disease is apparently non-specific since viral antibodies of different specificities may be produced intrathecally, in a similar pattern, in these two completely different CNS diseases. The explanation proposed by Roström et al. (1981) is that structural brain components liberated as a result of brain damage induce polyclonal B-cell activation. In AM, severe damage to the CNS parenchyma is rare, and this is the probable explanation for the infrequent intrathecal "bystander" antibody production in this benign disease.

Cell-mediated immunity

Adoption of the protein-A plaque assay for counting of immunoglobulin-producing cells has revealed that the dominating immunoglobulin class-specificity in peripheral blood from patients with AM is IgA, just as in healthy individuals, while in the CSF there is a shared predominance of IgA- and IgG-producing cells. A decrease, as expected, was registered for cells producing different classes of immunoglobulins in peripheral blood and CSF over the course of disease, often in parallel with decreasing concentrations of free immunoglobulins. It is, on the other hand, quite obvious that enumeration of immunoglobulin-producing cells in CSF is a more sensitive indicator of the intrathecal immune status than determination of free immunoglobulins. Patients with AM have higher T- and lower B-cell values as well as higher values of active T-cells in CSF than in peripheral blood. In convalescence, increasing numbers of total T-cells and decreasing numbers of active T-cells have been found in the CSF, probably reflecting the dynamics involved in the normalization of intrathecal immune processes. Stimulation in vitro with mitogens has revealed that CSF lymphocytes from AM patients show a lesser response than the corresponding PBL, while in patients with mumps meningitis there is a greater proliferative response of CSF lymphocytes compared to PBL, on stimulation with mumps virus; the latter finding indicates the expansion inside the diseased organ of specifically sensitized lymphocytes. In mixed lymphocyte culture, CSF lymphocytes from patients with AM were regularly reactive, sometimes even at higher levels than PBL. These data argue for the presence of immunocompetent lymphocytes in the CNS compartment of patients with AM.

Future perspectives

Exact definition of immunoregulation during the course of AM, adopting inter alia monoclonal antisera for lymphocyte typing and functional tests for effector, helper and suppressor activities, is essential for our understanding of the ordinary intrathecal immune response occurring within the CSF–CNS compartment in a self-limiting disease, such as AM. Introduction of highly sensitive methods for the determination of immunoglobulin class-specific viral antibodies in CSF and serum has already improved the diagnosis of herpes simplex encephalitis and will be used routinely within the next few years, yielding quicker and safer diagnosis of viral CNS diseases. The development of a method based on the hemolysis-in-gel, plaque-forming cell assay of Jerne, however, which allows the analysis of not only class-specific immunoglobulins as in the protein-A plaque assay in its present modification, but also of specific antibodies on the single cell level, will probably have an even greater impact on our ability to establish the etiologic diagnosis of viral CNS diseases and also on our understanding of the pathogenesis of such diseases.

ACKNOWLEDGEMENTS

The studies presented in this paper have been supported by grants from the Swedish Medical Research Council (Project 3381), "Förenade Liv" Mutual Group Life Insurance Company, Stockholm, Sweden, and the Swedish Multiple Sclerosis Society.

REFERENCES

Frydén, A. (1977) B and T lymphocytes in blood and cerebrospinal fluid in acute aseptic meningitis. *Scand. J. Immunol.*, 6: 1283–1288.

Frydén, A. and Link, H. (1978) Mitogen stimulation of cerebrospinal fluid lymphocytes in aseptic meningitis. *Acta neurol. scand.*, 57: 8–18.

Frydén, A., Link, H. and Möller, E. (1978a) Demonstration of cerebrospinal fluid lymphocytes sensitized against virus antigens in mumps meningitis. *Acta neurol. scand.*, 57: 396–404.

Frydén, A., Link, H. and Norrby, E. (1978b) Cerebrospinal fluid and serum immunoglobulins and antibody titers in mumps meningitis and aseptic meningitis of other etiology. *Infect. Immun.*, 21: 852–861.

Frydén, A. and Link, H. (1979) Predominance of oligoclonal IgG type in CSF in aseptic meningitis. *Arch. Neurol.*, 36: 478–480.

Frydén, A., Kam-Hansen, S., Link, H. and Maller, R. (1980) Active and total T cells in blood and cerebrospinal fluid during the course of aseptic meningitis. *Acta neurol. scand.*, 61: 306–312.

Gronowicz, E., Coutinho, A. and Melchers, F. (1976) A plaque assay for all cells secreting Ig of a given type or class. *Europ. J. Immunol.*, 6: 588–590.

Hapel, A.J. (1975) The protective role of thymus-derived lymphocytes in arbovirus-induced meningo-encephalitis. *Scand. J. Immunol.*, 4: 267–278.

Henriksson, A., Kam-Hansen, S. and Andersson, R. (1981) Immunoglobulin-producing cells in CSF and blood from patients with multiple sclerosis and other inflammatory neurological diseases enumerated by Protein-A plaque assay. *J. Neuroimmunol.*, 1: 299–309.

Hood, L.E., Weissman, J. and Wood, W.B. (1978) In *Immunology*, Benjamin/Cummings, Menlo Park, CA.

Jerne, N.K. and Nordin, A.S. (1963) Plaque formation in agar by single antibody producing cells. *Science*, 140: 405.

Johnson, R.T. and Mims, C.A. (1968) Pathogenesis of viral infections of the nervous system. *New Engl. J. Med.*, 278: 23–30, 84–92.

Kam-Hansen, S., Frydén, A. and Link, H. (1978) B and T cells in cerebrospinal fluid and blood in multiple sclerosis and acute mumps meningitis. *Acta neurol. scand.*, 58: 95–103.

Kam-Hansen, S. (1980) Distribution and function of lymphocytes from the cerebrospinal fluid and blood in patients with multiple sclerosis. *Acta neurol. scand.*, 62, Suppl. 62: 1–81.

Kam-Hansen, S., Andersson, R. and Link, H. (1982) Positive response of CSF lymphocytes from patients with multiple sclerosis and aseptic meningo-encephalitis in mixed lymphocyte culture. *J. Neuroimmunol.*, in press.

Laterre, E.C., Callewaert, A., Heremans, J.F. and Sfaello, Z. (1970) Electrophoretic morphology of gamma globulins in cerebrospinal fluid of multiple sclerosis and other diseases of the nervous system. *Neurology*, 20: 982–990.

Laurenzi, M.A., Mavra, M., Kam-Hansen, S. and Link, H. (1980) Oligoclonal IgG and free light chains in multiple sclerosis demonstrated by thin-layer polyacrylamide gel isoelectric focusing and immunofixation. *Ann. Neurol.*, 8: 241–247.

Laurenzi, M.A. (1981) Immunochemical characterization of immunoglobulins and viral antibodies synthesized within the central nervous system in patients with multiple sclerosis and controls. *Acta neurol. scand.*, 63, Suppl. 84: 1–84.

Link, H. and Zettervall, O. (1970) Multiple sclerosis: disturbed kappa/lambda light chain ratio of immunoglobulin G in cerebrospinal fluid. *Clin. exp. Immunol.*, 6: 435–438.

Link, H. and Müller, R. (1971) Immunoglobulins in multiple sclerosis and infections of the nervous system. *Arch. Neurol.*, 25: 326–344.

Link, H., Laurenzi, M.A. and Frydén, A. (1981) Viral antibodies in oligoclonal and polyclonal IgG synthesized within the central nervous system over the course of mumps meningitis. *J. Neuroimmunol.*, 1: 287–298.

Nanra, S.K. and Boettcher, B. (1980) Correlation between mixed lymphocyte culture and phytohaemagglutinin stimulation responses of human lymphocytes. *Clin. exp. Immunol.*, 41: 173–175.

Notkins, AL.L. (1974) Immune mechanisms by which the spread of viral infections is stopped. *Cell. Immunol.*, 11: 478–483.

46

Roström, B. (1981) Specificity of antibodies in oligoclonal bands in patients with multiple sclerosis and cerebrovascular disease. *Acta neurol. scand.*, 63, Suppl. 86: 1–84.

Roström, B., Link, H., Laurenzi, M.A., Kam-Hansen, S., Norrby, E. and Wahren, B. (1981) Viral antibody activity of oligoclonal and polyclonal immunoglobulin synthesized within the central nervous system in multiple sclerosis. *Ann. Neurol.*, 9: 569–574.

Roström, B., Link, H. and Norrby, E. (1981) Antibodies in oligoclonal immunoglobulins in CSF from patients with acute cerebrovascular disease. *Acta neurol. scand.*, 64: 225–240.

Shore, S.L., Nahmias, A.J., Starr, S.E., Wood, P.A. and McFarlin, D.E. (1974) Detection of cell-dependent cytotoxic antibody to cells infected with herpes simplex. *Nature (Lond.)*, 251: 350–352.

Sköldenberg, B., Kalino, K., Carlström, A., Forsgren, M. and Halonen, P. (1981) Herpes simplex encephalitis: a serological follow-up study. *Acta neurol. scand.*, 63: 273–285.

Tibbling, G., Link, H. and Öhman, S. (1977) Principles of albumin and IgG analyses in neurological disorders. I. Establishment of reference values. *Scand. J. clin. Lab. Invest.*, 37: 385–390.

Vandvik, B., Norrby, E., Nordal, H.J. and Degré, M. (1976) Oligoclonal measles virus-specific IgG antibodies isolated from cerebrospinal fluids, brain extracts and sera from patients with subacute sclerosing panencephalitis and multiple sclerosis. *Scand. J. Immunol.*, 5: 979–992.

Vandvik, B., Norrby, E., Steen-Johnsen, J. and Stensvold, K. (1978) Mumps meningitis: prolonged pleocytosis and occurrence of mumps virus-specific oligoclonal IgG in the cerebrospinal fluid. *Europ. Neurol.*, 17: 13–22.

Immunology of Nervous System Infections, Progress in Brain Research, Vol. 59, edited by P.O. Behan, V. ter Meulen and F. Clifford Rose

Immunosuppressive Effects of Virus Infection

A.M. DENMAN

Connective Tissue Diseases Research Group, Clinical Research Centre, Harrow, Middlesex (U.K.)

INTRODUCTION

The outcome of virus infections in man is determined by several factors and involves the interaction of viruses of varying virulence with host responses of varying efficiency. There has been considerable speculation that persistent virus infections may be partly or wholly responsible for demyelinating disorders of the central nervous system (CNS). Accordingly, there have been continued attempts to isolate viruses from the affected tissues of such patients or to demonstrate defects in handling ubiquitous viruses. So far, evidence in support of this concept is provided principally by animal models of persistent virus infection accompanied by demyelination. Infection by retroviruses of the visna-maedi group is a notable example. As yet there are few convincing observations in human demyelinating diseases such as multiple sclerosis to incriminate a viral etiology. Nevertheless, the immunological abnormalities reported in multiple sclerosis (Knight et al., 1981) are compatible with those induced by virus infections in both man and experimental animals. Thus it is reasonable to examine the mechanisms by which viruses affect immune function since such studies may provide indirect evidence for a viral etiology in human demyelinating diseases.

There are 3 general questions to be answered about the effects of virus infections on immune function. The first concerns the possibility that virus infection affects the specific immune response to the invading virus, thereby aiding and abetting its own dissemination and persistence. There is little evidence to this effect, and specific defects in immune responses to viral antigens are rarely gross and usually contentious. The second question concerns the possibility that virus infection interferes with immune responses to unrelated viruses, encouraging the development of secondary viral and bacterial infections. This is well accepted and viruses have been shown to interfere with several forms of host immunity. There is, however, a third more subtle possibility, which is that virus infection could initiate auto-immune reactions against antigenic components of the CNS (Denman, 1981), inducing both acute and chronic immunopathological disorders. Linked to this suggestion is the possibility that virus infections persist in lymphocytes and that the formal traffic patterns of infected cells encourage viral dissemination to distant sites (Summers et al., 1978). This hypothesis needs more extensive investigation.

This chapter is concerned mainly with the immunosuppressive effects of some viruses which are pathogenic for man. It also reviews the evidence that certain abnormalities of lymphocyte behaviour in human inflammatory diseases associated with abnormalities of the central nervous system may be attributable to persistent virus infection analogous to those induced by the experimental infection of lymphocytes in vitro.

[47]

MECHANISMS OF VIRAL IMMUNOSUPPRESSION

Several mechanisms have been proposed by which viruses induce immunosuppression (Table I). The most direct possibility is that virus grows in lymphocytes engaged in specific immune responses and directly inactivates such cells. Another possibility is that virus infection induces the production of interferon or other immunoregulatory substances which suppress the immune function of uninfected cells. Since many virus infections induce the proliferation of specific and non-specific suppressor cells, these could also interfere with the generation and expression of immune reactions. There are also several ways in which viruses may transiently interfere with lymphocyte function without necessarily infecting these cells. Thus, effects on lymphocyte membrane glycoproteins could affect such functions as antigen recognition and circulation patterns (Denman, 1979).

TABLE I

PROPOSED MECHANISMS OF VIRUS-INDUCED IMMUNOSUPPRESSION

(1) Direct inactivation of susceptible lymphocytes
(2) Activation of suppressor cells
    suppressor T-lymphocytes
    monocyte–macrophages
(3) Production of suppressor factors
    α, γ interferon
    other factors

The effects of virus infections on several forms of immune response have been assessed in experimental animals; these studies have considered the in vivo effects of virus infections on immune responses and also their in vitro effect on lymphocyte responses. Most in vivo observations in man have been confined to analyzing the effects of natural virus infection or immunization on the composition of circulating lymphocyte sub-populations. These kinds of observation have to some extent been supplemented by examining the effects of virus infection on in vitro lymphocyte function. Most of these experiments, however, concern the effect of virus infection on non-specific in vitro reactions to mitogens such as phytohaemagglutinin and concanavalin A. There are several problems in analyzing the results of such in vitro experiments. Non-specific lymphocyte activation does not resemble the selective responses of lymphocytes to defined antigens. There are also a number of non-specific factors, such as cell concentration, which make the interpretation of these assays very difficult (Farrant and Knight, 1979). These problems are compounded by attempts to measure suppressor or inducer activity by conventional methods in which in vitro mixtures are made of lymphocyte populations with allegedly specific functions (Farrant and Newton, 1981). Cultures stimulated with lectins are also unsuitable for measuring the extent and distribution of virus growth in the cultured cells because of the ease with which virus can pass from cell to cell, given the extent of lymphocyte activation and, with some lectins, cell clumping. There are advantages in selecting a form of in vitro immune response which reflects more faithfully the interactions between different lymphocyte populations engaged in the generation of specific immune responses. The introduction of techniques for inducing specific antibody responses in vitro provided a suitable assay for such studies. Suitable methods measure antibody production induced by diphtheria toxoid (Platts-Mills and Ishizaka, 1975) and influenza viral antigens (Callard,

1979). These responses involve synergistic reactions between monocytes, inducer T-lymphocytes, and B-lymphocytes. Such assays are not dependent on in vivo stimulation immediately before lymphocyte function is assayed, although this can be done to influence the pattern of responses after further exposure to antigen in vitro.

The effects of herpes simplex viruses types I and II, measles virus, and influenza viruses on specific antibody responses have been examined in detail. Herpes simplex virus suppresses antibody responses during the first stage of their induction (Pelton et al., 1976). Antibody responses are almost completely suppressed if the responding cultures are infected within the first 72 h of culture, but are unaffected if virus infection is further delayed. This indicates that not all lymphocytes are inactivated. Virological assays show that only a small percentage of T-lymphocytes are susceptible to infection. This conclusion is based upon experiments in which defined lymphocyte populations are separated by conventional methods after exposure to virus before or after the separation procedure. The isolated populations are assayed for virus growth by measuring virus infectivity titers, carrying out infectious center assays on the lymphocytes, or seeking evidence of infection by immunofluorescence and ultrastructural techniques. The results show clearly that T-inducer cells are not only the population most susceptible to infection, but is also the only population which is functionally affected. Limited virus growth is observed in monocytes and B-lymphocytes, but this infection does not have functional consequences (Pelton, 1980).

Experiments of this nature are still open to criticism because wild strains of herpes simplex virus that grow at 37°C can spread during the course of the experiment from lymphocytes initially infected by virus to other cells. This difficulty has been overcome by carrying out similar experiments with temperature sensitive (ts) mutants of herpes simplex virus. Lymphocytes are infected at a reduced temperature which allows these mutants to complete a limited part of their growth cycle; after this, the cells are cultured at the conventional temperature (37°C). At this temperature no productive virus infection is possible, but the immune responses of the infected lymphocytes can proceed optimally (Pelton et al., 1980). It should be stressed that such shifts in temperature do not affect the ability of uninfected lymphocytes to respond normally in functional assays of this nature. The results show that antibody responses are suppressed by those ts mutants which suppress protein synthesis in the non-productively infected cells. Mutants which infect cells without abolishing host cell protein synthesis do not interfere with the immune responses of the infected cells. Biological assays confirm that only a very small percentage of inducer T-lymphocytes are infected ($< 0.1\%$), and that there is no delayed infection of other lymphocytes in culture due to breakthrough of the ts mutants at 37°C. Furthermore, ts mutants allow one to study the immune function of lymphocytes in combination with uninfected cells under circumstances which preclude the possibility that continued virus growth might account for any of the experimental results. Thus it is possible to examine the proposition that suppressor cells induced by virus infection could account for some of the observed immunosuppression. Moreover, this approach allows a variety of experimental possibilities involving the co-culture of lymphocytes from donors immunized with antigen and lymphocytes challenged with further antigen in vitro. No evidence has so far been obtained, however, to show that suppressor cells are involved in the suppression of specific antibody responses by herpes simplex virus. Lymphocytes from cultures whose specific inducer cell function has been ablated by ts mutants of HSV do not affect the titre and kinetics of antibody production by uninfected lymphocytes with which the non-productively infected cells are mixed. Similar considerations govern the proposition that interferon and other lymphocyte mediators account for the depression of antibody synthesis. The medium in which infected lymphocytes are cultured does not affect the antibody response of fresh, uninfected lymphocytes to the same antigen, even if these uninfected cells are cultured exclusively in such a medium (Pelton, 1980). More directly, specific anti-interferon antibody does not prevent viral immunosuppression.

The results obtained with measles virus follow a similar pattern. This virus is of particular interest in the context of degenerative disorders of the CNS because of its association with sub-acute sclerosing pannencephalitis and because of the repeated suggestion that measles virus may be involved in the pathogenesis of multiple sclerosis. Moreover, there is ample evidence that measles virus produces a latent infection in circulating lymphocytes in man (Lucas et al., 1978) and this infection accounts for the depression of cell-mediated immune responses which accompanies natural infection by this virus (Whittle et al., 1978). The well-known observation that measles virus interferes with lymphocyte responses to phytomitogens suggests, but does not prove, that this immunosuppression is a direct consequence of virus growth in lymphocytes. Examining the effects of measles virus infection on specific antibody synthesis by human lymphocytes in vitro allows this conjecture to be examined more critically. Measles virus suppresses antibody synthesis if the responding cells are infected within the first 72 h of exposure to antigen (Pelton et al., 1981). Only a small percentage of lymphocytes are infected during this period, judged by virological techniques, but unlike the situation in cultures infected with herpes simplex virus, infection is not confined to inducer T-lymphocytes: B-lymphocytes and monocytes are also susceptible. However, there is a discrepancy between the ability of defined lymphocyte populations to support virus growth and the effect of this infection on lymphocyte function. Inducer T-lymphocytes are both infected and functionally inactivated. Monocytes and B-lymphocytes are infected but function normally. Similarly, human blood lymphocytes synthesizing antibody spontaneously after in vivo immunization consequent upon lympho-proliferative disorders are functionally unaffected by virus infection. Many attempts have been made in this system to show that suppressor cells induced by measles virus contribute to this immunosuppression, but these have been unsuccessful. In addition there is little difficulty in showing that interferon is produced by the infected cultures, but this does not confer immunosuppression on uninfected lymphocytes challenged with the same antigens. Nor is the immunosuppression blocked by anti-interferon antiserum.

The results obtained with herpes simplex and measles viruses show a consistent picture of selective virus growth leading to immunosuppression. Experiments with influenza virus produce a more complicated picture. Herpes simplex virus and measles virus invariably grow in appropriately stimulated cultures of lymphocytes from normal donors within a relatively consistent and reproducible range. In contrast, both type A and type B influenza viruses grow poorly in lymphocytes. Absorption, penetration, and uncoating of virus particles can readily be shown (Hackman et al. 1974), and there is some production of virus-coded polypeptides (Brownson et al., 1979). There is, however, very limited production of new infectious particles (Hackman et al., 1974). This non-productive infection has a variable effect on the immunological competence of the infected cells (Pelton, 1980). Specific antibody production is little affected in cultures of lymphocytes from most normal donors, but variable, statistically significant enhancement or suppression of both specific antibody production and IgM and IgG synthesis is observed in cultures from other donors: no obvious factors have been discovered which explain these differences. It is difficult therefore to invoke a simple correlation between virus growth and immunosuppression with respect to this virus. Equally, there is no correlation between interferon production used in these cultures and the effect of virus infection on immune function; suppressor T-cells, suppressor monocytes, or suppressor diffusible factors have not been detected to account for the immunosuppression when it is observed.

INDIRECT MECHANISMS FOR VIRAL-INDUCED IMMUNOSUPPRESSION

The experiments described above relate to selected viruses and their immunosuppressive effects on one form of immune response. Although these results indicate that these viruses are immunosuppressive because of their effects on the lymphocytes in which they grow, there are other situations in which it is reasonable to invoke other mechanisms. Moreover, it is hard to explain why the immunosuppressive effects of herpes simplex virus and measles virus infection should be so profound if only a small minority of cells are susceptible. Animal experiments have provided strong evidence that suppressor cells contribute at least in part to viral-induced immunosuppression. Evidence to this effect is still fragmentary and concerns non-specific effects on responses to mitogens in vitro. Suppressor mechanisms have been described in infections by other human herpes viruses, namely Epstein–Barr (EB) virus and cytomegalovirus infections (Ho, 1981). The mechanisms of immunosuppression in cytomegalovirus mononucleosis have been particularly fully investigated (Carney and Hirsch, 1981). Cells of the monocyte-macrophage series have been shown to have either helper or suppressor properties, thus raising the possibility that indirect mechanisms of immunosuppression may be operating in patients with this disorder. Since lymphocytes isolated from patients at the height of this complaint are relatively unresponsive to stimulation with concanavalin A, it is possible that the suppressor effects operate in vivo at this stage. Similar considerations apply to acute EB virus infection. However, the non-specific effects of cell concentration in vitro, make assays of this kind hard to evaluate (Farrant and Knight, 1979). Further indirect evidence for invoking suppressor mechanisms in human virus infections comes from analyzing circulating lymphocyte populations with monoclonal antibodies (Reinherz et al., 1980). There is little information about the extent to which changes in the relative numbers of inducer and suppressor cells, detected by monoclonal antibodies, in virus infections reflects the suppression of specific antibody responses. Such doubts are reinforced by observations that profound virus-induced changes in blood lymphocyte populations judged by conventional markers are not necessarily associated with functional immunosuppression. For example, in one study immunization with a killed influenza virus infection produced a profound T-lymphocytopenia and a less severe B-lymphocytopenia, but did not prevent a brisk antibody response to the immunizing virus (Faguet, 1981). Certainly, there is little evidence that the alleged activation of suppressor cells in Epstein–Barr or cytomegalovirus infections predisposes to secondary infections of clinical consequence. This contrasts with severe measles infection in which secondary bacterial infections are commonly encountered.

In infectious mononucleosis there is a reported increase in the number of activated T-lymphocytes with the phenotype of suppressor cells, and these cells allegedly suppress the response of autologous T-lymphocytes to the non-specific mitogens phytohaemagglutinin and concanavalin A, and also to specific antigens such as tetanus toxoid and mumps antigen. The response of autologous B-lymphocytes to pokeweed mitogen is also suppressed (Reinherz et al., 1980). Such experiments, however, do not take into account the possibility that normally reactive T-lymphocytes and other populations may be present in the blood in vivo but are diluted out in vitro and are therefore underestimated in assays where unseparated blood mononuclear cells are cultured at a single concentration. The unseparated mononuclear cells isolated from the blood by simple density techniques consist predominantly of cytotoxic T-cells directed at target cells infected with Epstein–Barr virus. Indeed, earlier studies have shown that the small lymphocytes in the blood of patients with infectious mononucleosis behave more normally if isolated and assayed at optimal concentrations (Denman and Pelton, 1974).

VIRUS PERSISTENCE IN LYMPHOCYTES

If experiments showing that a virus selectively infects and inactivates lymphocytes in vitro are pathogenetically important, it can be predicted that persistent infection of lymphocytes will be a factor in human immunopathological disorders induced by persistent virus infections (Table II). It is now apparent that many common viruses persist in human lymphocytes for longer periods than had hitherto been imagined. There are several technical reasons why this has not been hitherto appreciated. Often the virus is only rescued if the lymphocytes co-cultivated with indicator cells are first stimulated with phytohaemaglutinin. There has also been confusion about the site of virus persistence when crude populations of mononuclear cells isolated from the blood have not been subjected to further separation before attempts at virus rescue. Finally there is the problem that virus may persist in defective or altered form and may not be detectable by conventional co-cultivation.

TABLE II

VIRUS GROWTH IN HUMAN MONONUCLEAR CELLS

? denotes uncertain or conflicting data. Inverted commas mean that the infected cells have not been fully characterized

Virus	Experimental in vitro infection	In vivo association
Cytomegalovirus	Monocytes	Monocytes?
Herpes simplex	Predominantly inducer T-lymphocytes also B-lymphocytes and monocytes	T-lymphocytes?
EB virus	B-lymphocytes	B-lymphocytes
Measles	T- and B-lymphocytes, monocytes	T- and B-lymphocytes
Rubella	T- and B-lymphocytes	"Lymphocytes"
Influenza	Mainly incomplete; in T- and B-lymphocytes, monocytes	Lymphocytes?
Mumps	"Lymphocytes"	"Lymphocytes"
Dengue	Monocytes	Monocytes

Measles virus has been recovered from the blood lymphocytes of patients with sub-acute sclerosing panencephalitis, thereby establishing that this virus may persist for far longer periods than had hitherto been imagined (Wrzos et al., 1979); in earlier studies measles virus had only been recovered from these cells in the acute or convalescent stage of infection. Similarly, rubella virus has been isolated from the blood lymphocytes of individuals up to 2 years after adult immunization (Chantler et al., 1981). Moreover, there are recent reports of rubella isolation from the joints of patients with chronic or recurrent arthritis in individuals lacking any history of previous rubella immunization or obvious natural infection by this virus (Grahame et al., 1981). Although the clinical features of these patients distinguish their disease from classical juvenile chronic arthritis or adult rheumatoid arthritis (Grahame et al., 1982) and they lack rheumatoid factor, the arthritis is none the less erosive, the immunopathological features of the inflamed synovial membrane resemble those observed in chronic arthritis of unknown etiology, and some auto-antibodies such as anti-nuclear factor are detectable.

There are several possible explanations for viral persistence in the lymphocytes of patients with chronic disorders of the central nervous system or articular system. This persistence may reflect a primary defect in the elimination of infectious virus in the initial infection. Whilst there is little evidence in human disease that the extent of virus growth in lympho-reticular cells determines the virulence of the infection in the short- or longer-term, there is evidence to this effect in experimental systems. For example, the extent of viral replication and persistence in lympho-reticular tissues determines the extent of resistance to vesicular stomatitis virus (Fultz et al., 1981). There are also indications that the susceptibility of lympho-reticular cells to virus infection may be determined by ancillary factors such as efficient interferon production in response to the initial infection (Haller et al., 1981). The extent to which virus persists in human lymphocytes is likely to depend upon the initial balance between the extent to which virus replicates in these cells and host defense factors. Whilst there are some indications that the efficiency of some forms of immune defense such as cytotoxic T-lymphocyte reactions is genetically determined, there is little information about the other factors which determine such susceptibility.

Given that virus persistence in lymphocytes can be correlated with the long-term immuno-pathological consequences of the infection, there are several ways in which this association could arise. The susceptibility of lymphocytes to persistent infection may not be peculiar to these cells but could reflect a general susceptibility allowing unusual persistence in other tissues. There is so far little evidence to support the more obvious deduction that viral infection of lymphocytes interferes with the specific immune response to the infecting agent, and hence to its persistence. Another possibility is that lymphocytes which continue to support virus growth are a source of virus which is continually released and thereafter circulates as infectious complexes of virus and antibody. These infectious complexes could be deposited in the usual sites of predilection for antigen–antibody complexes. There is also the intriguing possibility that virus-infected lymphocytes continue to provide the stimulus for auto-immune reactions directed at neural antigens. Some caution is also necessary in interpreting the significance of virus isolation from the lymphocytes of patients with chronic degenerative diseases. These may be accounted for by the reactivation of viruses associated with lymphocytes participating in a primary lympho-proliferative disorder. This is the most likely explanation for the variable and unpredictable pattern of rising anti-viral antibody titres encountered in such disorders as systemic lupus erythematosus and chronic active hepatitis. Such caveats apply equally to diseases of the central nervous system. Recently, an infectious cytopathic paramyxovirus was rescued from the blood leucocytes of a patient with sub-acute sclerosing panencephalitis (Robbins et al., 1981) and was at first believed to be a measles-like virus similar to those repeatedly rescued from other patients with this disease. However, subsequent investigations showed that the virus was distinct from measles virus and was more closely related to Simian virus 5. This observation emphasizes that paramyxoviruses other than measles virus may be associated with lymphocytes as an entirely non-specific finding.

MECHANISMS FOR EVADING HOST RESPONSES

An increasing number of mechanisms have been recognized by which virus-infected cells may escape elimination by the host response. Some of these involve interference of one form of immune response with another, notably interference by antibody with cell-mediated immune responses (Oldstone, 1979). The best known of such mechanisms is antibody modulation of viral antigens on the surface of infected cells so that these are no longer susceptible to destruction by cytotoxic T-lymphocytes. There are also special reasons why defective virus infection of lymphocytes may allow the viral genome to persist without productive infection or even the expression of surface viral antigens. Thus lymphoblastoid cell lines that are defective in the enzymes needed to cleave measles F protein fail to place the active F1 protein on their surfaces (Fujinami and Oldstone, 1981). The antibody response to persistent virus may also generate anti-idiotype antibody which in turn suppresses the production of antibodies directed at viral proteins. This possibility has been suggested by experiments in which the serum of mice immunized with measles virus has been shown to cross-react with common idiotypes in monoclonal antibodies raised against measles virus antigens (Gheuens et al., 1981). Ts mutants of neurotropic viruses produce modified immunopathological effects in experimental animals. The role of such mutations in CNS infections in man is also now recognized (Hodes, 1981).

EVIDENCE FOR VIRUS INFECTION IN CONNECTIVE TISSUE DISEASES ASSOCIATED WITH DISORDERS OF THE CENTRAL NERVOUS SYSTEM

Some inflammatory connective tissue disease, invariably associated with auto-immune phenomena, are associated also with disorders of the central nervous system. Notably, a variety of neurological features are seen in patients with systemic lupus erythematosus (Sergent et al., 1975). These manifestations include grand mal fits, aseptic meningitis, a variety of focal neurological abnormalities, and psychoses without other evidence of neurological disease. The pathogenesis of the neurological disease is unknown, but is usually attributed to either immune complex deposition or to auto-immune reactions, albeit on slender evidence. Another disease characterized by inflammatory vasculitis with a typical picture of organ involvement is Behcet's syndrome. This disorder is also associated with neurological abnormalities (O'Duffy and Goldstein, 1976), which include aseptic meningitis, transient cranial nerve palsies, cerebellar signs, and spinal long tract involvement.

These diseases have many of the features of chronic immunopathological disorders induced by virus infections (Lehner and Barnes, 1979), but direct attempts to prove a viral etiology have been unsuccessful. The observation that growth in lympho-reticular cells is an obligatory stage in the dissemination of many experimental and human virus infections prompted a search for indirect evidence that these diseases might be accompanied by persistent infection of lymphocytes (Denman et al., 1976). The technique employed has been to look for evidence of viral interference; by this principle it can be anticipated that latent infection of lymphocytes will block the growth of the same or closely related viruses. Some virusss grow invariably in appropriately activated cultures of normal human lymphocytes; these viruses include herpes simplex viruses types 1 and 2, measles virus, polio virus, vesicular stomatitis virus, and rubella virus. The majority of these viruses also grow normally in similar lymphocyte cultures established from the blood of patients with systemic lupus erythematosus and Behcet's syndrome and other forms of inflammatory connective tissue disease.

Herpes simplex virus growth in normal lymphocytes can be used as a clinical assay; a multiplicity of infection of 0.1 virus particles per lymphocyte produces between 4.2 and 6.4 log PFU per 1.0×10^6 cultured lymphocytes, 3–5 days after infection (Denman et al., 1980). Herpes simplex virus, however, often fails to grow in activated lymphocytes from patients with these disorders. The blood lymphocytes of patients with rheumatoid arthritis also supports the growth of herpes simplex virus to normal titres, but lymphocytes isolated from rheumatoid synovial effusions are not permissive for this virus (Appleford and Denman, 1979a). Non-permissiveness for herpes simplex virus replication is not a constant feature in these patients and varies erratically in the same individual in whom virus growth is studied over a period of years (Denman et al., 1976; Denman et al., 1980). The fluctuations in herpes virus growth do not correlate with clinical activity. Non-permissiveness has been noted in patients whose systemic lupus erythematosus and Behcet's syndrome are associated with lesions of the central nervous system.

Simple explanations for this non-permissiveness have as far as possible been excluded. Cultures established from normal donors and assayed at the same time as cultures from these patients have invariably supported virus growth in a normal fashion. Since lymphocytes must be appropriately activated if they are to support the growth of herpes simplex virus, defective response to stimulation is a possible explanation for non-permissiveness in disease. No correlation has been observed, however, between the extent of lymphocyte proliferation judged by standard techniques and the fate of herpes simplex virus in the stimulated cultures (Denman et al., 1980; Appleford and Denman, 1979a). Nor is there any correlation between the number and function of inducer T-lymphocytes in these cultures, the lymphocyte population primarily susceptible to herpes simplex virus infection (Pelton et al., 1976), and virus growth. Cultures with very poor responsiveness to immunological stimulation judged by these criteria may support the growth of virus to normal titres, whereas conversely, no growth may be observed in cultures which produce a brisk proliferative response. The effects of treatment with immunosuppressive drugs on virus growth in lymphocytes from such patients support the contention that the extent of herpes replication does not simply reflect lymphocyte function as conventionally measured (Hollingworth et al., in preparation). In a comparative study of patients with inflammatory connective tissue diseases treated with steroids in isolation or with intensive immunosuppression, the effects of treatment on virus growth were systematically studied. Before treatment, virus growth was erratic and unpredictable in lymphocytes cultured from patients with all forms of inflammatory connective tissue disease in all stages of activity including those with systemic lupus erythematosus and Behcet's syndrome. In general, treatment with steroids or intensive immunosuppression, namely a combination of high-dose steroids, azathioprine and anti-lymphocyte globulin, restored a normal pattern of virus growth, although virus titres were higher in patients treated with intensive immunosuppression.

The failure of herpes simplex virus to grow in some cultures reflects anti-viral host immunity. The susceptible, non-permissive cultures contain potentially susceptible T-lymphocytes which in isolation are able to support the growth of herpes simplex virus to titres comparable with those obtained in unseparated blood mononuclear cell cultures from normal donors. These permissive cells can be isolated by a variety of techniques including velocity sedimentation, density gradient separation, and rosette formation followed by physical methods of separation (Appleford and Denman, 1979b). Non-permissiveness can again be conferred on these susceptible cells by admixture with other cell populations. The cells responsible for conferring non-permissiveness are medium- or large-sized, non-adherent cells with B-lymphocyte characteristics. The effect is not mediated by immunoglobulin, antibody, interferon, or diffusible substances and requires cell-to-cell contact. Moreover, the inhibiting cells do not have the characteristics of conventional natural killer (NK) cells, killer (K) cells, or suppressor cells. Furthermore, the inhibiting cells only prevent herpes simplex virus growth in lymphocytes from the same individual and are ineffective in cultures of histocompatible lymphocytes from normal donors or from other patients with the same disease. These observations have been made in non-permissive lymphocyte cultures isolated from rheumatoid synovial effusions (Denman et al., 1980), the blood of patients with Behcet's syndrome, and the blood of patients with other inflammatory connective tissue diseases (Denman et al., 1976). The main argument for invoking viral interference to explain this non-permissiveness is that only herpes simplex virus shows this abnormal behaviour; other RNA and DNA viruses grow equally well in lymphocytes from patients with these disorders and from normal controls. So far, however, attempts to rescue defective herpes simplex virus or other viruses from these cells have been unsuccessful.

Some indirect evidence for persistent viral infection has been obtained in cytogenetic studies of lymphocytes from patients with Behcet's syndrome. Detailed analysis of chromosome preparations taken from lymphocytes of patients with Behcet's syndrome have shown chromosome abnormalities often with specificity for certain chromosomes (Denman et al., 1980). These abnormalities have not been observed in similar preparations from control subjects, nor in patients with a variety of viral and bacterial inflammatory diseases, or other connective tissue disorders. It should be emphasized that the samples have been coded before analysis, that appropriate controls have been included in each batch, and that culture conditions have been selected which minimize artefacts such as familial hyperfragility. Remarkably, chromosome abnormalities are not consistently detected and show the same unpredictable fluctuations in sequential observations as the periods of non-permissiveness for herpes simplex virus. However, there is a statistical correlation between the appearance of chromosome abnormalities in lymphocytes and non-permissiveness of these cells for herpes simplex virus (Denman et al., 1980). It is noteworthy also that treatment with steroids and other immunosuppressive measures also eliminates lymphocytes with chromosome abnormalities. It is obviously important to see whether there is any familial pattern of chromosome abnormality inheritance in these patients. It is well recognized that features of Behcet's syndrome are found in one or more first degree family members of 5% of probands with definite Behcet's syndrome (Chamberlain, 1978). A family study currently in progress (Chamberlain et al., in preparation) suggests that similar chromosome abnormalities and non-permissiveness for herpes simplex virus are found in a significantly higher percentage of clinically normal relatives of patients with Behcet's syndrome, than in those of control subjects.

The explanation for these observations is unknown but persistent virus infection of lymphocytes is a feasible explanation; this infection could be asymptomatic in some family members but produce immunopathological consequences in those with obvious clinical disorders. It should also be pointed out that herpes simplex virus shows intermittent non-permissiveness in blood lymphocytes of patients with multiple sclerosis, although this is a less frequent finding, and the possibility has not been excluded that these fluctuations may be attributable to the periods of depressed lymphocyte responsiveness to mitogens which are characteristic of this disorder (Knight et al., 1981), (Table III).

TABLE III

HERPES SIMPLEX VIRUS GROWTH IN BLOOD LYMPHOCYTES FROM PATIENTS
WITH MULTIPLE SCLEROSIS

Under standard conditions lymphocytes from normal donors replicate herpes simplex virus (HSV) in vitro to titres indicated in the table (details in Denman et al., 1980). Cultures from patients which fail to support virus growth (< 3.0 log pfu/10^6 cells) are termed non-permissive

Number of patients studied	20
Total number of estimations	62
Mean HSV titre (log pfu/10^6 cells)	3.75 ± 1.37 S.D.
Number of patients non-permissive	9
Normal range (log pfu/10^6 cells)	4.2–6.4

CONCLUSIONS

It is accepted that several virus infections of man induce clinically significant immuno-suppression. The mechanism of this immunosuppression has not been elucidated, but in vitro experiments show that some viruses inactivate functionally important inducer T-lymphocytes. Whilst there are many observations in experimental animals implicating suppressor cells and related mechanisms, there is so far little evidence that these are concerned in the immuno-suppression which accompanies virus infections of man. The availability of more refined systems for measuring immune function in human lymphocyte cultures will make it easier to examine such hypotheses than was possible with the crude indicators of immune function which involve non-specific proliferative response induced by mitogens. There is also little evidence that virus infections precipitate exaggerated immune responses to conventional antigens or auto-antibody responses, but there are some hints from in vitro systems that this may be the case. It is also attractive to postulate that the fluctuations in immune functions which accompany, or even precede, relapses of chronic inflammatory and demyelinating diseases are attributable to periodic reactivation of latent virus associated with lymphocytes. Whilst this is still speculative, there is increasing evidence that viruses circulate in blood lymphocytes for prolonged periods following primary infection. There is also indirect evidence that the blood lymphocytes of patients with inflammatory connective tissue diseases associated with abnormalities of the central nervous system express abnormalities which may result from persistent virus infection of these cells. There are other explanations for these observations, however, and the problem needs further critical examination.

ACKNOWLEDGEMENTS

The author is grateful for the continuing help and advice of his collaborators, Drs. Diane Appleford, Teresa Bacon, B.K. Pelton and D.A.J. Tyrrell. He also wishes to acknowledge the expert help of Mrs. Jenny O'Connor in preparing the manuscript.

REFERENCES

Appleford, D.J.A. and Denman, A.M. (1979a) Fate of herpes simplex virus in lymphocytes from inflammatory joint effusions. I. Failure of the virus to grow in cultured lymphocytes. *Ann. Rheum. Diseases,* 38: 443–449.

Appleford, D.J.A. and Denman, A.M. (1979b) Fate of herpes simplex virus in lymphocytes from inflammatory joint effusions. II. Mechanisms of non-permissiveness. *Ann. Rheum. Diseases,* 38: 450–455.

Brownson, J.M., Mahy, B.W.J. and Haxleman, B.L. (1979) Interactions of influenza A virus with human peripheral blood lymphocytes. *Infect. Immun.,* 25: 749–756.

Callard, R.E. (1979) Specific in vitro antibody response to influenza virus by human blood lymphocytes. *Nature (Lond.),* 282: 734–736.

Carney, W.P. and Hirsch, M.S. (1981) Mechanisms of immunosuppression in cytomegalovirus mononucleosis. II. Virus–monocyte interactions. *J. Infect. Dis.,* 144: 47–54.

Chamberlain, M.A. (1978) A family study of Behcet's syndrome. *Ann. Rheum. Diseases,* 37: 459–465.

Chamberlain, A., Yazici, H., Fialkow, P.J., Schroeder, I. and Denman, A.M. (1982) in preparation.

Chantler, J.K., Ford, D.K. and Tingle, A.J. (1981) Rubella-associated arthritis: rescue of rubella virus from peripheral blood lymphocytes two years postvaccination. *Infect. Immun.,* 32: 1274–1280.

Denman, A.M. (1979) Lymphocyte function and virus infection. *J. clin. Path.,* 32, Suppl. (Roy. Coll. Path), 13: 39–47.

Denman, A.M. (1981) Viruses and autoimmune diseases. In E.J. Holborow, (Guest Ed.), *Autoimmunity,* W.B. Saunders, London pp. 17–39.

58

Denman, A.M. and Pelton, B.K. (1974) Control mechanisms in infectious mononucleosis. *Clin. exp. Immunol.*, 18: 13–25.

Denman, A.M., Pelton, B.K., Appleford, D. and Kingsley, M. (1976) Virus infections of lympho-reticular cells and auto-immune disease. *Transplant Rev.*, 31: 79–115.

Denman, A.M., Fialkow, P.J., Pelton, B.K., Salo, A.C., Appleford, D.J. and Gilchrist, C. (1980) Lymphocyte abnormalities in Behcet's syndrome. *Clin. exp. Immunol.*, 42: 175–185.

Faguet, G.B. (1981) The effect of killed influenza virus vaccine on the kinetics of normal human lymphocytes. *J. infect. Dis.*, 143: 252–258.

Farrant, J. and Knight, S.C. (1979) Help and suppression by lymphoid cells as a function of cellular concentration. *Proc. nat. Acad. Sci. U.S.A.*, 76: 3507–3510.

Farrant, J. and Newton, C. (1981) Relative ability to provide help: an explanation for Con A-induced suppression. *Clin. exp. Immunol.*, 45: 504–513.

Fujinami, R.S. and Oldstone, M.B.A. (1981) Failure to cleave measles virus fusion protein in lymphoid cells. *J. exp. Med.*, 154: 1489–1499.

Fultz, P.N., Shadduck, J.A., Kang, C.Y. and Streilein, J.W., (1981) Involvement of cells of hematopoietic origin in genetically determined resistance of syrian hamsters to vesicular stomatitis virus. *Infect. Immun.*, 34: 540–549.

Gheuens, J., McFarlin, D.E., Rammohan, K.W. and Bellini W.J. (1981) Idiotypes and biological activity of murine monoclonal antibodies against the hemagglutinin of measles virus. *Infect. Immun.*, 34: 200–207.

Grahame, R., Simmons, N.A., Wilton, J.M.A., Armstong, R., Mims, C.A. and Laurent, R. (1981) Isolation of rubella virus from synovial fluid in five cases of seronegative arthritis. *Lancet*, ii: 649–652.

Grahame, R., Simmons, N.A., Wilton, J.M.A., Armstrong, R., Mims, C.A. and Laurent, R. (1983) Chronic arthritis associated with the presence of intrasynovial rubella virus following rubella infections. *Ann. Rheum. Diseases*, 42: 2–13.

Hackeman, M.M.A., Denman, A.M. and Tyrrell, D.A.J. (1974) Inactivation of influenza virus by human lymphocytes. *Clin. exp. Immunol.*, 16: 583–591.

Haller, O., Arnheiter, H., Gresser, I. and Lindenmann, J. (1981) Virus-specific interferon action. *J. exp. Med.*, 154: 199–203.

Ho, M. (1981) The lymphocyte in infections with Epstein–Barr virus and cytomegalovirus. *J. infect. Dis.*, 143: 857–862.

Hodes, D.S. (1981) Temperature sensitivity of isolates of echovirus Type II causing chronic meningoencephalitis in an agammaglobulinemic patient. *J. infect. Dis.*, 144: 377.

Hollingworth, P., Hylton, W., Pelton, B.K. and Denman, A.M. (1983) Immunosuppression restores a normal pattern of HSV growth in lymphocytes from patients with connective tissue diseases. *Ann. Rheum Dis.*, in preparation.

Knight, S. C., Harding, B., Burman, S. and Mertin, J. (1981) Cell number requirements for lymphocyte stimulation in vitro: changes during the course of multiple sclerosis and the effects of immunosuppression. *Clin. exp. Immun.*, 46: 61–69.

Lehner, T. and Barnes, C.G. (1979) Criteria for diagnosis and classification of Behcet's syndrome. In T. Lehner and C.G. Barnes (Eds.), Academic Press, 1–9.

Lucas, C.J., Ubels-Postma, J., Rezee, A. and Galama, J.M.D. (1978) Activation of measles virus from silently infected human lymphocytes. *J. exp. Med.*, 148: 940–952.

O'Duffy, J.D. and Goldstein, N.P. (1976) Neurologic involvement in seven patients with Behcet's disease. *Amer. J. Med.*, 61: 170–178.

Oldstone, M.B.A. (1979) Immune responses, immune tolerance, and viruses. In H. Fraenkel-Conrat and R.R. Wagner (Eds.), *Comprehensive Virology*, Vol. 15, Plenum Press, New York, pp. 1–36.

Pelton, B.K., Imrie, R.C. and Denman, A.M. (1976) Susceptibility of human lymphocyte populations to infection by herpes simplex virus. *Immunology*, 32: 803–810.

Pelton, B.K., Duncan, I.B. and Denman, A.M. (1980) Herpes simplex virus depresses antibody production by affecting T-cell function. *Nature (Lond.)*, 284: 176–177.

Pelton, B.K., Hylton, W. and Denman A.M. (1981) Selective immunosuppressive effects of measles virus infection. *Clin. exp. Immunol.*, 47: 19–26

Pelton, B.K. (1980) *Virus Repliction in Sub-Populations of Human Lymphocytes*. PhD thesis, University of London.

Platts-Mills, T.A.E. and Ishizaka, K. (1975) IgG and IgA diphtheria antitoxin responses from human tonsil lymphocytes. *J. Immunol.*, 114: 1058–1064.

Reinherz, E.L., O'Brien, C., Rosenthal, P. and Schlossman, S.F. (1980) The cellular basis for viral-induced immunodeficiency: analysis by monoclonal antibodies. *J. Immunol.*, 125: 1269–1274.

Robbins, S.J., Wrzos, H., Kline, A., Tenser, R.B. and Rapp, F. (1981) Rescue of a cytopathic paramyxovirus from peripheral blood leukocytes in subacute sclerosing panencephalitis. *J. infect. Dis.*, 143: 396–403.

Sergent, J.S, Lockshin, M.D., Klempner, M.S. and Lipsky, B.A. (1975) Central nervous system disease in systemic lupus erythematosus. *Amer. J. Med.,* 58: 644–654.

Summers, B.A., Greisen, H.A. and Appel, M.J.G. (1978) Possible initiation of viral encephalomyelitis in dogs by migrating lymphocytes infected with distemper virus. *Lancet,* 2: 187–189.

Whittle, H.C., Dossetor, J., Oduloju, A., Bryceson, P.D.M. and Greenwood, B.M. (1978) Cell-mediated immunity during natural measles infection. *J. clin. Invest.,* 62: 678–684.

Wrzos, H., Kulczycki, J., Laskowski, Z., Matacz, D. and Brzosko, W.J. (1979) Detection of measles virus antigen(s) in peripheral lymphocytes from patients with subacute sclerosing panencephalitis. *Arch. Virol.,* 60: 291–297.

Immunology of Nervous System Infections, Progress in Brain Research, Vol. 59, edited by P.O. Behan, V. ter Meulen and F. Clifford Rose

Analysis of Antigens in the Circulating Immune Complexes of Patients with Coxsackie Infections

WIAAM AL KADIRY, R.G. GOLD, P.O. BEHAN[1] and J.F. MOWBRAY

Department of Immunopathology, St. Mary's Hospital Medical School, London W2 1PG, and [1]Department of Neurology, Glasgow University, Glasgow, Scotland (U.K.)

INTRODUCTION

The Coxsackie group of viruses causes a wide variety of different diseases in man, both acute and chronic. These viruses exhibit myotropism and also a tendency to infect the central and peripheral nervous systems. They are usually considered to cause acute disease but clinical evidence also implicates them in chronic illness, particularly of muscle. For a review of their role in disease see Grist et al. (1978). We have studied two groups of patients showing chronic disease: the first, from the Newcastle area, had pericarditis-myocarditis, and the second, from the Glasgow area, had epidemic myalgic encephalomyelitis (EME). Among the latter, some subjects had been ill for up to 20 years.

The purpose of this investigation was to study the role of the circulating immune complexes which can be found in these patients, and to try to detect the nature of the infecting agent in these persistent viral illnesses. This work was prompted by previous studies from our laboratory where we had shown a particular pattern of therapeutic response to gamma-globulin therapy in the pericarditis-myocarditis group. Here we record the clinical response of patients with EME to similar gamma-globulin therapy.

MATERIALS AND METHODS

Patients

Patients with pericarditis or myocarditis secondary to Coxsackie infection were obtained from the Newcastle area, where they were under the care of R.G.G. Patients with EME from Glasgow, were under the care of P.O.B. The diagnosis was established in all patients only after full investigation. Coxsackie antibody titres were measured at the time that patients were first seen. Serial samples for the study of immune complexes were obtained during periods of both disease activity and remission, but the immune complexes in this present study were all taken from patients at a time when the disease was active. Serum samples were stored at $-70°C$ until needed.

Detection of circulating complexes

The detailed method for the detection of immune complexes by the PEG precipitation technique has been previously described (Kazatchkine et al., 1980). This technique relies on precipitation of the complexes from serum with polyethylene glycol, followed by measurement of the precipitated proteins by single radial immunodiffusion.

[61]

Measurement of cross-reaction between IgG antibody and antigens in circulating immune complexes

To study the nature of the complexed antigens in these sera, it was not possible to use the techniques which we have previously described (Dambuyant et al., 1978, 1979). This was because the methods are unsuitable if acid-labile reactants are present (Kazatchkine et al., 1980). Many of the complexes in patients with pericarditis contain only immunoglobulin M antibodies (IgM) and no immunoglobulin G (IgG), but IgM antibodies are labile at a pH 3.5 or lower. Thus we have found (Abdallah and Mowbray, unpublished observations) that in systems in which acid is used to dissociate antigen–antibody complexes (Dambuyant et al., 1980), or where pepsin digestion of the complexes is used to prepare a $F(ab)_2$ fragment (Dambuyant et al., 1978), the acid lability of IgM antibodies precludes their detection. For this reason, we developed a new system in which peroxidase-labeled IgG antibodies are allowed to react with the complexes in 10 mM EDTA at 4°C, over a period of days. If the antibodies cross-react with the antigenic specificities in the complexes in the serum samples, some of the labeled antibody becomes bound. After allowing equilibrium to occur, the immune complexes are precipitated in the usual way, with polyethylene glycol at a final concentration of 2 % in 10 mM EDTA, usually after 5 days. The amount of label which is precipitated is then a measure of the degree of cross-reaction when it is compared to control values for labeled antibody in serum not containing complexes. The precipitation is carried out in undiluted serum and it has been found that rheumatoid factor and other anti-immunoglobulins do not produce significantly high backgrounds, because their binding to the small amount of complexed immunoglobulin appears to be effectively prevented by the excess of immunoglobulin present in the serum.

The results are expressed as the percentage of the peroxidase-labeled immunoglobulin which is bound to the complex, and hence precipitated. Full details of this technique and its validation will be published elsewhere (Zewdie et al., 1983).

RESULTS

Fig. 1 shows the cross-reaction observed between the sera of patients of each disease group and a peroxidase-labeled globulin of a patient with high titre antibody to Coxsackie B4. There is a significant increase in binding in both the pericarditis-myocarditis and the EME groups, showing that both have the same, or cross-reacting antigens complexed in the circulation. The controls are from patients who had immune complexes due to other conditions, predominantly bacterial endocarditis. These were used, rather than sera from normal individuals, because the background binding of immunoglobulin was found to be about 20 % higher in immune-complex-positive sera than in normals, possibly due to a minor residual reaction with rheumatoid factors.

In comparison to the above, Fig. 2 shows the cross-reaction between the complexed antigens of the patients in the two groups, and the enzyme-labeled globulin of pooled normal IgG. It will be seen that although there is a significant difference between the cross-reactions of patients with pericarditis and a group of 23 patients with immune complex glomerulonephritis, there is no difference between the latter and the patients with Coxsackie-associated neurological disease. Thus, it seems that the pericarditis patients have complexed antigens which are commonly 'seen' by the normal population, whereas the neurological patients' antigens are less frequently 'seen'.

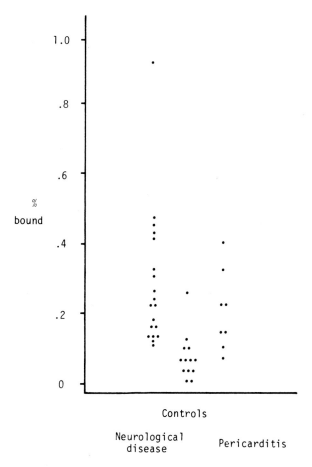

Fig. 1. Comparison of binding of labeled IgG from a patient with high titre anti-Coxsackie B4 antibody to complexes of patients with Coxsackie-associated diseases, and controls.

The antibody of contacts, plasma IgG from individual non-contact donors, or pooled normal IgG was given to the pericarditis patients, with the results as shown in Table I. The intrafamilial plasma produced a good result, unlike that seen with plasma from single blood donors who were not contacts. This suggests that only a few of the general population have been exposed to the putative antigen and have developed protective antibody. This hypothesis is supported by the high frequency of remission induced by the pooled IgG given, compared to the lack of any observable benefit after the 4 infusions from single donors. Also, if the ability of the pooled normal IgG to react with the antigens of the complex were a determinant in the production of sustained remission, it would be expected that a greater effect would be obtained in the pericarditis group (which share complexed antigens with the general population), than in patients with immune-complex glomerulonephritis or Coxsackie-associated neurological disease.

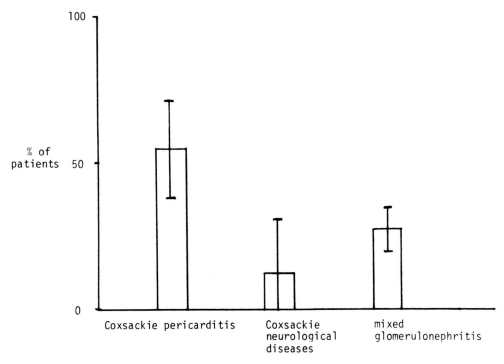

Fig. 2. Comparison of the cross-reactions between pooled normal IgG and the serological complexes from patients with either chronic glomerulonephritis or Coxsackie infections.

TABLE I

REMISSION OBTAINED AFTER TREATMENT OF PATIENTS WITH PERICARDITIS OR MYOCARDITIS WITH PLASMA FROM 3 SOURCES

Two values are shown for patients who have been treated twice. PF, familial plasma; PB, plasma from National Blood Transfusion Service

Treatment	Number of patients	Weeks remission	Fraction in remission after treatment
PF	3	16	3/4
		32	
		9	
		0	
PB	4	0	0/4
		0	
		0	
		0	
IgG	11	28	11/12
		3	
		12	
		13	
		28 7+	
		0 5+	
		12+	
		12+	
		9+	
		11+	
		3+	

Fig. 3 shows the effect of treatment with plasma transfusion in patients with chronic pericarditis and/or erythema multiforme. The results are compared to those in patients with glomerulonephritis. The patients with chronic pericarditis/erythema multiforme had demonstrated previously a high degree of cross-reaction between the antigens of their immune complexes and pooled normal IgG (see Fig. 2). The results show that in patients studied for 2 years, this treatment produced periods of remission for up to 15 months, whereas before treatment the remissions obtained were, on average, one month. In contrast, patients with EME failed to respond to normal IgG, although some showed a beneficial effect after plasma exchange and intravenous pooled IgG (50 mg/kg/day given on 9 alternate days). Thus the results are in agreement with our hypothesis.

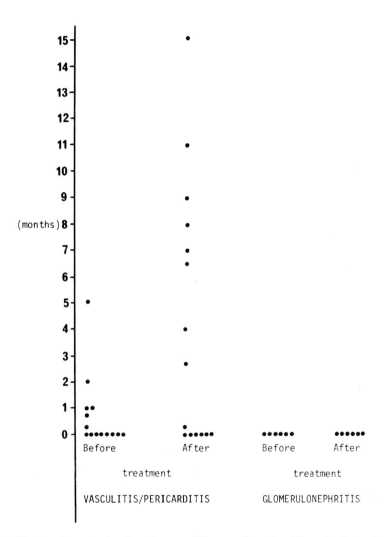

Fig. 3. Effect of treatment on patients with erythema multiforme and/or pericarditis, and patients with glomerulonephritis. All subjects were tested with plasma from one unit of blood from a familial donor. The maximum length of remission obtained before and after treatment is shown.

DISCUSSION

These results suggest that there is considerable antigenic homogeneity between the circulating immune complexes of patients who have different Coxsackie infections, manifest as pericarditis-myocarditis or as neurological disease. There are symptoms common to Coxsackie infections in both these categories, such as exhaustion, emotional lability and exacerbation of weakness by exercise. Thus it is interesting to find that there is a common antigenic component in their immune complexes, irrespective of the specificity of the Coxsackie antibody (Fig. 1). The use of a specific Coxsackie antibody to identify the circulating antigen present in the complexes from these patients shows a much tighter antigenic configuration than would be expected from study of anti-Coxsackie antibodies. The distribution of antibodies is quite varied in the Newcastle region, although we would assume that the endemic nature of the disease suggests a single agent. We have detected a few examples where more than one member of a family was affected, and where the raised Coxsackie antibody titres were of different Coxsackie B specificities.

The difference between the response of the two groups of patients to the administration of plasma or IgG is striking. In many of the pericarditis patients, significant remission was obtained following transfusion with pooled normal IgG or IgG from an extrafamilial source, but transfusion of single units of plasma from unrelated donors did not prove of benefit. This would lead one to suggest that family members who are unaffected do, nonetheless, have protective antibodies which are so uncommon in the general population that a single donor is unlikely to provide protection. A pool of IgG from many donors means a high likelihood that the antibody is present. The small amount of IgG required to produce a remission also militates against the suggestion that a very rare antibody donor has been included in a pool of hundreds of donors: if this were so, the antibody would probably be too diluted in the pool for 750 mg of IgG to be effective.

When the neurological patients are considered, however, a very different pattern is seen. None of these patients apparently responded to pooled IgG when it was given in amounts similar to those of the pericarditis patients, but 4 showed a good response to plasma exchange of 12 litres and replacement by fresh plasma. Plasma exchange, as well as having the potential effect of removal of noxious substances from the blood, is also accompanied by the administration of more than 30 g of IgG. This represents an amount two orders of magnitude greater than that which had failed as a simple IgG injection, and its effect has to be considered in the beneficial response.

Since many of the patients with either form of disease have circulating complexes not containing IgG, it seems possible that it is the inability of the patient to make IgG antibody that is related to his or her disease. Thus, the persistence of the virus infection may follow the lack of specific T-cells to the virus, such that there is neither cytotoxic T-cell activity, nor IgG antibody for K-cells, so that an effective attack on the reservoir of virus cannot be made.

It can be postulated that the problems related to antibody diffusion across the blood–brain barrier result in much greater amounts of antibody being necessary to produce an effect in patients with neurological diseases than are required in patients with pericarditis or myocarditis. Whatever the reason, the roles of IgG transfusion and plasma exchange need to be separated in this group to find out whether the observable benefit is due to transfusion or plasma exchange. We have done this in a previous study where we compared the remission obtained with plasma exchange and replacement with fresh plasma, to that obtained by plasma exchange and replacement with plasma protein fraction (PPF), which is free of antibody (Mowbray and Burton, 1977). This investigation is continuing.

CONCLUSION

These preliminary findings implicate immunological factors in the pathogenesis of the muscle and nervous tissue damage which follows Coxsackie infections.

ACKNOWLEDGEMENTS

We are grateful to the Regional Virus Laboratory, Ruchill Hospital, Glasgow and the Newcastle Public Health Laboratory, for the measurement of Coxsackie antibodies in the patients of this study.

REFERENCES

Burton-Kee, J., Morgan-Capner, P. and Mowbray, J.F. (1980) Nature of circulating immune complexes in infective endocarditis. *J. clin. Pathol.*, 33: 653–659.

Burton-Kee, E.J., Mowbray, J.F. and Lehner, T. (1980) Different cross-reacting circulating immune complexes in Behcet's syndrome and recurrent oral ulcers. *J. lab. clin. Med.*, 97: 559–568.

Dambuyant, C., Burton-Kee, J. and Mowbray, J.F. (1978) The use of the preparation of F(ab)$_2$ antibody from soluble immune complexes to determine the complexed antigens. *J. immunol. Meth.*, 24: 31-38.

Dambuyant, C., Burton-Kee, J. and Mowbray, J.F. (1979) Demonstration of two disease specific antigens in circulating immune complexes. *Clin. exp. Immunol.*, 37: 424-431.

Dambuyant, C., Thivolet, J., Guillet, G. and Doutre, M.S. (1980) Circulating immune complexes in bullous pemphigoid. In J. Thivolet and D. Schmitt (Eds.). *Cutaneous Immunopathology*, INSERM, Paris, pp. 305–312.

Grist, N.R., Bell, E.J. and Assaad, F. (1978) Enteroviruses in human disease. *Progr. Med. Virol.*, 24: 114–157.

Kazatchkine, M.D., Sultan, Y., Burton-Kee, J. and Mowbray, J.F. (1980) Circulating immune complexes containing anti-VIII antibodies in multi-transfused patients with haemophilia A. *Clin. exp. Immunol.*, 39: 315-320.

Mohammed, I., Ansell, B.M., Holborow, E.J. and Bryceson, A.D.M. (1977) Circulating immune complexes in subacute infective endocarditis and post-streptococcal glomerulonephritis. *J. clin. Pathol.*, 30: 308–311.

Mowbray, J.F. (1979) Identification of antigens in immune complexes. In J. Thivolet and D. Schmitt (Efs.). *Cutaneous Immunopathology*, INSERM, Paris, pp. 275–280.

Mowbray, J.F. and Burton, E.J. (1977) Clinical relevance of the determination of circulating immune complexes. In J.L. Tourane, J. Traeger and R. Triau (Eds.). *Transplantation and Clinical Immunology*, Simep-Editions, Villeurbanne, France, pp. 35–43.

Zewdie, Debrework and Mowbray, J.F. (1983) A technique for studying the antigens in immune complex without the use of dissociating agents, (in preparation).

Immunology of Nervous System Infections, Progress in Brain Research, Vol. 59, edited by P.O. Behan, V. ter Meulen and F. Clifford Rose
© *1983 Elsevier Science Publishers B.V.*

Complement Deficiency Syndromes and Bacterial Infections

J. VEITCH[1], C. LOVE[2], A.K.R. CHAUDHURI[3] and K. WHALEY[1]

[1]*University of Glasgow Department of Pathology, Western Infirmary, Glasgow G11 6NT,* [2]*Department of Infectious Diseases, Ruchill Hospital, Glasgow, and* [3] *Monklands District General Hospital, Airdrie, Lanarkshire, Scotland (U.K.)*

INTRODUCTION

The complement system plays a major role in the elimination of bacteria from the body. There are several ways in which the complement system deals with bacterial infections, but before they can be discussed in detail, a description of the constituent proteins, and their patterns of activation is required.

The constituent proteins

At least 20 proteins constitute the complement system (Table I). These proteins can be divided into 4 groups on the basis of their known action. There are two pathways for activation, the classical and the alternative, which form enzymes which activate the terminal group of proteins. Finally a group of proteins regulates complement activation.

The classical pathway

The classical pathway (Fig. 1) is activated by antigen–antibody complexes of the IgM class or IgG1, 2 or 3 subclasses, (Whaley and Ferguson, 1981). The antibody part of the complex binds to the C1q subcomponent of C1, a trimolecular complex, which exists in plasma as an inactive precursor molecule. Following the binding of C1 to the complex, C1r becomes

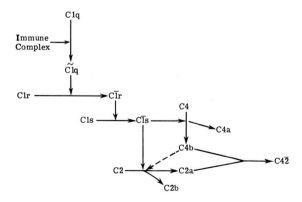

Fig. 1. Molecular interactions of the classical pathway. A line over a symbol indicates that it has undergone a conformational change. (From Whaley and El Ghobarey, (1981), reproduced with permission.)

TABLE I

COMPLEMENT PATHWAY PROTEINS

1, classical pathway components; 2, alternative pathway components; 3, terminal sequence; 4, control proteins.

Component	Molecular weight	Electrophoretic mobility	Serum concentration ($\mu g/ml$)	Polypeptide chain structure	Genetic polymorphism	Cleavage products		
1 C1q	400,000	α	250	18 (6×3)	−	−		
C1r	90,000	β	100	1	?	H & L chains		
C1s	90,000	β	80	1	?	H & L chains		
C4	204,000	β	430	3	+	C4a	C4b	
C2	100,000	β	20	1	+	C2a	C2b	
2 B	93,000	β	150	1	+	Ba	Bb	
D̄	25,000	α	2	1	?	−		
P	22,000	γ	30	4	?	−		
3 C3	190,000	β	1300	2	+	C3a	C3b	C3c
						C3d	C3e	
C5	185,000	β	75	2	−	C5a	C5b	
C6	128,000	β	60	1	+	−		
C7	121,000	β	60	1	+	−		
C8	153,000	γ	80	3	+	−		
C9	79,000	β	50	1	−	−		
4 C1-inhibitor	105,000 90,000	α	180	1	+	−		
C4 binding protein	540,000 590,000	β	?	8	?	−		
C3b inactivator	90,000	β	50	2	−	−		
β1H	150,000	β	300	1	?	−		
S-protein	88,000	α	?	1	?	−		
Anaphylotoxin Inactivator	300,000	α	?	8	?	−		

activated to form $C\bar{1}r^*$, which enzymatically activates C1s to $C\bar{1}s$. $C\bar{1}s$ has two natural substrates, C4 and C2, and produces a limited proteolytic cleavage in each molecule. In the presence of Mg^{2+}, a bimolecular complex, $C\bar{4}\bar{2}$ is formed, which is the classical pathway C3 convertase. This enzyme cleaves C3 into C3a and C3b. C3a is a small peptide cleaved from the N-terminus of the chain, C3b comprises the residual chain and the intact B chain.

The alternative pathway

The alternative pathway (Fig. 2) is phylogenetically older than the classical pathway, and is activated when complex polysaccharides such as those found on the surface of bacteria, are added to serum.

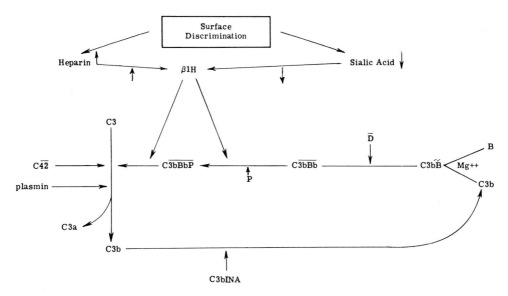

Fig. 2. Molecular interactions of the alternative pathway. The ability of surface constituents to dictate turnover is represented. Reducing surface sialic acid restricts β1H activity and therefore enhances turnover. Increasing surface heparin enhances β1H activity and turnover is restricted. (From Whaley and Ferguson, (1981), reproduced with permission.)

C3b, or C3 which has been altered to acquire C3b-like properties (Isenman et al., 1981), binds to factor B, to form a complex $\bar{D}$, the alternative pathway analogue of $C\bar{1}$, then cleaves B to form the unstable alternative pathway C3 convertase, $C\overline{3bBb}$. The term unstable is applied to this enzyme because Bb decays rapidly from the complex. Properdin, after binding to C3b stabilizes the enzyme by retarding the decay of Bb (Fearon and Austen, 1975). The enzyme $C3\overline{bBb}P$ is thus referred to as the properdin-stabilized alternative pathway C3 convertase. As C3b is an integral part of the enzyme which cleaves C3, the alternative pathway is a positive feedback loop, the turnover of which is kept controlled by two proteins, C3b inactivator and β1H globulin (see below).

The terminal sequence is initiated when C3 is cleaved. C3b has a short-lived hydrophobic binding site by which it binds to membranes and to antibody. C3b molecules which bind in close proximity to the C3 convertase transform the specificity of the enzyme to that of a C5

---

* A bar over a symbol indicates that the component is in its active form.

convertase. C3b acts as a C5 acceptor, and the enzymatic site on C2a or Bb cleaves C5 in a similar manner to which C3 is cleaved. C5a is a small peptide released from the N-terminus of the α-chain of C5, and C5b consists of the remainder of the α-chain and the intact β-chain. C5b has a labile binding site which permits it to bind to cell membranes.

Cleavage of C5 is the last enzymatic step during complement activation. Following formation of C5b, C6 binds to C5b, C7 to C5b6, C8 to C5b67, and finally C9 to C5b678. The C5b-9 complex is termed the membrane attack complex (MAC): it is hydrophobic, and inserts itself into the lipid portion of cell membranes to create a transmembrane channel through which water and electrolytes pass, and cells lyse osmotically (Mayer, 1972). The C5b-8 complex will induce lysis, but the incorporation of C9 into the complex increases the speed of the lytic process.

Control of complement activation

Control of complement activation is achieved by two mechanisms. The first is the rapid decay rates of the classical and alternative pathway C3 convertases. The second rests upon the presence of a series of control proteins which exist naturally in plasma. C1-inhibitor stoichiometrically binds to C1s to limit cleavage of C4 and C2. C4-binding protein binds to C4b and accelerates the decay of C42 by displacing C2 from the complex (Gigli et al., 1980). C4-binding protein also acts as a cofactor for the enzyme C3b inactivator to facilitate cleavage of C4b into C4c and C4d.

C3b inactivator also acts on C3b to convert it to a haemolytically inactive product C3bi (Fig. 3). To produce the single cleavage in the α-chain of C3b to form C3bi, the cofactor β1H is required. β1H also binds to C3b to displace Bb from C3bBb or C3bBbP (Whaley and Ruddy, 1976).

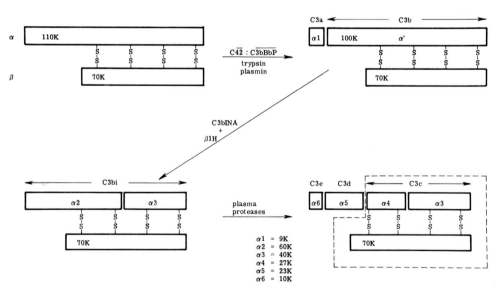

Fig. 3. Diagrammatic model depicting enzymatic cleavage products of the C3 molecule occurring during complement activation. (From Whaley and Ferguson (1981), reproduced with permission.)

Conversion of C3bi to C3c and C3d requires the action of other plasma proteases such as plasmin.

Absence of C3b inactivator or β1H results in uncontrolled turnover of the alternative pathway (Whaley and Thompson, 1978), the alternative pathway probably undergoing continuous low-grade activation as a result of the formation of C3b.C3bINA and β1H control activation by degrading C3b. When alternative pathway activating bacteria are added to serum, some of this spontaneously formed C3b binds to the bacterial surface and in some way becomes resistant to the actions of β1H, (Fearon and Austen, 1977). Thus this C3b is not degraded and can form $\overline{\text{C3bBbP}}$, which cleaves more C3 and the bacteria therefore become coated with C3b. This allows the bacteria to react with C3b receptors on macrophages and become phagocytosed, or with C5b to be lysed by the C5b-9 complex.

BIOLOGICAL ACTIVITIES

Proinflammatory

The peptides C4a, C3a and C5a are anaphylotoxins. They bind to receptors on the membranes of mast cells, basophils and smooth muscle. They induce histamine release from mast cells and basophils, which causes increased vascular permeability.

C5a is the most potent, and C4a has little anaphylotoxic activity. C5a is a potent chemotactic agent for both neutrophils and monocytes. Carboxypeptidase N, an enzyme present in plasma, removes the C-terminal arginine residue from anaphylotoxins, which results in loss of their anaphylotoxic activity. The chemotactic activity of $C5a_{desarg}$ (as the degraded form of C5a is known), retains reduced chemotactic activity. A plasma cofactor for $C5a_{desarg}$, however, enhances its chemotactic activity.

Cytolytic

The C5b-9 complex forms a transmembrane channel, causing lysis. $\overline{\text{C5b6}}$ can bind to cells which have not been sensitized by antibody; interaction with C7, C8 and C9 results in lysis (so-called bystander lysis).

Opsonic

C3b coating bacteria or complexes, allows them to bind to the membranes of cells possessing C3b receptors. If these cells are phagocytic, then phagocytosis is enhanced. The intracel-

TABLE II

BIOLOGICAL ACTIVITIES OF COMPLEMENT

Activity	Mediator	Action
Proinflammatory	C4a C3a C5a	Histamine release from mast cells. Increased vascular permeability
	C5a $C5a_{desarg}$	Chemotactic for PMN and monocytes
Cytolytic	C5b-9	Lysis of microorganisms
Opsonic	C3b (C4b C5b)	Facilitate interaction of microorganisms and complexes with phagocytic cells
Solubilization of antigen–antibody complexes	C3b	Reduced size of complexes and therefore facilitates their removal

lular killing of bacteria is also enhanced if the C3b receptor is triggered after bacteria have been internalized (Leigh et al., 1979). The intracellular degradation of antigen–antibody complexes is enhanced when complexes are coated with C3b. This is due to increased adherence to the macrophage cell membrane (Kjilstra et al., 1979).

Solubilization of antigen–antibody complexes

Antigen–antibody complexes are thought to be a potent cause of tissue injury. Interaction of complexes with the complement system, prevents them precipitating, and insoluble complexes are solubilized. An intact alternative pathway is an essential pre-requisite for this activity, but for optimal efficiency the classical pathway must also be intact (Takahashi et al., 1978). The effect is due to the intercalation of C3b into the antigen–antibody lattice, thus making the complexes smaller and more soluble (Czop and Nussenzweig, 1976). The advantage of this phenomenon is that smaller complexes are probably less tissue damaging and are probably more rapidly removed from the tissues than the larger insoluble complexes.

Complement and bacterial infections

Following on from the above description of the biological activities of complement, it is apparent that the complement system acts in several ways to promote the elimination of bacteria: (1) increasing vascular permeability and attracting phagocytic cells into the area of infection as a result of C5a generation; (2) cytolysis by the C5b-9 complex; (3) opsonization of bacteria by C3b, thus promoting their phagocytosis and killing by mononuclear phagocytes.

On the basis of these observations one would conclude that complement deficiency syndromes would be associated with an increased risk of bacterial infections.

Complement deficiency syndromes

Homozygous deficiency of all the classical pathway components, terminal components, $C\bar{1}$-inhibitor, C3b-inactivator, β1H and properdin have been reported (Table III). Not all deficiency states have been associated with a high incidence of bacterial infections, although patients with deficiencies of C3, C5, C6, C7, C8, C3b inactivator, properdin and perhaps C2 appear to be so predisposed.

There is now overwhelming evidence to suggest that patients with complement deficiency syndromes, especially those with defects of the classical pathway, are predisposed to the development of connective tissue diseases.

C7 DEFICIENCY

Case report 1

This patient had been healthy until the age of 17 years when she was admitted to the Infectious Diseases Unit in Strathclyde Hospital, Motherwell on April 20th, 1977 with a 3-days history of headache, vomiting, photophobia, and pyrexia. On admission she was found to have signs of meningeal irritation. Lumbar puncture produced turbid cerebrospinal fluid with 4100 cells (mostly polymorphs), elevated protein at 2.7 g/l and reduced glucose content at 0.9 mmol/l. Scanty gram-negative diplococci were seen on direct smear, but culture was sterile. White blood count was $31.6 \times 10^9/l$ with neutrophils 90%. She was treated with penicillin and sulphadimidine for 14 days and made an uneventful recovery.

TABLE III

GENETICALLY DETERMINED DEFICIENCIES OF COMPLEMENT COMPONENTS

References for: (1) properdin deficiency (A. Sjoholm, personal communication); (2) C5-C6 C7 and C8 deficiencies (Petersen et al., 1979); (3) β1H deficiency (Thompson and Winterborn, 1981); (4) Other component deficiencies (Whaley and Ferguson, 1981).

Component	Protein absent or non-functional	Mode of transmission	Heterozygotes detected	HLA linkage	Disease associations
C1q	Both	C1q deficiency unknown / C1q dysfunctional protein Codominant	No	No	Recurrent infection, glomerulonephritis / Recurrent infection, glomerulonephritis
C1r	Absent	Autosomal recessive	Yes	No	Glomerulonephritis, SLE
C1s	Absent	Autosomal recessive	Yes	No	Glomerulonephritis, SLE
C4	Absent	Autosomal recessive	Yes	Yes	SLE
C2	Absent	Autosomal recessive	Yes	Yes	SLE, juvenile rheumatoid polymyositis
Properdin	Absent	?	?	No	Recurrent neisserial bacteraemia
C3	Absent	Autosomal recessive	Yes	No	Recurrent pyogenic infections
C5	Absent	Autosomal recessive	Yes	No	Recurrent neisserial bacteraemia, SLE
C6	Absent	Autosomal recessive	Yes	No	Recurrent neisserial bacteraemia, Raynaud's phenomenon
C7	Absent	Autosomal recessive	Yes	No	Raynaud's phenomenon, ankylosing spondylitis, recurrent neisserial bacteraemia
C8	Both	Autosomal recessive	Yes	No / Neisserial	SLE, xeroderma pigmentosa, recurrent bacteraemia
C9	Absent	Autosomal recessive	Yes	No	Normal
C1-INH	Both	Autosomal dominant	Heterozygotes get disease	No	Hereditary angioedema, SLE
C3bINA	Absent	Autosomal recessive	Yes	No	Recurrent pyogenic infections
β1H	Trace	Autosomal recessive	Yes	?	Haemolytic uraemic syndrome
Anaphylotoxin inactivator	Levels 20% of normal ?		Reduced levels in other family members	?	

She remained well until two years later when on June 28th, 1979 she was admitted to Monklands District General Hospital with a two-days history of pyrexia, headache, photophobia, drowsiness and widespread purpuric eruption over arms and legs. Marked meningism was noted but there was no evidence of local CNS signs. WBC was $35.3 \times 10^9/l$ (neutrophils 97 %). CSF was turbid with polymorphonuclear pleocytosis (5400 cells/mm³), protein 3.1 g/l. Glucose was undetectable. Although direct smear of CSF showed gram-negative diplococci, the culture failed to yield n. meningitidis. However, countercurrent immunoelectrophoresis (CIE) examination of CSF identified group Y meningococcal antigen. She responded well to penicillin and sulphonamide and a repeat CSF examination at the end of therapy showed normal results.

Three months later on September 26th, 1979 she had to be readmitted to the hospital during the early hours of the morning with an 8-h history of headache, vomiting and pyrexia. By this time she was sufficiently familiar with these symptoms to be able to tell the attending General Practitioner that her "meningitis is coming on again". On examination she was pyrexial (37.8°C) with signs of meningeal irritation. There was polymorphonuclear leucocytosis with WBC $23.5 \times 10^9/l$. CSF was turbid with cells 11,750/mm³. As on the previous occasions gram-negative diplococci were seen on direct smear, but culture of CSF was sterile. Group W-135 meningococcal antigen was, however, demonstrated by CIE. She made a rapid recovery with penicillin and sulphonamide.

Apart from these recurrent episodes of meningococcal meningitis she had no undue predilection to other bacterial or viral infection. She had no history of head injury. Family history was not relevant as she was an adopted child and the identity of the real parents could not be disclosed.

The following investigations were carried out with normal results: chest X-ray, skull X-ray, sinus X-ray, computerized axial tomographic (CAT) scan, immunoglobulins, polymorphonuclear function test, T- and B-lymphocyte function tests, skin test with bacterial, viral and candida antigens.

Complement investigations

The assays used have been described previously (Whaley, 1982): total haemolytic complement (CH50) activity — zero; alternative pathway haemolytic activity (AP.CH50) — zero; C3-C9 assay — zero.

These results show that the defect is among the terminal components. Haemolytic assays of C1, C4, C2, C3, C5, C6, C8, C9 and factor B were all normal. C7 activity was not detected. Concentrations of C1q, C1s, C4, C3, C5, factor B, properdin, C1-inhibitor, C3b inactivator and β1H were measured by radial immunodiffusion and all were found to be within the normal range. C1r, C6, C8 and C9 were detected by double diffusion in agarose gels. C7 was not detected.

These results show that the patient was deficient in C7 activity, and that the defect was due to the absence of C7 and not to synthesis of a functionally inactive molecule.

The nature of the defect was confirmed in two ways: (1) the addition of purified C7 to the patient's serum restored the haemolytic activity; (2) the addition of the patient's serum to sera deficient in C5, C6 or C8 resulted in lysis. Lysis was not produced when her serum was added to known C7 deficient serum.

When IgM-coated sheep erythrocytes were incubated with the patient's serum they acquired the ability to form rosettes with peripheral blood lymphocytes and monocytes. This finding indicates that the patient's serum could sustain the formation of a C3 convertase and possessed C3.

Chemotactic activity was generated when the patient's serum was incubated with zymosan (37° C for 1 h). As the chemotactic activity is due to C5a$_{desarg}$, the defect must occur after the C5 stage.

We were unable to demonstrate that C7 deficiency in this patient was due to a genetic defect, as she had been adopted as a baby, and although her parents were alive, access to them could not be obtained.

C5 DEFICIENCY

Case report 2

The patient, a 22-year-old male, presented with headache, drowsiness, pyrexia, vomiting and a purpuric rash over his limbs. CSF analysis revealed purulent fluid. A direct smear showed gram-negative diplococci, and meningococci were isolated. The patient recovered following treatment with penicillin and sulphonamide.

Previous medical history revealed three previous attacks of meningococcal meningitis at the ages of 5 years, 6 years and 17 years. One of the patient's 3 brothers (who also turned out to be C5 deficient), had also had two attacks of meningitis. At the age of 2 years he had had a pyogenic meningitis from which no organism could be identified, and at age 7 he had had an attack of meningococcal meningitis.

The remainder of the family were healthy.

Complement investigations

Assays used: CH50 — zero; APCH50 — zero; C3-C9 assay zero. These findings show that the patient had a defect among the terminal components.

Haemolytic assay of C1, C4, C2, C3, C6, C7, C8, C9 and factor B showed normal levels of these components. C5 was not detected. Radial immunodiffusion assays for C1q, C1s, C4, C3, factor B, properdin, C1-inhibitor, C3b inactivator and β1H showed normal levels of these components. C5 was not detected. C1r, C2, C6, C7, C8 and C9 were detected by double-diffusion in agarose gel. The defect is therefore one of absence of C5, and not due to synthesis of a functionally inactive molecule.

We confirmed that the defect was due to deficiency of C5 by restoring haemolysis through the addition of purified C5 to the serum (Fig. 4). Addition of the patient's serum to C6, C7 and C8 deficient serum resulted in lysis, whereas lysis failed to occur when the patient's serum was mixed with known C5-deficient serum.

Other investigations

When IgM antibody-coated sheep erythrocytes were incubated at 37° C for 30 min with the patient's serum they acquired the ability to form rosettes with peripheral blood lymphocytes and monocytes. This observation confirms that the patient can form C3 convertases and has C3 in the patient's serum.

Chemotactic activity was not generated when the patient's serum was incubated with zymosan at 37° C for 1 h. As the chemotactic activity generated in serum is derived from C5a, this finding confirms that the patient lacks C5.

78

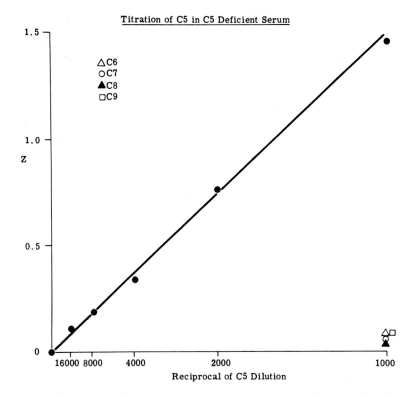

Fig. 4. Restoration of lysis activity of patients' serum by the addition of purified C5.

Family studies

We were able to investigate 3 generations of this family (Fig. 5), the parents, the three sibs, and one child. A history of consanguinity was not elicited and tissue typing confirmed this.

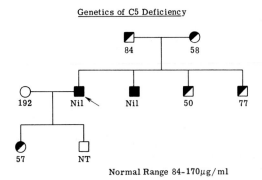

Fig. 5. Inheritance of C5 deficiency in a family. Filled squares, homozygous; half-filled circles and squares, heterozygous; open circle and square, normal. Figures indicate levels of C5 (normal range 84–170 μg/ml). Squares, female; circles, males.

Both parents had C5 levels at the lower limit of normal, suggesting that they were heterozygotes. Of the sibs, one brother had no detectable C5, indicating that he, although totally asymptomatic, was homozygous for C5 deficiency. The two other brothers appeared to be heterozygotes as they had C5 levels at the lower limit of normal. The wife of the patient had normal C5 levels, and the only child tested was heterozygous for C5 deficiency. HLA linkage was not present.

DISCUSSION

Recurrrent septicaemia with meningitis has been reported in patients with C2 (streptococcus pneumoniae, or haemophilus influenzae), C3 (meningococci, streptococcus pneumoniae or haemophilus influenza), C5, C6, C7 and C8 (meningococcal and gonococcal bacteraemias). Properdin deficiency has been shown to be associated with recurrent meningococcal meningitis (A. Sjoholm, personal communication). The bacterial complications of the complement deficiency syndromes have been reviewed recently (Rynes and Pickering, 1982). The data from these patients lend insight into the in vivo biological role of the complement system in handling bacterial infections. It would appear that only a small proportion of bacteria are handled by lysis. Indeed, it appears that with the exception of n. meningitidis and n. gonorrhoea, the principle means of elimination of bacteria is by the process of opsonization. Phagocytosis and killing by mononuclear phagocytes may be a more effective means of handling bacteria than complement lysis. The reason why neisseria must be killed by the complement system may be a reflection of their inability to be killed by macrophages. Certainly, smears on gonococcal or meningococcal pus show large numbers of intracellular organisms, perhaps indicating their intracellular growth.

A number of other important points emerge: (1) not all patients with complete deficiencies of C5, C6, C7 or C8 develop recurrent neisserial bacteraemias; (2) patients frequently do not develop clinical problems until they are in their teens; (3) heterozygotes are normal; (4) the observation that properdin deficiency predisposes to meningococcal meningitis (A. Sjoholm, personal communication) indicates that the cytolytic process is dependent upon the alternative pathway.

The management of these patients is difficult. Once a diagnosis has been reached, and the family investigated, patients should be advised of the risk of neisserial infections. Immunization with appropriate vaccines may be beneficial.

SUMMARY

A review of the mechanisms of activation of the complement system, and the biological activities generated as a result of complement activation, is presented.

Two patients with recurrent meningococcal meningitis are described. One patient had no C7 in her serum, the other lacked C5. Family studies on the C5-deficient patient showed that the disease was inherited as an autosomal recessive condition.

The relationship between complement deficiency syndromes and bacterial infections is discussed.

ACKNOWLEDGEMENTS

This study was supported by a grant from the Western Infirmary Research Support Group. Dr. R.A. Thompson performed the experiments in which both patients' sera were mixed with complement-deficient sera.

REFERENCES

Czop, J. and Nussenzweig, V. (1976) Studies on the mechanism of solubilization of immune precipitates by serum. *J. exp. Med.*, 143: 615–630.

Fearon, D.T. and Austen, K.F. (1975) Properdin: binding to C36 and stabilization of the C36-dependent C3 convertase. *J. exp. Med.*, 142: 856–863.

Fearon, D.T. and Austen, K.F. (1977) Activation of the alternative complement pathway due to resistance of zymosan-bound amplification convertase to endogenous regulatory mechanisms. *Proc. nat. Acad. Sci. U.S.A.*, 74: 1683–1687.

Gigli, I., Fujita, T. and Nussenzweig, V. (1980) Modulation of the classical pathway C3 convertase by the plasma proteins C4-BP and C3bINA. *J. Immunol.*, 124: 1521 (abstr.).

Isenman, D.E., Kells, D.I.C., Cooper, N.R., Muller-Eberhard, H.J. and Pangburn, M.K. (1981) Nucleophilic modification of human complement protein C3: correlation of conformational changes with acquisition of C3b-like functional properties. *Biochemistry*, 20: 4458–4467.

Kjilstra, A., van Ess, L.A. and Daha, M.R. (1979) The role of complement in the binding and degradation of immunoglobulin aggregates by macrophages. *J. Immunol.*, 123: 2488–2493.

Leigh, P.C.J., Van den Barselaar, M.Th., Van Zwet, T.L., Daha, M.R. and Van Furth, R. (1979) Requirement of extracellular complement and immunoglobulin for intracellular killing of microorganisms by human monocytes. *J. clin. Invest.*, 63: 772–784.

Mayer, M.M. (1972) Mechanism of cytolysis by complement. *Proc. nat. Acad. Sci. U.S.A.*, 69: 2954–2958.

Petersen, B.H., Lee, T.J., Snyderman, R. and Brooks, G.F. (1979) Neisseria meningitides and Neisserie gonorrhoea bacteremia associated with C6, C7 or C8 deficiency. *Ann. Intern. Med.*, 90: 917–920.

Takahashi, M., Takahashi, S., Brade, V. and Nussenzweig, V. (1978) Requirements for the solubilization of immune aggregates by complement. The role of the classical pathway. *J. clin. Invest.*, 61: 349–358.

Rynes, R. and Pickering, R. (1982) Complement deficiency syndromes. In K. Whaley (Ed.), *Complement in Disease*, Churchill Livingstone, in press.

Thompson, R.A. and Winterborn, M.H. (1981) Hypocomplementaemia due to a genetic deficiency of β1H globulin. *Clin. exp. Immunol.*, 46: 110–119.

Whaley, K. (1982) Measurement of complement. In K. Whaley (Ed.), *Complement in Disease*. Churchill Livingstone, in press.

Whaley, K. and El-Ghobarey, A.F. (1981) Complement. In W.C. Dick (Ed.), *Immunological Aspects of Rheumatology*, MTP Press, pp. 93–122.

Whaley, K. and Ferguson, A. (1981) Molecular aspects of complement activation. *Molec. Asp. Med.*, 4: 209–213.

Whaley, K. and Ruddy, S. (1976) Modulation of the alternative complement pathway by β1H globulin. *J. exp. Med.*, 144: 1147–1163.

Whaley, K. and Thompson, R.A. (1978) Requirements for β1H globulin and C3b inactivator in the control of the alternative complement pathway in human serum. *Immunology*, 35: 1045–1049.

Immunology of Nervous System Infections, Progress in Brain Research, Vol. 59, edited by P.O. Behan, V. ter Meulen and F. Clifford Rose

Viruses and Immunodeficiency Diseases

A.D.B. WEBSTER

Clinical Research Centre, Harrow, Middlesex (U.K.)

INTRODUCTION

Patients with primary immunodeficiency diseases can be broadly divided into those with defects in lymphocytes, the complement system, or neutrophils. As far as is known, primary neutrophil dysfunction does not predispose to severe viral infection. Defects in the complement system usually lead to bacterial infection, although some workers have suggested that low levels of the early components (C1, C2) might predispose to the formation of soluble immune complexes containing viral antigens. I will not discuss this further as this is still only a hypothesis.

From the clinical standpoint, severe or unusually prolonged viral infections are not a common problem in most of the primary lymphocyte disorders. However, there are a few rare syndromes where certain virus infections are a frequent cause of death and these will be discussed in some detail. On the other hand, severe virus infections may not always be secondary to an underlying defect in immunity, and there is now good evidence that EB virus infection itself can cause permanent immunodeficiency.

Before describing these conditions, it is necessary to briefly classify (Table I) and describe the known primary immunodeficiency diseases so that the reader gains an overall impression of the clinical features.

TABLE I

CLASSIFICATION OF PRIMARY IMMUNODEFICIENCY DISEASES

This list is not intended to be a comprehensive classification and only concerns those diseases discussed in this chapter.

Antibody deficiency syndromes
  (a) X-linked hypogammaglobulinaemia
  (b) late onset hypogammaglobulinaemia
  (c) functional antibody deficiency

T-cell defects
  (a) thymic aplasia
  (b) purine nucleoside phosphorylase deficiency

Combined immunodeficiency
  (a) severe combined immunodeficiency (adenosine deaminase deficiency accounts for about 20%)
  (b) short-limbed dwarfism with immunodeficiency
  (c) ataxia telangiectasia
  (d) Wiskott–Aldrich syndrome
Interferon deficiency
  –diseases not yet defined

CLINICAL FEATURES OF PRIMARY LYMPHOCYTE DISORDERS

Antibody deficiency syndromes

This is a heterogeneous group of conditions, the best known and investigated patients having severe hypogammaglobulinaemia (Asherson and Webster, 1980). A subgroup have X-linked (Bruton's) hypogammaglobulinaemia, but a commoner variety is late onset hypogammaglobulinaemia where there is no family history. There are also some patients who fail to make functional antibody but have normal serum immunoglobulin levels. All these patients are prone to upper and lower respiratory tract infection with organisms such as h.influenzae and pneumococci. Patients with severe hypogammaglobulinaemia are also prone to mycoplasma infection of the joints and urinary tract and to parasitic infections of the gut. They recover uneventfully from most common viral infections but are prone to self-limiting herpes zoster and potentially fatal echovirus infection.

T-lymphocyte defects

Patients with selective defects of T-lymphocytes are extremely rare. There are two known causes: absence of the thymus caused by abnormal foetal development of the third and fourth pharyngeal pouch or a deficiency of the purine enzyme, nucleoside phosphorylase (PNP). There is very little long-term follow-up information on athymic children, but those with PNP deficiency are prone to severe vaccinial and cytomegalovirus infections (Ammann, 1979). Other infections do not seem to be a major problem.

Mixed humoral and cellular immunodeficiency

Both cellular and humoral immunity is severely affected in the syndrome of severe combined immunodeficiency which affects infants and young children. A defect of the purine enzyme, adenosine deaminase (ADA), accounts for about 20% of cases. These children are prone to bacterial, fungal and viral infections, but there is not much information about their susceptibility to individual viruses. Nowadays, these children are usually given a bone marrow graft as soon as possible and most of the infection problems are due to a combination of graft-vs-host disease and immunosuppressive therapy (Bortin and Rimm, 1977).

Miscellaneous syndromes

There are some very rare autosomal recessive syndromes where there is a partial defect in T- and B-lymphocyte function associated with severe virus infections. The most striking is the syndrome of short-limbed dwarfism with cartilage hair hypoplasia. This disease has a relatively high frequency in the old-order Amish and some of these children have died of fatal varicella infection (McKusick and Cross, 1966). Ataxia telangiectasia is another autosomal recessive condition with severe central nervous system involvement and selective IgA deficiency. The disease is based on a defect in DNA repair and there is a high incidence of lymphoreticular malignancy. There is some indirect evidence that affected patients may be susceptible to chronic virus infection; this concept will be further explored in the section dealing with EB virus infection and immunodeficiency. The Wiskott–Aldrich syndrome is associated with defects in IgM production, partial T-lymphocyte abnormalities, and a high incidence of lymphomas. A few of these patients have died of herpes simplex infection, but they seem to handle most viruses normally (St. Geme et al., 1965).

Defects in interferon production

There are a few anecdotal reports of children with severe persistent herpes virus infections whose lymphocytes are unable to produce interferon. Interferon deficiency may also predispose to recurrent upper respiratory viral infections in some children.

THE RELATIONSHIP OF SPECIFIC VIRUS INFECTIONS TO IMMUNODEFICIENCY

I shall now take individual viruses separately and review the primary host defence defects that predispose to severe or persistent infection.

Enteroviruses

Echovirus infection

It is appropriate to consider echovirus infection first because this is responsible for a particularly interesting chronic 'slow' virus disease in patients with primary hypogammaglobulinaemia. In fact, it mainly occurs in boys with X-linked hypogammaglobulinaemia who have a complete failure to make antibody but have normal cell-mediated immunity. This in itself is important information because it tells us that the elimination of established echovirus infection probably requires specific antibody. The disease has a characteristic chronic and insidious course which may last for up to 10 years. The clinical manifestations involve the subcutaneous tissues, muscles, the brain and sometimes the liver (Wilfert et al., 1977). A few patients present acutely with drowsiness, headache and convulsions, although in most these are late symptoms. The most common initial signs involve the lower legs which become swollen, sometimes with a transient erythematous rash. The subcutaneous tissues and muscles have a characteristic ligneous quality. In some cases the arms are also affected and there may be muscle contractures of the elbows and knees producing a characteristic stooped posture (Asherson and Webster, 1980). This was the first sign of the disease in one of our patients (MR) who remained generally healthy until 8 years later when symptoms of central nervous system disease appeared.

Ultimately, nearly all affected patients develop severe and usually fatal central nervous system disease. The usual symptoms are deafness due to eighth nerve involvement, frequent severe headaches, drowsiness and grand mal epilepsy. Some patients also experience transient sensory aura involving one side of the body. This stage of the disease may last for several years, although there is usually a steady deterioration until death occurs due to involvement of a vital center. For instance, two of our patients died suddenly with respiratory center failure.

Diagnosis

The clinical features described above are virtually pathognomonic of chronic echovirus infection when they occur in a patient with primary hypogammaglobulinaemia. The diagnosis can be confirmed, regardless of the stage of the disease, by aspirating cerebrospinal fluid (CSF) which usually contains a high lymphocyte count, raised protein and echovirus, the latter being easy to culture with standard procedures. It is particularly interesting that virus can nearly always be isolated from the CSF for many years before there are any signs of central nervous system involvement.

When the muscles are involved, the histology may show a florid myositis with many infiltrating mononuclear cells and some muscle cell atrophy. In the later stages there may be considerable muscle fibrosis. The muscle fiber destruction is not as severe as that seen in other forms of acute myositis and this probably accounts for the normal creatinine phosphokinase levels in the serum of most patients. Echovirus can sometimes be isolated from the muscle, and occasionally from the blood of affected patients. In one of our patients (MR) and another in the literature (Wilfert et al., 1977), a different echovirus serotype was found in the muscle from that found in the CSF.

Characteristic changes are not seen on the electroencephalogram. Patients with a history of seizures do show focal abnormalities although in their absence the EEG is usually normal.

Affected patients are often suspected of having a cerebral abscess because of their underlying immunodeficiency. Physicians are therefore tempted to ask for cerebral arteriography. However, two of our patients rapidly deteriorated following this procedure, one developing status epilepticus leading to coma and the other requiring artificial ventilation for about a week due to respiratory center failure. Arteriography should therefore be avoided in these patients and computer-aided tomography is the investigation of choice.

CNS pathology

The brains of two of our patients who died of respiratory center failure have been examined (Table III). In one (AG), there was gross thickening and chronic inflammation of the leptomeninges of the brain and spinal cord. There was patchy cortical scarring together with astrocyte proliferation, microcalcification and some perivascular lymphocyte infiltration. There was a decrease in the number of Purkinje cells and of the cells in the central grey matter, dentate nuclei and olives. In contrast, the brain in the second patient (WF) showed only granular ependymitis.

Treatment

The patients usually develop chronic echovirus infection while receiving gammaglobulin replacement therapy. Up to now this has taken the form of intramuscular gammaglobulin injections which raise the serum IgG level to about 250 mg/100 ml (normal > 600 mg/100 ml). Such treatment is clearly ineffective in preventing echovirus infection, probably because it contains no antibody to the relevant echovirus serotype. The prevalent echovirus serotype in the community changes from year to year, and since gammaglobulin is prepared about two years before being used it is unlikely to contain the relevant antibody.

Research into echovirus infections in neonates shows that antibodies are important in preventing the systemic spread of infection from the mucosa. It is also likely that failure of specific antibody production underlies the rare cases of fatal echovirus infection in neonates, particularly when a new strain enters the community (Modlin et al., 1981). Therefore, the obvious treatment in our patients was to give specific antibody against the relevant echovirus serotype. To this end we prepared a vaccine from the viruses isolated from the CSF and raised antibodies by immunizing sheep (Webster, 1979). The sheep produced an antibody titre of > 1:512 and this was given intravenously at a dose of 200 ml of neat serum every week. Such treatment can only be tolerated by antibody deficient patients as others would develop serum sickness reactions. There was a clinical impression in all 3 patients that the myositic element of the disease improved, and in one patient this was supported by improvement in the muscle biopsy. There were no changes, however, in the numbers of cells or the protein concentration in the CSF. Serial sampling of CSF in one of our cases (AG) showed that we were not always able to isolate the virus (Webster et al., 1978) and this has been a mysterious feature of another of our patients (MR). The sequence of events in this patient is illustrated in Table II. In brief, his illness has lasted at least 6 years and for the past 4 years his CSF has consistently shown a

TABLE II

PATIENT MR (NOW AGED 22 YEARS)

Date	Treatment	Clinical features		Investigation
September 1977	i.m. gammaglobulin	Flexion deformities in elbows and knees. Muscles feel hard and tight	CSF	Protein 6 g/l Cell 5×10^8/1 (mononuclear cells) Echo 17 isolated
February 1978	Hyperimmune sheep serum, 200 ml/2 weeks for 3 months	No change		Muscle biopsy Marked chronic inflammatory infiltrate. Echo 3 isolated
July 1978		Muscles feel better		Muscle biopsy Improved–no cellular infiltrate. Minor changes in muscle fibers
			CSF	No change but *no* virus isolated
November 1980	i.v. gammaglobulin, 10 g/week for 5 months	Transient attack of numbness down left side Increasing deafness, severe headaches, drowsiness	CSF	No change. Still *no* virus isolated
March 1981	i.m. gammaglobulin only	Well for previous 3 months–no CNS features	CSF	No change
September 1981	Starts i.v. gammaglobulin again	Deteriorating. Drowsy, severe headaches, sensory aura again		Muscle biopsy Severe inflammatory infiltrate; fibrosis with muscle fiber atrophy
			CSF	No change. No virus isolated

raised protein and cell count. However, virus was only isolated from the first two CSF samples, and the CSF has since been negative on culture despite the development of central nervous system features. One possibility is that the hyperimmune sheep serum altered the virus so that it could no longer be cultured with standard in vitro techniques.

TABLE III

ECHOVIRUS INFECTION

These 3 male patients with echovirus infection account for about 20 % of all the cases of X-linked hypogammaglobuli-naemia known to us in the South of England.

Age when symptoms noted	Clinical features	Outcome
24	Oedema of legs, rash, deafness, headaches, sensory aura	Died (aged 27 years) after bone marrow transplantation
11	Deafness, oedema of arms, convulsions, hydrocephalus	Died 13 years
17	Flexion deformities of knees and elbows, deafness, headaches, drowsiness	Still alive. Improved on i.v. gamma

Another promising approach is to give large quantities of human gammaglobulin intravenously. Commercial preparations can now be given safely and will raise the serum IgG concentration to well above normal. Mease et al. (1981) described a man with hypogammaglobulinaemia and progressive central nervous system echovirus disease who was apparently cured after the administration of high dose i.v. gammaglobulin. The gammaglobulin contained a relatively low titre (1:32) of antibody to the specific serotype involved although enough was given to produce a measurable titre in the patient's serum. We have tried i.v. gammaglobulin (Sandoglobulin — about 10 g per week for 4 months) in our only living patient with echovirus infection (Table II); he improved dramatically after about a month and relapsed when this was discontinued. We have recently started him on a further course of i.v. gammaglobulin and he seems to be improving again. The mystery is that the gammaglobulin used contains no antibody to the original echovirus 17 serotype isolated. One explanation is that he has been infected with a different agent, although this seems unlikely as these patients are not prone to other neurotropic viruses. Alternatively, the apparent beneficial effects of i.v. gammaglobulin may not only be due to the presence of specific antibody; for instance, the increase in plasma C1 levels after such therapy may be important.

In conclusion, the best available treatment at the moment is to give i.v. gammaglobulin, preferably containing antibody to the serotype involved, at intervals of about a week and at a dose of between 10 and 20 g until there are signs of improvement. In patients who do not respond, there may be a case for injecting specific IgG or interferon intrathecally, although neither has yet been tried.

Poliovirus

There is no evidence for a raised incidence of natural infection in patients with various immunodeficiency syndromes. However, patients with primary hypogammaglobulinaemia or severe combined immunodeficiency (SCID) are prone to vaccine-related disease (Wright et al., 1977). Patients who only have hypogammaglobulinaemia develop a self-limiting non-paralytic disease, whereas paralysis and death occur in SCID children. In one SCID patient the vaccine strain of virus apparently reverted to a more virulent type (Davis et al., 1977). There are no reports of the disease occurring in vaccinated patients already receiving gammaglobulin replacement therapy, but two such patients continued to excrete the vaccine strain in the stools for 3 or 4 weeks after vaccination (Medical Research Council Report, 1971).

Herpes viruses

Herpes simplex

Severe herpes simplex infection is not a particular feature of any of the known immunodeficiency disorders. Fatal herpes simplex encephalitis has been described in a few patients with severe combined immunodeficiency and in one patient with the Wiskott–Aldrich syndrome. It is interesting that herpes simplex infections around the mouth and on the labia are very rare in patients with primary hypogammaglobulinaemia, and there is an impression that these occur much less frequently than in the general population.

Cytomegalovirus

Although cytomegalovirus infection is a well-known complication in patients on immunosuppressive drugs following organ transplantation, there is no definite association with any of the immunodeficiency disorders except for purine nucleoside phosphorylase deficiency. Two such patients developed chronic cytomegalovirus infection, one dying from giant cell pneumonia (Biggar et al., 1978; Carapella de Luca et al., 1978). There also seems to be a high incidence in patients with thymoma and hypogammaglobulinaemia, although some of these patients had additional complications such as systemic lupus erythematosus and many were on immunosuppressive drugs (Asherson and Webster, 1980). It is unclear whether it is common in infants with severe combined immunodeficiency, and this question cannot now be answered since such infants receive bone marrow transplantation early.

Epstein–Barr virus

There is no evidence that EB virus infection complicates any of the known immunodeficiency disorders. It has been suggested that herpes viruses may induce the lymphomas that are common in the Wiskott–Aldrich syndrome and ataxia telangiectasia, although there is no real evidence to support this idea. In ataxia telangiectasia autopsy specimens from many organs have shown large cells with giant hyperchromatic nuclei and cytoplasmic vacuolation, a finding which is compatible with a virus infection (Strich, 1966).

On the other hand, there is good evidence that EB virus infection can induce permanent immunodeficiency. Purtilo et al. (1975) first described this in a family where some members died of acute glandular fever, others developed malignant lymphoma and some developed hypogammaglobulinaemia. The condition was X-linked. Since then a few similar families have been described (Provisor et al., 1975) and there are also sporadic cases where the hypogammaglobulinaemia seems to have followed an episode of glandular fever. The primary defect in these patients presumably involves an inability to control EB virus. Serum antibody to EB virus is usually absent in these patients, although their T-lymphocytes can effectively kill autologous or heterologous EB virus-infected B-lymphocytes in vitro. The question remains why this system is not effective in vivo (Purtilo et al., 1979). The hypogammaglobulinaemia in these cases is usually not very severe and the patients retain some ability to make antibody to antigens other than EB virus. They have normal numbers of circulating B-lymphocytes which may contain EB virus nuclear antigen (EBNA) and which spontaneously form cell lines in vitro. Some patients have an expanded population of T-suppressor lymphocytes in their circulation but there is no evidence that these cells suppress immunoglobulin production in vivo.

Varicella

Severe and sometimes fatal varicella zoster infection may occur in patients with severe T-lymphocyte deficiencies. A particularly high incidence is seen in the syndrome of short limbed dwarfism with immunodeficiency, these patients having low numbers of T-lymphocytes in their peripheral blood which function poorly in vitro (McKusick and Cross, 1966). Some of these patients also fail to make antibody and essentially have a severe combined immunodeficiency. One patient with T-cell deficiency due to purine nucleoside phosphorylase deficiency developed severe varicella infection, although he eventually recovered (Biggar et al., 1978). These findings, together with the obvious susceptibility of children on immunosuppressive drugs to severe varicella, indicates that T-lymphocytes are important in the control of this disease. Patients who fail to make antibodies but have normal T-cell function recover uneventfully from varicella infection. At all events, life-threatening varicella is not such a feared complication nowadays in immunodeficient patients because Acyclovir is a very effective treatment.

Rubella

This virus is a cause of immunodeficiency and Soothill et al. (1966) found 4 patients out of 22 affected children with low serum IgG and IgA. There may also be partial defects of cell-mediated immunity. The IgM is usually raised, however, and specific antibody to rubella is usually present. The virus can be cultured from the throat and urine for up to two years, after which there may be spontaneous improvement in the hypogammaglobulinaemia. Since the immunodeficiency is relatively mild, infections are not usually a problem, and the other features of the disease such as deafness, cataracts, cardiac and neurological abnormalities are the over-riding clinical problems.

Miscellaneous viruses

Hepatitis viruses

There is no evidence of an increased incidence of viral hepatitis in patients with immunodeficiency, although sporadic cases have been reported in patients with cell mediated or humoral immunodeficiency. Only one patient out of about 200 with primary hypogammaglobulinaemia known to us has developed hepatitis, and this was unusual in that he had 9 recurrences during a 3 year period with complete recovery between attacks. His serum was HBsAg-positive on one occasion. Other forms of viral hepatitis do not seem to be associated with antibody deficiency despite the frequent use of fresh frozen plasma infusions as replacement therapy.

Vaccinia

Immunization against smallpox is contra-indicated in any patient with suspected immunodeficiency. A number of children with severe combined immunodeficiency have died from vaccinial infection and two children with T-cell defects due to PNP deficiency had disseminated vaccinia, and one died. Like varicella zoster, T-cells seem important for the control of this infection. A number of patients with only antibody deficiency have been immunized without complication.

Interferon deficiency

Patients with severe or chronic viral infections may have interferon deficiency. This diagnosis is not straightforward, however, since there are many different types of interferon, each requiring different assays. Furthermore, interferon production may be secondarily inhibited by virus infections, so that tests should be repeated if and when the patient recovers (Virelizier and Griscelli, 1981).

One patient has been reported with chronic EB virus infection who appeared to have a primary defect in interferon production, although this did not clinically involve the CNS (Virelizier et al., 1978). Another patient had a severe adenovirus infection (Virelizier and Griscelli, 1981). Furthermore, a failure to produce interferon-α may be partly responsible for the increased susceptibility of some young children to recurrent rhinovirus infection (Isaacs et al., 1981).

CONCLUSION

A clinical study of the primary immunodeficiency diseases shows us that patients with T-lymphocyte defects are prone to severe cytomegalovirus and pox virus infections. It is not clear, however, which aspect of T-cell function is required for controlling these infections. Antibody-deficient patients are prone to insidious and chronic echovirus infections of the CNS. This is important because it increases the likelihood that other chronic CNS diseases are due to viruses to which susceptible patients fail to make specific antibody.

REFERENCES

Ammann, A.J. (1979) Immunological aberrations in purine nucleoside phosphorylase deficiencies. In *Ciba Foundation Symposium Series, No. 68,* Elsevier, Amsterdam.

Asherson, G.L. and Webster, A.D.B. (1980) *Diagnosis and Treatment of Immunodeficiency Diseases,* Blackwell Scientific Publications.

Biggar, W.D., Giblett, E.R., Ozere, R.L. and Grover, B.D. (1978) A new form of nucleoside phosphorylase deficiency in two brothers with defective T-cell function. *J. Pediat.,* 92: 354.

Bortin, M.M. and Rimm, A.A. (1977) Severe combined immunodeficiency disease, characterization of the disease and results of transplantation. *J. Amer. Med. Ass.,* 238, 591.

Carapella de Luca, E. Aiuti, F., Lucarelli, P., Bruni, L., Baroni, C.D., Imperato, C., Roos, D. and Astaldi, A. (1978) A patient with nucleoside phosphorylase deficiency, selective T-cell deficiency, and autoimmune hemolytic anemia. *J. Pediat.,* 93: 1000.

Davis, L.E., Bodian, D., Price, D., Butler, I.J. and Vickers, J.H. (1977) Chronic progressive poliomyelitis secondary to vaccination of an immunodeficient child. *New Engl. J. Med.,* 297: 241.

Isaacs, D., Clarke, J.R., Tyrrell, D.A.J., Webster, A.D.B. and Valman, H.B. (1981) Deficient production of leucocyte interferon (Interferon α) in vitro and in vivo in children with recurrent respiratory infection. *Lancet,* 2: 950.

Mease, P.J., Ochs Hans, D. and Wedgwood, R.J. (1981) Successful treatment of echo viral meningoencephalitis and myositis-fasciitis with intravenous immune globulin therapy in a patient with X-linked agammaglobulinemia. *New Engl. J. Med.,* 304: 1278.

McKusick, V.A. and Cross, H.E. (1966) Ataxia-telangiectasia and Swiss-type agammaglobulinemia. Two genetic disorders of the immune mechanism in related Amish sibships. *J. Amer. Med. Ass.,* 195: 739.

Medical Research Council Special Report Series (1971) *Hypogammaglobulinaemia in the United Kingdom.* 310.

Modlin, J.F., Polk, B.F., Horton, P., Etkind, P., Crane, E. and Spiliotes, A. (1981) Perinatal echovirus infection: risk of transmission during a community outbreak. *New Engl. J. Med.,* 305: 368.

Provisor, A.J., Iacuone, J.J., Chilcote, R.R., Neiburger, R.G., Crussi, F.G. and Baehner, R.L. (1975) Acquired agammaglobulinemia after a life-threatening illness with clinical and laboratory features of infectious mononucleosis in three related male children. *New Engl. J. Med.,* 293: 62.

Purtilo, D.T., Cassel, C., Yang, J.P.S., Stephenson, S.R., Landing, B.H. and Vawter, G.F. (1975) X-linked recessive progressive combined variable immunodeficiency (Duncan's disease). *Lancet,* 1: 935.

Purtilo, D.T., Paquin, L., De Florio, D., Virzi, F. and Sakhuja, R. (1979) Immunodiagnosis and immunopathogenesis of the X-linked Recessive Lymphoproliferative Syndrome. *Seminars in Hematology,* 16: 309.

Soothill, J.F., Hayes, K. and Dudgeon, J.A. (1966) The immunoglobulins in congenital rubella. *Lancet,* i: 1385.

St. Geme, J.W., Prince, J.T., Burke, B.A., Good, R.A. and Krivit, W. (1965) Impaired cellular resistance to herpes-simplex virus in Wiskott–Aldrich syndrome. *New Engl. J. Med.,* 273: 229.

Strich, S.J. (1966) Pathological findings in 3 cases of ataxia-telangiectasia. *J. Neurol. Neurosurg. Psychiat.,* 29: 489.

Webster, A.D.B., Tripp, J.H., Hayward, A.R., Dayan, A.D., Doshi, R., MacIntyre, E.H. and Tyrrell, D.A.J. (1978) Echovirus encephalitis and myositis in primary immunoglobulin deficiency. *Arch. Dis. Childh.,* 53: 33.

Webster, A.D.B. (1979) Infections in immunodeficient patients. In D.A.J. Tyrrell (ed.) *Aspects of Slow and Persistent Virus Infections,* Martinus Nijhoff, p. 255.

Wilfert, C.M., Buckley, R.H., Mohanakumar, T., Griffith, J.F., Katz, S.L., Whisnant, J.K., Eggleston, P.A., Moore, M., Treadwell, E., Oxman, M.N. and Rosen, F.S. (1977) Persistent and fatal central nervous system echovirus infections in patients with agammaglobulinemia. *New Engl. J. Med.,* 296: 1485.

Wright, P.F., Hatch, M.H., Kasselberg, A.G., Lowry, S.P., Wadlington, W.B. and Karzon, D.T. (1977) Vaccine-associated poliomyelitis in a child with sex-linked agammaglobulinemia. *J. Pediat.,* 91: 408.

Virelizier, J.L., Lenoir, G. and Griscelli, C. (1978) Persistant Epstein–Barr virus infection in a child with hyper-gammaglobulinaemia and immunoblastic proliferation associated with a selective defect of immune interferon secretion. *Lancet,* 2: 231.

Virelizier, J.L. and Griscelli, C. (1981) Défaut sélectif de sécrétion d'interféron associé à un déficit d'activité cytotoxique naturelle. *Arch. Fr. Pediatr.,* 38: 77.

Virelizier, J.L. (1982) Testing immunity to viral infections, *Clin. Immunol. Allergy,* 1: 669.

Immunology of Nervous System Infections, Progress in Brain Research, Vol. 59, edited by P.O. Behan, V. ter Meulen and F. Clifford Rose

Autoimmune Disease and Viral Infection

J.O. FLEMING and L.P. WEINER

University of Southern California, School of Medicine, 2025 Zonal Ave, Los Angeles, CA 90033 (U.S.A.)

INTRODUCTION

The relationship between host responses to self-antigens and viral infection continues to be a perplexing problem in the understanding of "autoimmune" diseases of man. In diseases such as multiple sclerosis, post-infectious encephalomyelitis, Guillain–Barre Syndrome and polymyositis the target antigen has not been defined. In each case, viruses have been implicated in the pathogenesis of the disease. In myasthenia gravis, the target antigen has been identified, but the chain of events leading to the disease process has not been deciphered.

In this chapter we will attempt to define the mechanism by which viruses could induce "autoimmune" diseases, discuss models of viral-induced immunopathology, and review possible host antigens which could and do serve as targets in nervous system disease.

MECHANISMS

Johnson and Weiner (1972) reviewed possible mechanisms by which viruses could induce an immune mediated demyelinating process. The most obvious mechanism is that a virus might share an antigenic determinant with normal host cell membrane constituents. Panitch et al. (1979) have perhaps given credence to this mechanism, having demonstrated cross-reactivity between measles virus and myelin basic protein. Wroblewska et al. (personal communication) have recently shown that an anti-herpes hybridoma antibody exhibits a cross-reactivity between viral and cellular components.

A second mechanism by which autoimmune responsiveness may be associated with virus infection involves viral infection leading to the release of host cell antigens with which immunocytes have never previously interacted. These may be internal antigens which are released following viral-induced cell lysis or "neo-antigens" which, because of the viral infection, have become "unmasked" and are expressed on the cell surface. Such antigens have probably not been expressed since an early stage of development, and hence are not recognized as self. Paterson (1980) described additional mechanisms of virus-augmented neuroimmunologic disease. These include viral activation of neuro-reactive lymphoid cells, increased vulnerability of CNS target tissue through enhanced vascular permeability, and finally, the induction of the "bystander effect".

The so-called "bystander effect" has been applied to the possibility that myelin may be destroyed incidental to an immune reaction to nearby, but unrelated antigens. The theoretical basis for this phenomenon derives from the observations of Ruddle and Waksman (1968) who showed non-specific cytolysis of cells in the presence of heterologous antigen and sensitized lymphoid cells. Wisniewski and Bloom produced CNS demyelination in previously sensitized guinea pigs following local injection of tuberculin-purified protein derivative (Wisniewski and Bloom, 1975). Such a mechanism has been suggested in the Theiler's virus-induced demyelination (Lipton and Dal Canto, 1976) and in the peripheral demyelination induced by the herpes infection of chickens (Marek's disease) (Stevens et al., 1981). The virus serves as the target antigen and myelin is non-specifically destroyed by the antiviral immune response. The mechanism for the "bystander effect" has been attributed to the liberation of proteolytic enzymes. Cammer et al. (1978) have shown myelin fragmentation in the presence of neutral proteases secreted by activated macrophages. Dal Canto et al. (1975) have further suggested that the vesicular disruption of myelin seen by electron microscopy in demyelinating models may be due to lysosomal enzymes. Dal Canto and Rabinowitz (1982) have recently commented on the attractiveness of this theory, suggesting a mechanism by which similar pathological patterns in white matter could be produced by different and often unrelated viruses.

VIRAL MODELS AND IMMUNOPATHOLOGY

The relationship between viral models and "autoimmune" disease remains tenuous. The immunopathology may be due to direct infection of immune cells producing probable disruption of immune cell regulation, or to the interaction of viral antigen with specific host cell antigens (Weiner and Stohlman, 1978). There are a number of models in which virus, host cell antigens and the immune response combine to produce an immunopathologic process.

Lactic dehydrogenase virus

Lactic dehydrogenase virus (LDV) is an RNA-enveloped virus which produces interesting immunologic abnormalities in NZB mice. The NZB strain of mice is known to have immune complex nephritis. During LDV infection, there is an exaggerated humoral response to some antigens and depression to other antigens (Oldstone et al., 1974). The graft-host reaction, induction of tolerance, and phagocytosis are depressed (Notkins et al., 1978). A number of immune derangements seem to be taking place. The exaggerated humoral response results in incomplete neutralizing activity which could be due to blocking factors such as antigen–antibody complexes, or inhibitory immunoglobulin. It might also be due to a failure of macrophage function or viral destruction of suppressor T-cells. Certainly T-cells are destroyed by LDV. The T-cell destruction in LDV-infected animals, coupled with an increase in the number of germinal centers and plasma cells in thymus-dependent areas of spleen and lymph nodes, may account for the Ig enhancement and for the defects in cell-mediated immunity. The findings in LDV are not unlike those seen in autoimmune processes in which IgG levels are increased in conjunction with defects in cell-mediated immunity (Rowson and Mahy, 1975).

Aleutian disease

Aleutian disease (AD) of mink is due to a naturally occurring, temperature-sensitive, parvovirus infection. The virus contains a single-stranded DNA. Aleutian disease virus (ADV) replicates in macrophages of mink and lesions are not noted immediately. When lesions first appear, they coincide with an exaggerated antiviral antibody response and hypergammaglobulinemia. The IgG levels can reach 11 g/100 ml. Late in the disease, ADV circulates as infectious antigen–antibody complexes and smaller complexes are deposited in glomeruli and arteries causing severe inflammatory lesions. Both host and viral genotype influence the severity of the arteritis (Porter et al., 1980). Thus, non-aleutian mink have persistent infection without lethal disease. One group of pastel mink has no viremia, but does have a transient increase in serum gamma-globulin and a relatively low ADV antibody.

In the Aleutian mink there is hyperplasia of the B-lymphoid cell system. Lymphocytes and plasma cells infiltrate many organs. Both the percentage of gamma-globulin and the total serum protein is increased during AD. Thus far no immunologic differences have been shown between IgG of normal and AD mink. The IgG does show some restriction of mobility, and after one year 10 % of animals developed monoclonal gammopathy (Porter et al., 1980). The relationship of antigen–antibody complexes to disease appears to depend on viral antigen, but it is not known how much of the IgG is indeed virus specific antibody. Peak ADV antibody titers are reached before the maximal increase in serum IgG is present, suggesting most of IgG is not specific antibody (Bloom et al., 1975). The question of autoimmune processes is further complicated by the occasional finding of nuclear antigens and antinuclear antibodies in the serum of AD mink.

Lymphocytic choriomeningitis

Lymphocytic choriomeningitis (LCM) and other arenaviruses produce an immunopathology which has been well studied in regard to T-lymphocyte-mediated killing of virus-infected target cells (Cole and Nathanson, 1974), activation of natural killer (NK) cells in acute infection (Welsh, 1978) viral antigen–antibody complex-induced disease (Oldstone and Dixon, 1971), and associated H-2 restriction (Zinkernagel and Doherty, 1974). It is the H-2 restriction in both LCM and, more recently, in influenza virus studies (Frankel et al., 1979), that has suggested that T-cell recognition is directed against some association of viral and H-2 glycoproteins, which has led to the "altered self" concept. An antibody to a sufficiently stable association of viral or H-2 glycoproteins, or the presence of the particular antibody attachment sites sufficiently close to a neo-antigen (formed by the nexus of viral and H-2 molecules) to sterically block the function of cytotoxic T-cells, might be involved.

Theiler's virus

Theiler's virus (TV), a murine picornavirus, has been associated with immunopathology. TV produces a chronic CNS infection in which viral antigen can be localized to neuronal terminals, astrocytes, and inflammatory cells, particularly macrophages, around white matter lesions (Dal Canto and Lipton, 1982). The pathology consists of primary demyelination with disruption of myelin and stripping of myelin sheaths by mononuclear cell processes. These changes are similar to EAE (Dal Canto and Lipton, 1975). Oligodendrocytes in and around the myelin breakdown are free of viral antigen, suggesting that the myelin degeneration is not a direct viral-induced oligodendrocytolysis. Immunosuppression with cyclophosphamide results in a marked decrease in the white matter lesions, suggesting that demyelination is dependent on the host immune response (Lipton and Dal Canto, 1976). Of interest are the large amounts of viral antigen in macrophages, but a role for these cells has not yet been defined. The mechanisms underlying host-mediated virus-induced demyelination in the Theiler's model is still unknown, but a "bystander effect" has been postulated.

Herpes viruses

Herpes viruses have also been implicated in autoimmune disease. Both cytomegalovirus (Schmitz and Enders, 1977) and Epstein–Barr virus (EBV) have been associated with Guillain–Barre syndrome (Birnbaum, 1973). Marek's disease, an avian herpes virus, has been suggested as an experimental model for GBS (Stevens et al., 1981). The virus consistently induces lymphocytic infiltration and subsequent demyelination of peripheral nerves in domestic chickens. Latent infection can be established in satellite cells, non-myelinating Schwann cells and lymphocytes of spinal ganglia and associated nerves. In reactivation experiments, virus was not found in neurons or myelinating Schwann cells (Stevens et al., 1981). Studies in chickens show that infected birds develop specific cellular immune responses to chicken peripheral nerve (Schmahl et al., 1975). Stevens et al. (1981) have postulated that in "bystander" demyelination in which latent infection of non-myelinating Schwann cells and satellite cells are the proposed target of a cellular immune response, lymphotoxins and proteolytic enzymes actually produce the demyelination. Released myelin, possibly with viral antigens acting as adjuvants, sensitizes the host and results in an ongoing autoimmune demyelinating process.

There is, however, an alternate hypothesis which needs to be explored. Most cells infected with herpes viruses express a protein which binds to the Fc region of IgG. The Fc cellular receptors have been demonstrated on lymphocyte and tumor cell membranes (Kerbel and Davies, 1974), staphylococcus aureus cell walls (Forsgren and Sjoquist, 1966), and a variety of non-lymphoid cells. The affinity for the Fc region seems to be a non-specific phenomenon, but probably has an important role in immune regulation, persistent and latent infection and, perhaps, autoimmune disease. Cowan et al. (1980) recently reviewed the role of Fc and immune complexes and indicated that MHC antigens, transfer factor and immune interferon, as immune regulatory or modulator molecules, are either associated with Fc receptors or alter Fc receptor-mediated immunity. They further suggest that Fc receptors may provide a link between antigen specific, immune complex-mediated, intercellular interactions and intracellular regulation of gene expression. These latter factors appear to be important in immune regulation, cellular differentiation, viral replication, and malignant transformation. Cells infected with herpes viruses express a protein which binds the Fc fragment. This has been shown in HSV-I, -II, zoster-varicella and cytomegalovirus and includes cultured epithelioid, fibroblasts, and neural cells (Watkins, 1964; Westmoreland and Watkins, 1974; Rahman et al., 1976; Coster et al., 1977; Adler et al., 1978). Spear and her colleagues, in a series of papers, demonstrated that the receptor for Fc in HSV-I-infected cells is a viral-specified glycosylated membrane protein (Baucke and Spear, 1979; Para et al., 1980, 1982). They have designated this protein as glycoprotein E (gE), and detected it also in virion preparations isolated from infected cells. An antiserum prepared against this glycoprotein selectively precipitated gE from a variety of cell types infected with HSV-I and neutralized HSV-I infectivity in the presence of complement. F (ab)$_2$ fragments interfered with Fc binding activity. The inhibition of the Fc receptor function by the F (ab)$_2$ fragments of anti-gE antibodies supports the hypothesis that g E and the Fc receptor on herpes-infected cells are the same protein (Para et al., 1982).

The physiological role of the Fc binding receptor is unknown, but it has been postulated that IgG binding might interfere with cytotoxic antibodies or lymphocytes. Lehner et al. (1975) have suggested that anti-HSV antibodies which bind to both Fc receptor and HSV cell surface antigens would make the Fc portion of these antibodies unavailable for complement or cytotoxic cells. Although most investigators postulate a role for Fc-binding in the establishment of latency, it is certainly possible that the gE expression and subsequent binding may play an important part in non-specific IgG binding and in the subsequent immune cytolysis which is complement-dependent. Rager-Zisman et al. (1976) have shown that cross-linking of effector and target cells through aggregated immunoglobulins bound to Fc receptor present on HSV-infected cells is the mechanism of selective, nonspecific killing.

CONCLUSION

The role of viruses in autoimmune human disease is still not defined. The epidemiology of multiple sclerosis suggests a viral etiology, and the pathology is most consistent with an immunopathologic process. Antigen or antigens have not been demonstrated, but we have set out the theoretical and experimental evidence which implicates a virus in the pathogenesis of the disease. We have discussed the interaction of virus with host cell antigens, described the presence of the Fc receptor in herpes infection, and indicated the possibility of a "bystander" effect in the pathogenesis of autoimmune disease.

REFERENCES

Adler, R., Glorioso, J.C., Cossman, J. and Levine, M. (1978) Possible role of Fc receptors on cells infected and transformed by herpes virus: escape from immune cytolysis. *Infect. Immun.*, 21: 442–447.

Baucke, R. and Spear, P.G. (1979) Membrane proteins specified by herpes simplex viruses. V Identification of Fc-binding glycoprotein. *J. Virol.*, 32: 779–789.

Birnbaum, G. (1973) Guillain–Barre Syndrome. Increased lymphoproliferation potential. *Arch. Neurol.*, 28: 215–218.

Bloom, M.E., Race, R.E., Hadlow, W.J. and Chesebro, B. (1975) Aleutian disease of mink: antibody response of sapphire and pastel mink to aleutian disease virus. *J. Immunol.*, 115: 1034–1037.

Cammer, W., Bloom, B.R., Norton, W.T. and Gordon, S. (1978) Degradation of basic protein in myelin by neutral proteases secreted by stimulated macrophages: a possible mechanism of inflammatory demyelination. *Proc. Nat. Acad. Sci. U.S.A.*, 75: 1554–1558.

Costa, J., Rabson, A.S., Yee, C. and Tralka, T.S. (1977) Immunoglobulin binding to herpes virus-induced Fc receptors inhibits virus growth. *Nature (Lond.)*, 269: 251–252.

Cole, G.A. and Nathanson, N. (1974) Lymphocytic choriomeningitis. *Prog. Med. Virol.*, 18: 94–110.

Cowan, F.M., Klein, D.L., Armstrong, G.R., Stylos, W.A. and Pearson, J.W. (1980) Fc receptor mediated immune regulation and gene expression. *Biomedicine*, 32: 108–110.

Dal Canto, M.C., Wisniewski, H.M., Johnson, A.B., Brostoff, S.W. and Raine, C.S. (1975) Vesicular disruption of myelin in autoimmune demyelination. *J. Neurol. Sci.*, 24: 313–319.

Dal Canto, M.C. and Rabinowitz, S.G. (1982) Experimental models of virus-induced demyelination of the central nervous system. *Ann. Neurol.*, 11: 109–127.

Dal Canto, M.C. and Lipton, H.L. (1982) Ultrastructural immunohistochemical demonstration of Theiler's virus in acute and chronic Theiler's demyelinating encephalomyelitis. *Amer. J. Path.*, 106: 20–29.

Dal Canto, M.C. and Lipton, H.L. (1975) Primary demyelination in Theiler's virus infection: an ultrastructural study. *Lab. Invest.*, 33: 626–637.

Forsgren, A. and Sjoquist, J. (1966) Protein A from S. aureus. I. Pseudo-immune reaction with human γ-globulin. *J. Immunol.*, 97: 822–827.

Frankel, M., Effros, R.B., Doherty, P.C. and Gerhard, W.V. (1979) A monoclonal antibody to viral glycoprotein blocks virus-immune effector T cells operating at H-2D[d] but not at H-2K[d]. *J. Immunol.*, 123: 2438–2440.

Johnson, R.T. and Weiner, L.P. (1972) The role of viral infections in demyelinating diseases. In F. Wolfgram, G. Ellison, J. Stevens and J. Andrews (Eds.), *Multiple Sclerosis*, Academic Press, New York, 1972, pp. 245–264.

Kerbel, R.S. and Davies, A.J.S. (1974) The possible biological significance of Fc receptors on mammalian lymphocytes and tumor cells. *Cell*, 3: 105–112.

Lehner, T., Wilton, J.M.A. and Shillitoe, E.J. (1975) Immunological basis for latency, recurrences and putative oncogenecity of herpes simplex virus. *Lancet*, 2: 60–62.

Lipton, H.L. and Dal Canto, M.C. (1976) Theiler's virus-induced demyelination. Prevention by immunosuppression. *Science*, 192: 62–64.

Notkins, A.L., Mergenhagen, S.E. and Howard, R.J. (1970) Effect of virus infections on the function of the immune system. *Ann. Rev. Microbiol.*, 24: 525–538.

Oldstone, M.B.A. and Dixon, F.J. (1971) Immune complex disease in chronic viral infections. *J. Exp. Med.*, 134: 32–40.

Oldstone, M.B.A., Tishon, A. and Chiller, J.M. (1974) Chronic virus infection and immune responsiveness. II. Lactic dehydrogenase virus infection and immune response to non-viral antigens. *J. Immunol.*, 112: 370–375.

Panitch, H.S., Swoveland, P. and Johnson, K.P. (1979) Antibodies to measles virus react with myelin basic protein. *Neurology*, 29: 548–549.

Paterson, P.Y. (1980) Immune responses implicated in immunopathological disorders of the central nervous system. In A. Boese (ed.), *Search for the Cause of Multiple Sclerosis and Other Chronic Diseases of the Central Nervous System*, Chemie Verlag, Weinheim, pp. 173–183.

Para, M.F., Baucke, R.B. and Spear, P.G. (1982) Glycoprotein gE of Herpes simplex type I: Effects of anti-gE on virion infectivity and on virus-induced Fc binding receptors. *J. Virol.*, 41: 129–136.

Para, M.F. Baucke, R.B. and Spear, P.G. (1980) Immunoglobulin G (Fc)-binding receptors on virions of herpes simplex virus type I and transfer of these receptors to the cell surface by infection. *J. Virol.*, 34: 512–520.

Porter, D.D., Larsen, A.E. and Porter, H.G. (1980) Aleutian disease of mink. *Advanc. Immunol.*, 29: 261–285.

Rahman, A.A., Teschner, M., Sethi, K.K. and Brandis, H. (1976) Appearance of IgG (Fc) receptor(s) on cultured human fibroblasts infected with human cytomegalovirus. *J. Immunol.*, 117: 253–258.

Rager-Zisman, B., Grose, C. and Bloom, B.R. (1976) Mechanism of selective nonspecific cell-mediated cytotoxicity of virus-infected cells. *Nature (Lond.)*, 260: 369–370.

Rowson, K.E. and Mahy, B.W.J. (1975) Lactic dehydrogenase virus. *Virol. Monograph*, 13: 1–121.

Ruddle, N.H. and Waksman, B.H. (1968) Cytotoxicity mediated by soluble antigen and lymphocytes in delayed hypersensitivity. Part I (characterization of the phenomenon). *J. exp. Med.*, 128: 1237–1254.

Schmahl, W., Hoffman-Fezer, G. and Hoffman, R. (1975) Zur Pathogenese der nervenlasionen bei Marekscher krankheit des huhnes. I. Allergische hautreaktion gegen myelin peripherer nerven. *Z. Immunitaetsforsch.*, 150: 175–183.

Schmitz, H. and Enders, G. (1977) Cytomegalovirus as a frequent cause of Guillain–Barre' syndrome. *J. Med. Virol.*, 1: 21–27.

Stevens, J.G., Pepose, J.S. and Cook, M.L. (1981) Marek's Disease: A natural model for the Landry–Guillain–Barre' Syndrome. *Ann. Neurol.*, 9 (Suppl.): 102–106.

Watkins, J.F. (1964) Adsorption of sensitized sheep erythrocytes to HeLa cells infected with herpes simplex virus. *Nature (Lond.)*, 202: 1364–1365.

Weiner, L.P. and Stohlman, S.A. (1980) Viral-induced immunological incompetence as an etiologic factor in multiple sclerosis. In K. Tritsch, (Ed.), *Progress in Multiple Sclerosis*, Heidelberg: Springer, (1978) Heidelberg, pp. 40–45.

Welsh, R.M. (1978) Cytotoxic cells induced during lymphocytic choriomeningitis virus infection of mice. I. Characterization of natural killer cell induction, *J. exp. Med.*, 148: 163–181.

Westmoreland, D. and Watkins, J.F. (1974) The IgG receptor induced by herpes simplex virus: studies using radioiodinated IgG. *J. gen. Virol.*, 24: 167–178.

Wisniewski, H.M. and Bloom, B.R. (1975) Primary demyelination as a non-specific consequence of a cell-mediated immune reaction. *J. exp. Med.*, 141: 346–359.

Zinkernagel, R.M. and Doherty, P.C. (1974) Immunological surveillance against altered self components by sensitized T lymphocytes in lympocytic choriomeningitis. *Nature (Lond.)*, 251: 547–548.

Immunology of Nervous System Infections, Progress in Brain Research, Vol. 59, edited by P.O. Behan, V. ter Meulen and F. Clifford Rose

Interferon in Acute and Chronic Viral Infections

D. BRIGDEN and D.S. FREESTONE

The Wellcome Research Laboratories, Beckenham, Kent BR3 3BS (U.K.)

INTRODUCTION

Relatively little information about the clinical use of interferon has been generated since Isaacs and Lindeman (1957) first described a biological mediator responsible for virus interference some 24 years ago. Improvements in large-scale cell culture and the recent demonstration that it is possible to produce human interferon from genetically manipulated bacteria have led to quantities of interferon becoming available for larger scale clinical evaluation. Considerable advances have also been made in the purification process. Interferons most widely used until recently have been in the main less than 1 % pure with the rest of the material being made up largely of uncharacterized protein. Interferon can now be manufactured consistently in excess of 80 % purity and frequently up to 95 % pure. The increase in availability and purity warrants a new look at interferon as a therapeutic substance.

CLASSIFICATION AND SOURCE

Human interferons are a heterogenous group of proteins that are now classified broadly into Hu-IFNα (leukocyte, lymphoblastoid), Hu-IFN-β (fibroblast) and Hu-IFN-γ (immune interferon). A large part of the clinical work has been conducted with Hu-IFN-α, although Hu-IFN-β has also been used. Hu-IFN-α can be obtained from primary leukocytes, from lymphoblastoid cell lines and from genetically engineered bacteria. Because of the potential limit on the quantity of donor leukocytes, this does not seem likely to be a suitable source for large-scale manufacture. The techniques of cell or bacterial culture are, on the other hand, capable of being scaled up to supply the demand. There are now believed to be at least 8-10 different human α-interferons, each being coded by a different gene. These are likely to differ somewhat in their biological activity. It may, of course, be an advantage to be able to select for a desired activity. At the present time, however, it is not known what that activity should be in relation to most clinical usage, so that there may be some advantage in conducting clinical work with preparations containing a mixture of interferons. Allen and Fantes (1980) have shown that human lymphoblastoid interferon prepared by the techniques of Finter and Fantes (1980) contains at least 8 different α-interferons.

The main part of the clinical work has been conducted with Hu-IFN-α obtained from primary leukocytes. The studies discussed here used such material unless stated otherwise.

[97]

PHARMACOKINETICS

Interferon has usually been given to man as an i.m. injection. Cantell et al. (1974) showed that doses in adults of 5 million units (1×10^5/kg) achieved mean blood levels between 1 and 12 h of 50 units/ml serum. Emodi et al. (1975) compared different routes and showed that following an i.v. infusion of 30 million units over 5 min the half-life was about 15 min during the first hour and about 90 min between the first and fourth hours. The interferon was essentially cleared within 6 h. The same dose given as an infusion over 8 h produced a rising blood level during the 8 h to reach a peak between 10^2 and 10^3 units/ml, but the blood level had declined to insignificant levels by 24 h. Following an i.m. injection of 1 million units in some 20 subjects, the peak was seen at 2 h and the level remained around 100 units for 6 h. The pattern following s.c. injection was very similar to the i.m. pharmacokinetic profile. In a careful study carried out with lymphoblastoid interferon, Priestman (1980) demonstrated that doses of 5 mega units/m^2 maintained an average blood level of 150 units over 24 h. No interferon was detected in the cerebrospinal fluid (CSF).

Interferon does not easily penetrate the intact blood–brain barrier. Jablecki et al. (1981) in patients with amyotrophic lateral sclerosis were only just able to detect interferon levels in the CSF after 6 million units were given by either s.c. or bolus i.v. injection. High and prolonged CSF levels, however, have been demonstrated following intrathecal injection in monkeys by Habif et al. (1975) and Hilfenhaus et al. (1981). Because of these findings, direct intrathecal administration in man has been used in serious infections of the CNS. De Clercq et al. (1975) reported the administration of 600,000 units intrathecally to a neonate. Merigan (1977) reported the cases of two additional neonates given 50,000 units per day.

ANTIVIRAL ACTIVITY IN MAN

Model human experiments

The first demonstration of the antiviral effects of interferon in man were reported by the British Medical Research Council's Interferon Scientific Committee in 1962. In a double-blind controlled trial, interferon produced in rhesus monkey kidney cells, or saline were administered intradermally at two separate sites to 38 healthy human volunteers. Twenty-four hours later the subjects received a smallpox vaccination into each site. Vaccination takes were present in 24 saline pre-treatment sites but not in the corresponding interferon pre-treatment sites, while the reverse applied in one subject. In the 13 subjects who had takes at both sites, the reaction rates were greater with saline in 8, and equivalent at both sites in 5.

Merigan et al. (1973) at the Medical Research Council's Common Cold Unit, Salisbury, U.K., administered a total of 8×10^5 U of interferon intranasally to 22 healthy volunteers in the 24 h post-challenge with an influenza B-strain again given intranasally. There were no differences in symptomatology, virus shedding or antibody development between the 11 treated and the 11 control subjects, possibly due to the lack of pre-challenge treatment and to the relatively low dose of interferon administered. When these workers gave a total dose of 1.4×10^7 U of interferon, again administered intranasally, in 39 doses over the 4 days from 24 h before to 72 h after challenge, this time with a rhinovirus type 4 in a similar controlled experiment, significant reductions in clinical symptoms, virus shedding and antibody response were found in the treated subjects. Recently, however, Scott et al. (1980) did not obtain any effects with fibroblast interferon in an almost identical experiment, again carried out at the

MRC Common Cold Unit, against a rhinovirus type 4 challenge. This experiment differed in that approximately 5 mega units of interferon were applied 3 times daily to treated volunteers over the 24 h before and 72 h after challenge. These negative results might be explained by the less frequent administration of interferon, allowing nasal mucociliary clearance systems to operate, to the lower total dose of interferon used, or to different activities of leukocyte and fibroblast interferons.

Finally, in a very small controlled study of 4 treated and 4 controls (rubella seronegative subjects, who were vaccinated subcutaneously with RA27/3 strain rubella vaccine), Best and Banatvala (1975) in London found that pre-treatment with interferon in a total dose of 3.25×10^5 U delayed post-vaccination virus shedding.

These clinical experiments, therefore, show evidence of antiviral activity of interferon against vaccinia virus, rhinovirus type 4, and probably rubella virus.

Hepatitis B virus (HBV)

The most extensive studies have been carried out by Merigan and his colleagues at Stanford University. They have recently published (Scullard et al., 1981) a summary of their results over many years. Thirty-two patients were treated by antiviral therapy. Five out of 16 treated with interferon became HBV DNA polymerase (DNAP)-negative and 4 (25%) of these remained so. Thirteen out of 16 became DNAP-negative on an alternating cycle of interferon and adenine arabinoside 7 (44%) and remained negative. Results on the infectivity of these patients' serum, and on liver function and histology, are awaited. Others have confirmed that interferon will reduce DNAP levels (Kato et al., 1979), although usually this has only been temporary (Scullard et al., 1979; Weimar et al., 1980). Work is continuing to define the role of antiviral drugs including interferon, in this complex disease.

Varicella zoster virus (VZV)

Merigan et al. (1978) conducted several small placebo controlled trials in cancer patients with localized herpes zoster infections. Essentially, he has demonstrated that interferon can limit the spread within the primary dermatome and can reduce cutaneous and visceral dissemination. An initial dose of 42,000 units/kg followed at 12 hourly intervals by a dose of 21,000 units/kg was ineffective. An initial dose of 170,000 units/kg, however, followed by 85,000 units/kg at 12 hourly intervals was clearly effective, and a higher dose of 255,000 units/kg (12.75 million units in a 50 kg patient) at 12 hourly intervals for 4 doses, followed by 127,000 units/kg 12 hourly thereafter, was apparently even more effective, though this may have been due to earlier entry of the patients. In the two higher dose groups there was a significant reduction in the incidence of post-herpetic neuralgia. In all these studies the duration of therapy was 8 days. A further study where Merigan et al. (1981) carried out a two-day course of treatment only at the higher dose of 255,000 units/kg 12 hourly, demonstrated less impressive results. There was still, however, an effect on cutaneous dissemination and post-herpetic neuralgia. Emodi and Rufli (1977) carried out a placebo controlled trial in which they claimed that viral clearance was accelerated, crust formation enhanced and pain reduced, by a dose of 1 million units given daily for 5 days.

Arvin et al. (1978) reported on a trial of interferon in primary varicella in children with cancer. Two doses of interferon were used: 42,000 units/kg and 255,000 units /kg. The numbers were extremely small, with 9 patients on interferon and 9 patients on placebo. No difference was observed in the duration of new lesions, although there was a statistically significant difference in the incidence of visceral complications in favour of treatment with interferon.

Cytomegalovirus infections (CMV)

Cheeseman et al. (1979) demonstrated a delay in excretion of CMV in renal transplant recipients produced by 3 mega units given on the day of transplantation, the following day, and twice weekly thereafter for 6 weeks. This was a relatively low total dose but they were limited by haematological toxicity. They were unable to show an effect on herpes simplex virus. Weimar et al. (1978) had previously demonstrated that human fibroblast interferon (Hu-IFN-β) in doses of 3 mega units twice weekly did not influence clinical or subclinical infections with cytomegalo or herpes simplex viruses. Meyers et al. (1980) gave doses of 2×10^4–6.4×10^5 units/kg/day to bone marrow transplant patients with lung biopsy positive CMV pneumonia. All the patients died, although less toxicity was experienced than had been expected, and the authors thus concluded that prophylactic interferon might be successful.

Herpes simplex virus (HSV)

An elegant study conducted by Pazin et al. (1979) clearly demonstrated that 7×10^4 U/kg of interferon for 5 days starting the day before microsurgical trigeminal nerve decompression prevented reactivation of labial herpes simplex. However, in a follow-up study, Haverkos et al. (1980) showed that this had not prevented later recurrences.

Both Coster et al. (1977) and Sundmacher et al. (1978) have clearly demonstrated that topically applied interferon in combination with debridement is able to improve the outcome of a herpes simplex ulcer in the eye. However, the development of more effective anti-herpes simplex agents has led to a reduction in the relative value of interferon in infections due to this virus.

TOXICITY

The use of interferon is limited by toxicity. The studies previously discussed essentially demonstrate that the main limiting toxicities that systemic interferon exhibits are suppression of bone marrow function, which recovers on cessation of therapy or dose reduction, and a fairly severe influenza-like syndrome consisting of malaise, fever and frequently, rigors. This latter problem appears to diminish after a few days, allowing an increase in dosage. These toxic reactions appear to be due to the interferons themselves, as in general an increase in purity has not led to a reduction of these effects.

Therapeutic interferon and viral infections of the central nervous system

As was mentioned in the section on pharmacokinetics, little interferon appears to cross the intact blood–brain barrier, so that attempts to treat viral infections of the central nervous system are now concentrating on direct administration into the cerebrospinal fluid.

The diseases that theoretically could respond to interferon fall into two main groups, namely those known to be classical virus infections, such as rabies, or herpes encephalitis where the virus is known and its multiplication is responsible for cell destruction. Assuming one can get virus static concentrations of interferon to the site of infection early enough to prevent the spread of the infection significantly, then it is reasonable to suppose that interferon may have an effect on the clinical outcome of the disease. The second group of diseases are those where either the virus etiology is unproven, such as multiple sclerosis (MS) or where although a virus etiology is known, such as sub-acute sclerosing panencephalitis (SSPE), there is little evidence that the virus is still spreading from cell to cell and the tissue damage is probably due to inflammatory destruction. These latter diseases are probably less likely to respond to the antiviral effect of interferon, although one must remember that interferon has subtle immunological effects in addition to its other actions. These effects may be beneficial, or equally, they may have the opposite effect.

Rabies

Hilfenhaus et al. (1977) have demonstrated that combined intramuscular and intrathecal Hu-IFN-α is able to protect monkeys inoculated with rabies virus. Hattwick et al. (1972) have demonstrated that it is possible to cure rabies by intensive supportive care. It may therefore be possible to influence the 100 % mortality of established rabies encephalitis by a combination of interferon and intensive care.

Viral encephalitis

Several attempts have been made to treat herpes encephalitis, none with much success. Whitley et al. (1977) have claimed that adenine arabinoside has an effect in reducing the mortality in herpes encephalitis. Clinical trials are now well underway, exploring the use of the more active antiherpes compound acyclovir. It would seem unlikely that interferon would prove to be superior to these agents. It would seem likely, however, that the limitation on the success of such a highly potent antiherpes agent as acyclovir will be due to the progress of the disease at the time of therapy rather than inadequate potency.

The encephalitides produced by arboviruses, such as St. Louis encephalitis, are also diseases with a high mortality in which interferon could possibly have a therapeutic effect.

Subacute sclerosing panencephalitis

Attempts have been made to treat this slow virus disease with interferon, but with little success. Behan (1981) reported a complete lack of clinical effect in 3 patients treated with 3 mega units intravenously for 20–90 days. The effects of higher doses or different routes need to be explored.

Progressive multifocal leucoencephalopathy (PML)

Cheeseman et al. (1980) showed that interferon had no effect on the excretion in the urine of BK papovavirus in renal transplant patients. PML has been shown to be due to a related papovavirus. It would seem unlikely that interferon would prove effective in this very rare disease of immunocompromised patients.

There are other CNS diseases with either probable viral or "virus-like" etiology, i.e. kuru and Creutzfeldt-Jakob disease, and diseases which may have a virus etiology, i.e. multiple sclerosis and amyotrophic lateral sclerosis, which may respond to interferon. Progress will, however, be extremely difficult in these diseases.

CONCLUSION

Interferon is clearly an antiviral agent with demonstrated activity in man against the hepatitis B virus, vaccinia, rhinovirus type 4, varicella zoster, cytomegalovirus and herpes simplex. There is still a long way to go, however, before it will be possible to recommend therapy with interferon in any virus disease, and in particular, the course will be difficult in virus diseases of the central nervous system.

REFERENCES

Allen, G. and Fantes, K.H. (1980) A family of structural genes for human lymphoblastoid (leucocyte-type) interferon. *Nature (Lond.)*, 287: 408–411.

Arvin, A.M., Feldman, S. and Merigan, T.C. (1978) Human leukocyte interferon in the treatment of varicella in children with cancer: a preliminary controlled trial. *Antimicrob. Agents Chemother.*, 13: 605–607.

Behan, P., (1981) Interferon in treatment of subacute sclerosing panencephalitis. *Lancet, i*: 1059–1060.

Best, J.M. and Banatvala, J.E. (1975) The effect of a human interferon preparation on vaccine-induced rubella infection. *J. biol. Stand.*, 3: 107–112.

Cantell, K., Pyhälä, L. and Strander, H. (1974) Circulating human interferon after intramuscular injection into animals and man. *J. gen. Virol.*, 22: 453–455.

Cheeseman, S.H., Rubin, R.H., Stewart, J.A., Tolkoff-Rubin, N.E., Cosimi, A.B., Cantell, K., Gilbert, J., Winkle, S., Herrin, J.T., Black, P.H., Russell, P.S. and Hirsch, M.S. (1979) Controlled clinical trial of prophylactic human leukocyte interferon in renal transplantation. Effect on cytomegalovirus and herpes simplex virus infection. *New Engl. J. Med.*, 300: 1345–1349.

Cheeseman, S.H., Black, P.H., Rubin, R.H., Cantell, K. and Hirsch, M.S. (1980) Interferon and BK papovavirus — clinical and laboratory studies. *J. infect. Dis.*, 141: 157–161.

Coster, D.J., Falcon, M.G., Cantell, K. and Jones, B.R. (1977) Clinical experience of human leukocyte interferon in the management of herpetic keratitis. *Trans. Ophthal. Soc. U.K.,* 97: 327–329.

De Clercq, E., Edy, V.G., De Vueger, H., Eeckels, R. and Desmyter, J. (1975) Intrathecal administration of interferon in neonatal herpes. *J. Pediat.*, 86: 736–739.

Emodi, G., Just, M., Hernandez, R. and Hirt, H.R. (1975) Circulating interferon in man after administered ration of exogenous human leukocyte interferon. *J. nat. Cancer Inst.*, 54: 1045–1049.

Emodi, G. and Rufli, Th. (1977) Antiviral action of interferon in man: use of interferon in varicella zoster infections in man. *Tex. Rep. Biol. Med.*, 35: 511–515.

Finter, N.B. and Fantes, K.H. (1980) The purity and safety of interferons prepared for clinical use: the case for lymphoblastoid interferon. In I. Gresser (Ed.), *Interferon 2*, Academic Press, Oxford, pp. 65–80.

Habif, D.V., Lipton, R. and Cantell, K. (1975) Interferon crosses blood–cerebrospinal fluid barrier in monkeys. *Proc. Soc. exp. Biol. (N.Y.)*, 149: 287–289.

Hattwick, M.A.W., Weiss, T.T., Stechshuft, C.J., Baer, G.M. and Gregg, M.B. (1972) Recovery from rabies: a case report. *Ann. Int. Med.*, 76: 931–942.

Haverkos, H.W., Pazin, G.J., Armstrong, J.A. and Ho, M. (1980) Follow-up of Interferon treatment of herpes simplex. *New Engl. J. Med.*, 303: 699–700.

Hilfenhaus, J., Weinmann, E., Mager, M., Barth, R. and Jaeger, O. (1977) Administration of human interferon to rabies virus infected monkeys after exposure. *J. infect. Dis.*, 135: 846–849.

Hilfenhaus, J., Damm, H., Hofstaetter, T., Mauler, R., Ronneberger, H. and Weinmann, E. (1981) Pharmacokinetics of human interferon β in monkeys. *J. Interferon Res.*, 1: 427–436.

Isaacs, A., Lindeman, J. (1957) Virus interference 1. The interferon. *Proc. roy. Soc. B*, 147: 258–267.

Jablecki, C., Cantell, K., Connor, J., Kingsbury, D., Hamburger, R., Westall, F. and Smith, R. (1981) Experimental treatment of ALS with interferon. *Ann. Neurol.*, Abstr. 10: 82.

Kato, Y., Kobayashi, K., Suyama, T. and Hattori, N. (1979) Effects of human leucocyte interferon therapy on hepatitis B virus in patients with chronic active hepatitis. *Gastroenterology*, 7/5: A21.

Medical Research Council Scientific Committee on Interferons (1962) The effect of interferon on vaccination in volunteers. *Lancet*, i: 873–5.

Merigan, T.C., Reed, S.E., Hall, T.S. and Tyrrell, D.A.J. (1973) Inhibiton of respiratory virus infection by locally applied interferon. *Lancet*, i: 563–567.

Merigan, T.C. (1977) Pharmacokinetics and side effects of interferon in man. *Tex. Reps. Biol. Med.*, 35: 541–547.

Merigan, T.C., Rand, K.H., Pollard, R.B., Abdallah, P.S., Jordan, G.W. and Fried, R.P. (1978) Human leukocyte interferon for the treatment of herpes zoster in patients with cancer. *New Engl. J. Med.*, 298: 981–987.

Merigan, T.C., Gallagher, J.G., Pollard, R.B. and Arvin, A.M. (1981) Short-course human leukocyte interferon in the treatment of herpes zoster in patients with cancer. *Antimicrob. Agents Chemother.*, 19: 193–195.

Meyers, J.D., McGuffin, R.W., Neiman, P.E., Singer, J.W. and Thomas, E.D. (1980) Toxicity and efficacy of human leukocyte interferon for treatment of cytomegalovirus pneumonia after marrow transplantation. *J. infect. Dis.*, 141: 555–562.

Pazin, G.J., Armstrong, J.A., Larn, M.T., Tarr, G.C., Jannetta, P.J. and Ho., M. (1979) Prevention of reactivated herpes simplex infection by human-leukocyte interferon after operation on the trigeminal root. *New. Engl. J. Med.*, 301: 225–30.

Priestman, T.J. (1980) Initial evaluation of human lymphoblastoid interferon in patients with advanced malignant disease. *Lancet*, ii: 113–118.

Scott, G.M., Reed, S., Cartwright, T. and Tyrrell, D. (1980) Failure of human fibroblast interferon to protect against rhinovirus infection. *Arch. Virol.*, 65: 135–139.

Scullard, G.H., Alberti, A., Wansborough-Jones, M.H., Howard, C.R., Eddleston, A.L.W.F., Zuckerman, A.J., Cantell, K. and Williams, R. (1979) Effects of human leucocyte interferon on hepatitis B virus replication and immune responses in patients with chronic hepatitis B infection. *J. clin. Lab. Immunol.*, 1: 277–282.

Scullard, G.H., Pollard, R.B., Smith, J.L., Sacks, S.L., Gregory, P.B., Robinson, W.S. and Merigan, T.C. (1981) Antiviral treatment of chronic hepatitis B virus infection. I. Changes in viral markers with interferon combined with adenine arabinoside. *J. infect. Dis.*, 143: 772–783.

Sundmacher, R., Cantell, K., Hang, P. and Neumann-Haefelin, D. (1978) Role of debridement and interferon in the treatment of dendritic keratitis. *Albrecht v. Graefes Arch. Ophthal.*, 207: 77–82.

Weimar, W., Schellekeus, H., Lameijer, L.D.F., Masurel, N., Edy, V.G., Billiau, A. and De Somer, P. (1978) Double-blind study of interferon administration in renal transplant recipients. *Europ. J. clin. Invest.*, 8: 255–258.

Weimar, W., Heijtink, R.A., ten Kate, F.J.P., Schalm, S.W., Masurel, N. and Schellekens, H. (1980) Double-blind study of leucocyte interferon administration in chronic HBsAG positive hepatitis. *Lancet*, i: 336–338.

Whitley, R.J., Soong, S.-J. and Odin, R. (1977) Adenine arabinoside therapy of biopsy-proven herpes simplex encephalitis: national institute of allergy and infectious diseases collaborative antiviral study. *New Engl. J. Med.*, 297: 289–294.

Immunology of Nervous System Infections, Progress in Brain Research, Vol. 59, edited by P.O. Behan, V. ter Meulen and F. Clifford Rose

Antigenic Modulation:
A Mechanism of Viral Persistence

ROBERT S. FUJINAMI and MICHAEL B.A. OLDSTONE

Scripps Clinic and Research Foundation, Department of Immunopathology, 10666 N. Torrey Pines Road, La Jolla, CA 92037 (U.S.A.)

INTRODUCTION

Several naturally occurring infections in man are associated with viral persistence in the face of a specific antiviral immune response. Some examples are herpes simplex virus, cytomegalovirus, hepatitis B virus and measles virus infection (Stevens et al., 1978). Measles virus is an interesting situation. In humans, infection by measles virus can take two vastly different forms. Generally, the infection is acute and the infected individual mounts an immune response that clears the virus from all tissues, i.e. a self-limiting disease. Low titers of antimeasles antibody, as well as immune lymphocytes that develop during convalescence, last throughout life. In contrast, on rare occasions, measles virus can cause a persistent infection known as subacute sclerosing panencephalitis (SSPE). These patients have high titers of antimeasles antibody in the circulation and cerebrospinal fluid (Ter Meulen et al., 1972; Ter Meulen and Hall, 1978). Further, these individuals have cytotoxic immune lymphocytes as well as functional complement systems (Ter Meulen et al., 1978; Joseph and Oldstone, 1975; Perrin et al., 1977; Kreth et al., 1975). Despite an antiviral immune response, measles virus persists and can be isolated from their central nervous systems and lymphoid tissues (Ter Meulen et al., 1972; Joseph and Oldstone, 1975).

To account for the events observed in SSPE, we have suggested that antibody to measles virus can "modulate or strip off" viral antigens from the surfaces of infected cells. This stripping effectively reduces the amount of foreign (viral) antigens on such cells rendering them resistant to lysis by immune lymphocytes or specific antibody and complement. The concept of antigenic modulation is not new in that it was first described by Boyse, Old and colleagues when studying the TL differentiation antigen on thymocytes and leukemia cells (Boyse et al., 1963, 1967; Old et al., 1968). They noted that TL antigens disappeared from the surfaces of cells cultured in the presence of specific antibody. This phenotypic suppression of TL antigen occurred both in vitro and in vivo. Subsequently, the suppression or removal of cell surface antigens of various retroviruses was also found whenever specific antibody was present (Aoki and Johnson, 1972; Ioachim et al., 1972; Calafat et al., 1976; Genovesi et al., 1977; Doig and Chesebro, 1978; Yagi et al., 1978; Doig and Chesebro, 1979). Antibody induced antigenic modulation of measles virus antigens occurs similarly on measles virus-infected cells (Joseph and Oldstone, 1975; Oldstone and Tishon, 1978). Additionally, under modulating conditions, nucleocapsids within cells infected in this way accumulate and become randomly distributed instead of neatly aligned under the plasma membrane, much like the disordered nucleocapsids in cells obtained by biopsies from patients with SSPE (Iwasaki and Koprowski, 1974; Lampert et al., 1976).

106

DISCUSSION

One can identify a total of 6 measles virus polypeptides from acutely infected HeLa cells: the large (L) protein with a molecular weight of 160,000; hemagglutinin (HA) with a molecular weight of 80,000; P with a molecular weight of 70,000; nucleocapsid (NC) protein with a molecular weight of 60,000; fusion (F) protein whose F1 subunit, shown here, has a molecular weight of 42,000; and membrane or matrix (M) protein with a molecular weight of 36,000 (Fig. 1). When the surfaces of cells infected with measles virus are labeled, however, the only proteins evident are the HA and F1 proteins which can be identified on the cells' exterior (Fig. 1) (Fenger et al., 1978; Sissons et al., 1979; Fujinami and Oldstone, 1980; Fujinami et al., 1981).

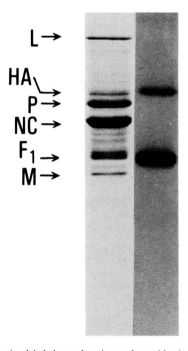

Fig. 1. The left lane is [^{35}S]methionine-labeled measles virus polypeptides immunoprecipitated from HeLa cells acutely infected during incubation for 18 h. The right lane is [^{125}I]-surfaced labeled infected HeLa cells from which only the HA and F1 were immunoprecipitated. Both sets of samples were run on 10.5% gels at 100 V for approximately 4 h. Gels were dried and X-ray film exposed to the gel. From these studies, it is clear that only HA and F measles virus polypeptides are expressed on the cells surface.

A new and unique component in our system is that the observer can quantify not only antimeasles antibody's capacity to strip viral antigens off the surface of infected cells, but also to alter the expression and synthesis of measles virus polypeptides inside these cells (Fujinami and Oldstone, 1979, 1980). During the initial or initiation phase of antibody-induced antigenic modulation — exposure to antibody for 24 h or less, the quantity of measles virus polypeptides obtained from infected cells cultured in the presence of antimeasles antibody decreases. Table I shows that treatment with either polyclonal antibody (containing specificities to all measles virus polypeptides) or monoclonal antibody (specific for measles virus HA) decreases the amount of viral polypeptides in cells infected with this virus as compared to those in untreated cells tested concurrently. The decrease in the polypeptides is particularly marked for the P, M, and F1 proteins. Similarly, when amounts of each of these viral polypeptides are compared to that of the NC protein within each group of cells, similar conclusions can be drawn. Therefore, infected cells cultured in the presence of either monoclonal antibody (anti-HA) or polyclonal antibody are dramatically altered in their expression of the measles virus polypeptides (Fujinami et al., 1981); Table I).

TABLE I

COMPARATIVE PERCENTAGES OF MEASLES VIRUS POLYPEPTIDES ON ANTIBODY-TREATED
CELLS AND UNTREATED CELLS INFECTED WITH MEASLES VIRUS

Data represent the percent of viral protein on antibody-treated cells relative to 100 % on untreated cells (no antibody).
Two monoclonal antibody directed against measles virus HA are shown.

Polypeptides	Treatment		
	No antibody (%)	Polyclonal antibody (%)	Monoclonal antibody (%)
HA	100	55	59 36
P	100	5	15 5
NC	100	65	55 39
F_1	100	19	40 22
M	100	38	26 18

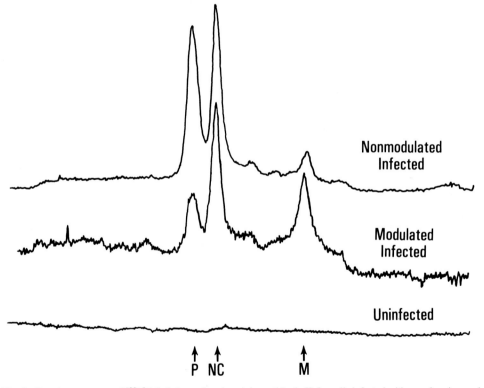

Fig. 2. Densitometer scan of [^{32}P]-labeled measles virus polypeptides in HeLa cells infected with measles virus and cultured with (modulated) or without (nonmodulated) measles virus antibody (from Fujinami and Oldstone, 1980). Note the marked decrease in P and the increase in M polypeptides.

Three of the internal viral polypeptides, P, M, and NC, are phosphorylated in infected cells. When these cells are incubated under modulating conditions, that is, in the presence of antiviral antibody, the incorporation of ^{32}P into the P protein drops, as expected, since amounts of P protein have decreased so that less of this acceptor is available. In contrast, the incorporation of ^{32}P into the M protein rises even though the $[^{35}S]$methionine counts decreased (Fig. 2 and Table I). There are two species of M protein in cells; a phosphorylated and a nonphosphorylated form. We suspect that the phosphorylated form is either dephosphorylated and/or the nonphosphorylated form is preferentially incorporated into the virion since little or no phosphorylated M protein is found in purified virions (Fujinami and Oldstone, 1980).

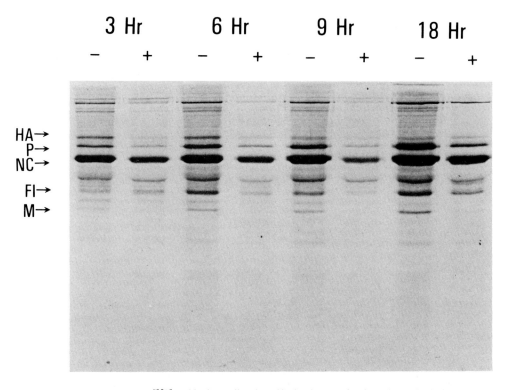

Fig. 3.   Negative (−) prelabeled ($[^{35}S]$methionine) cells cultured in the absence of antimeasles antibody. Positive (+) prelabeled cells cultured in the presence of antimeasles antibody; at 3 h, 6 h, 9 h, 18 h, cells were harvested and the labeled proteins analyzed on 10.5% SDS-gels. This study demonstrates that the P polypeptide is not preferentially degraded. In contrast to the P polypeptide, the M polypeptide is degraded or turned over.

The loss of the P, F1 and M proteins does not result from preferential degradation of these polypeptides (Fig. 3). Infected cells labeled with $[^{35}S]$methionine before culturing in either the presence or absence of antimeasles antibody containing media and harvested at various intervals bear P and F1 proteins that are turned over at the same rate as the other polypeptides according to electrophoretic analysis. M protein in general is degraded faster than the other viral polypeptides, so proportionately less M protein is present within 6 h.

Alterations in the expression of viral polypeptides could have several consequences. The first is failure of cell fusion. In this case antibody treatment causes a decrease in the amount of F protein being synthesized and available on the cell's surface. This decrease minimizes cell fusion. As a result, fewer giant cells or syncytia form so that viral spread is limited; cells appear normal and cell survival is enhanced (Graves et al., 1978). Nonetheless, the viral genome persists within. Infected cell survival and viral persistence in the presence of antibody was demonstrated previously by Rustigian (1966), Minagawa (1971), and Joseph and Oldstone (1975) for measles virus. Our experiments determine that the molecular basis for cell survival and lack of giant cell formation is due to a decrease in the numbers of F molecules. Recently, Merz et al. (1980) used a related paramyxovirus, SVS and showed similar results. Therefore, the infection of cells by any virus like measles virus, that does not effectively "shut off" host cell protein synthesis (Haspal et al., 1977) and allows continued cellular functions, can enter persistent infection if the fusion step is blocked or inhibited.

Secondly, a decrease in the amount of P protein could account for the generalized drop in measles viral polypeptides as seen in Table I. The P protein, L or polymerase, and NC proteins are thought to comprise the replication complex of the virus. Certainly, alterations in these 3 polypeptides would effect replicative events. For example, the NS protein of vesicular stomatitis virus is comparable to the P protein of measles virus. Emerson and Yu (1975) demonstrated clearly that transcription activity is dependent not only on the L protein but the NS protein as well. Although both proteins are necessary for transcription, they are not factors in the efficiency of transcription (Emerson and Yu, 1975). The identification and characterization of the transcriptase or polymerase of measles virus (Seifried et al., 1978) are just beginning, but similar prerequisites are probably necessary for synthesis of measles virus RNA. Again, decreased synthesis of viral products as observed would favor cell survival and possible persistence of the viral genome in infected cells.

Third, antimeasles antibody treatment of infected cells reduces the amount of M protein in these cells and alters the degree of M protein phosphorylation (Fujinami and Oldstone, 1979, 1980). The potential result is misalignment of nucleocapsids, often seen in SSPE brain cells (Iwasaki and Koprowski, 1974; Lampert et al., 1976), and the related failure to produce infectious virions. The occurrence of measles virus M protein in a fully phosphorylated and a less or nonphosphorylated species was initially reported by us (Fujinami and Oldstone, 1979, 1980) and by Hall et al. (1980) for the HeLa cell line. Phosphorylation of M protein from infected HeLa cells has recently been confirmed by Graves (1981). A decrease in the amount of M protein and/or more M protein in a phosphorylated form (intracellular) are consistent with the concept of directing an acute infection toward a persistent form.

We are currently undertaking experiments to understand mechanistically how such changes occur. Specifically, we are concerned with knowing how antibody binding to a surface component causes such drastic changes within the cells. Whatever the cause, the outcome is initiation and maintenance of viral persistence.

SUMMARY

Since viruses such as herpes, hepatitis B, cytomegalo and measles can persist in a host despite a vigorous immune response, we investigated the ability of antibody to measles virus to alter the expression of viral antigens on and within infected cells. The monoclonal antibody directed against the measles virus hemagglutinin (HA) used in these experiments bound to the surfaces of infected HeLa cells. As a result, expression of all the virus polypeptides decreased, particularly that of the phosphoprotein and membrane protein but also the fusion protein. This decrease was significant: it could be quantitated in densitometer tracings of autoradiograms

110

from infected cells treated with antibody compared to those left untreated or treated with antibody against viral polypeptides not expressed on the cells surface. Modifications of measles virus antigens by specific monoclonal antibody to virus HA prevented cellular events that would otherwise have led to the lysis and elimination of infected cells. This in turn favored the survival of these cells and was associated with viral persistence.

ACKNOWLEDGEMENTS

This is publication number 2604 from Scripps Clinic and Research Foundation, La Jolla, CA 92037. This research was supported by Grants NS 12428, AI 07007, NS 17214 and a grant from the Multiple Sclerosis Society, JF 2009-A-1. R.S.F. is a Harry Weaver Neuroscience Scholar of the National Multiple Sclerosis Society. The authors acknowledge the technical contribution of Ms. Alicia Cross and thank Mrs. Susan Edward for manscript preparation.

REFERENCES

Aoki, T. and Johnson, P.A. (1972) Suppression of gross leukemia cell-surface antigens: a kind of antigenic modulation. *J. nat. Cancer Inst.,* 49: 183–192.

Boyse, E.A., Old, L.J. and Luell, S. (1963) Antigenic properties of experimental leukemias. II. Immunological studies in vivo with C57BL/6 radiation-induced leukemias. *J. nat. Cancer Inst.,* 31: 987–995.

Boyse, E.A., Stockert, E. and Old, L.J. (1967) Modification of the antigenic structure of the cell membrane by thymus-leukemia (TL) antibody. *PNAS,* 58: 954–57.

Calafat, J., Hilgers, J., von Blitterswijk, W.J., Verbeet, M. and Hageman, P.C. (1976) Antibody-induced modulation and shedding of mammary tumor virus antigens on the surfaces of GR ascites leukemia cells as compared on the normal antigens. *J. nat. Cancer Inst.,* 56: 1019-1029.

Doig, D. and Chesebro, B. (1978) Antibody-induced loss of friend virus leukemia cell surface antigens occurs during progression of erythroleukemia in F1 mice. *J. exp. Med.,* 148: 1109–1121.

Doig, D. and Chesebro, B. (1979) Anti-Friend virus antibody is associated with recovery from viremia and loss of viral leukemia cell-surface antigens in leukemic mice. *J. exp. Med.,* 150: 10.

Emerson, S.U. and Yu, Y.-H. (1975) Proteins are required for in vitro RNA synthesis by vesicular stomatitis virus. *J. Virol.,* 15: 1348–1356.

Fenger, T.W., Smith, J.W. and Howe, C. (1978) Analysis of immunoprecipitated surface glycoproteins in measles virions and in membranes of infected cells. *J. Virol.,* 28: 292–299.

Fujinami, R.S. and Oldstone, M.B.A. (1979) Antiviral antibody reacting on the plasma membrane alters measles virus expression inside the cell. *Nature (Lond.),* 279: 529–530.

Fujinami, R.S. and Oldstone, M.B.A. (1980) Alterations in expression of measles virus polypeptides by antibody molecular events in antibody-induced antigenic modulation. *J. Immunol.,* 125: 78–85.

Fujinami, R.S., Sissons, J.G.P. and Oldstone, M.B.A. (1981) Immune reactive measles virus polypeptides on the cell's surface: turnover and relationship of the glycoproteins to each other and to HLA determinants. *J. Immunol.,* 127: 936–940.

Genovesi, E.V., Marx, P.A. and Wheelock, E.F. (1977) Antigenic modulation of Friend virus erythroleukemic cells in vitro by serum from mice with dormant erythroleukemia. *J. exp. Med.,* 146: 520–534.

Graves, M.C. (1981) Measles virus polypeptides in infected cells studied by immune precipitation and one-dimensional peptide mapping. *J. Virol.,* 38: 224–230.

Graves, M.C., Silver, S.M. and Choppin, P.W. (1978) Measles virus polypeptide synthesis in infected cells. *Virology,* 86: 254–263.

Hall, W.W., Lamb, R.A. and Choppin, P.W. (1980) The polypeptides of canine distemper virus: synthesis in infected cells and relatedness to the polypeptides of other morbilliviruses. *Virology,* 100: 433–449.

Haspel, M.V., Pellegrino, M.A., Lampert, P.W. and Oldstone, M.B.A. (1977) Human histocompatibility determinants and virus antigens: effect of measles virus infection on HLA expression. *J. exp. Med.,* 146: 146–156.

Ioachim, H.L., Dorsett, B., Sabbath, M. and Keller, S. (1972) Loss and recovery of phenotypic expression of Gross leukemia virus. *Nature New Biol.,* 237: 215–218.

Iwasaki, Y. and Koprowski, H. (1974) Cell to cell transmission of virus in the central nervous system. I. Subacute sclerosing panencephalitis. *Lab. Invest.,* 31: 187–196.

Joseph, B.S. and Oldstone, M.B.A. (1975) Immunologic injury in measles virus infection. II. Suppression of immune injury through antigenic modulation. *J. exp. Med.,* 142: 864–876.

Kreth, W.H., Kackell, M.Y. and ter Meulen, V. (1975) Demonstration of in vitro lymphocyte-mediated cytotoxicity against measles virus in SSPE. *J. Immunol.,* 114: 1042–1046.

Lampert, P.W., Joseph, B.S. and Oldstone, M.B.A. (1976) Morphological changes of cells infected with measles or related viruses. In H.M. Zimmerman (Ed.), *Progress in Neuropathology,* Grune and Stratton, New York, pp. 51–68.

Merz, D.C., Scheid, A. and Choppin, P.W. (1980) Importance of antibodies to the fusion glycoprotein of para-myxoviruses in the prevention of spread of infection. *J. exp. Med.,* 151: 275–288.

Minagawa, T. (1971) Studies on persistent infection with measles virus in HeLa cells. I. Clonal analysis of cells of carrier cultures. *Jap. J. Microsc.,* 15: 325.

Old, L.J., Stockert, E., Boyse, E.A. and Kim, J.H. (1968) Antigenic modulation. Loss of T1 antigen from cells exposed to TL antibody. Study of the phenomenon in vitro. *J. exp. Med.,* 127: 523–539.

Oldstone, M.B.A. and Tishon, A. (1978) Immunologic injury in measles virus infection. IV. Antigenic modulation and abrogation of lymphocyte lysis of virus-infected cells. *Clin. Immunol. Immunopath.,* 9: 55–62.

Perrin, L.H., Tishon, A. and Oldstone, M.B.A. (1977) Immunologic injury in measles virus infection. III. Presence and characterization of human cytotoxic lymphocytes. *J. Immunol.,* 118: 282–290.

Rustigian, R. (1966) Persistent infection of cells in culture by measles virus. II. Effect of measles antibody on persistently infected HeLa sublines and recovery of a HeLa clone persistently infected with complete virus. *J. Bact.,* 92: 1805.

Stevens, J.G., Todaro, G.J. and Fox, C.F. (Eds.) (1978) *Persistent Viruses,* Academic Press, New York.

Seifried, A.S., Albrecht, P. and Milstein, J.B. (1978) Characterization of a RNA-dependent RNA polymerase activity associated with measles virus. *J. Virol.,* 25: 781–787.

Sissons, J.G.P., Cooper, N.R. and Oldstone, M.B.A. (1979) Alternative complement pathway-mediated lysis of measles virus infected cells: induction by IgG antibody bound to individual viral glycoproteins and compara-tive efficacy of F(ab')$_2$ and F ab' fragments. *J. Immunol.,* 123: 2144–2149.

Ter Meulen, V. and Hall, W.W. (1978) Slow virus infections of the nervous system: virological, immunological and pathogenetic considerations. *J. gen. Virol.,* 41: 1–25.

Ter Meulen, V., Katz, M. and Muller D. (1972) Subacute sclerosing panencephalitis: a review. *Current Top. Microbiol. Immunol.,* 57: 1–38.

Yagi, M.J., Blair, P.B. and Lane, M.A. (1978) Modulation of mouse mammary tumor virus production in the MJY-alpha cell line. *J. Virol.,* 28: 611–623.

Immunology of Nervous System Infections, Progress in Brain Research, Vol. 59, edited by P.O. Behan, V. ter Meulen and F. Clifford Rose

Paramyxovirus and Morbillivirus Infections and their Relationship to Neurological Disease

W.C. RUSSELL

Division of Virology, National Institute for Medical Research, Mill Hill, London NW7 1AA (U.K.)

INTRODUCTION

The family of viruses grouped under the title of paramyxoviridae (Kingsbury et al., 1978) contains a number of different viruses which have been associated with neurological diseases. All of the viruses in this group have one large single-stranded RNA as genome and at least 6 virus-coded virion polypeptides. The RNA is negative stranded, is closely associated with 3 of the polypeptides (N, P, L), and is surrounded by a liproprotein envelope containing two virus-coded glycoproteins (G and F) which play an important role in many aspects of the infectious process. The remaining polypeptide (matrix) appears to be tightly associated with the inner side of the virus envelope and seems to be intimately involved in virion assembly (see Fig. 1). The family has been sub-divided into 3 genera: the morbilliviruses, the pneumoviru-

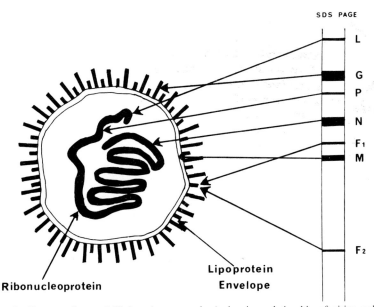

Fig. 1. Schematic diagram of a morbillivirus (paramyxovirus) showing relationship of virion polypeptides as revealed by SDS polyacrylamide gel electrophoresis to structural features of the virus.

[113]

ses and the paramyxoviruses proper. Most of the viruses in the family grow relatively poorly in tissue culture and accordingly, information on their properties has been mainly derived from two viruses of the paramyxovirus genus which grow quite well in tissue culture, viz. a murine virus — Sendai, and an avian one — Newcastle Disease Virus (NDV). One striking feature of many members is their propensity to form persistent infections in tissue culture and this raises the question of whether this property has a parallel in in vivo infections.

The relationship of the paramyxoviridae family to neurological disease is most firmly established in the case of the morbillivirus genus where there is compelling evidence that subacute sclerosing panencephalitis (SSPE) correlates with a systemic infection by a measles virus (MV) and the virus can be recovered from the brain and from lymph nodes (for a review see ter Meulen et al., 1978). The course of the disease is extremely varied (Risk and Haddad, 1979) and although the antibody response can also be variable, in most cases large titres of measles antibody can be found in both serum and CSF (Agnarsdottir, 1977). The virus, nevertheless, seems to persist in the presence of an apparently normal immune response and the progress of the disease presumably reflects the inability of the immunological response to counter the spread of virus infection. In the case of SSPE the disease mostly affects young people aged from 10 to 16 years, but there seems to be no clear-cut relationship either temporally or virologically between disease onset and primary measles infection. This disease therefore is distinct from measles encephalitis where there is a clear temporal relationship to a primary measles infection.

Lesions of the CNS have also been well-documented in association with another closely related member of the morbillivirus genus — canine distemper virus (CDV). The course of the disease is also very variable, ranging from an acute respiratory-associated infection in young dogs to a late chronic disease in older animals ("old dog" encephalitis) (Adams et al., 1975). A demyelinating encephalomyelitis can be obtained reproducibly with special strains of the virus in gnotobiotic dogs (McCullough et al., 1974), whereas other CDV strains can produce only a low incidence of demyelination in dogs (for a review see Appel and Gillespie, 1972). The other two members of this genus, viz. rinderpest virus (RV) and peste de petits ruminants (PPR) cause severe disease in cattle, sheep and goats, particularly in underdeveloped countries, and there have been reports from south India of associated neurological involvement (Shaila, personal communication).

Members of the paramyxovirus genus are mostly associated with respiratory infections although mumps virus can induce a self-limiting meningitis. There are, moreover, a number of studies demonstrating the ability of paramyxoviruses to persist in man (Gross et al., 1973; Parkinson et al., 1980) and there are reports that they can be isolated from various tissues derived from patients with multiple sclerosis (see below). Velogenic strains of NDV have also been studied in chickens as a model for paramyxovirus induced neurological disease (Stevens et al., 1976). In this paper some further aspects of the virology, serology and epidemiology of the paramyxovirus family are explored particularly in relation to possible persistence and their involvement in multiple sclerosis (MS). It should, however, be pointed out that this is not a comprehensive review of the literature on this subject and does not, of course, preclude the possibility that viruses other than those of the paramyxovirus family may play an important role in the etiology of MS or other neurological diseases.

EPIDEMIOLOGICAL STUDIES IMPLICATING VIRUSES IN NEUROLOGICAL DISEASE

A number of neurological syndromes have disease characteristics which could be consistent with a progressive virus infection. Thus, amyotrophic lateral sclerosis (ALS) is a major form of motor neuronal disease and is a progressive illness characterized by pyramidal tract and anterior horn destruction. However, standard virological investigations have failed to reveal any significant virus associations. Parallel epidemiological studies have, as yet, not revealed any geographic variation which cannot be explained by difference in diagnostic facilities (Kurtzke and Beebe, 1980); the disease, in general, affects older people (median age of onset of 66) with an annual incidence of about 2 per 100,000 (Juergens et al., 1980). The prevalence of ALS is of the order of 5 per 100,000, reflecting the rapid progress of the disease (average survival being 22 months after onset). It is interesting to compare ALS with multiple sclerosis (MS) where the incidence of the disease is only slightly greater, but because the median age of onset is very much younger (about 30) and the disease can follow a relapsing and remitting course, the prevalence rates are very much higher (30–50 per 100,000).

Multiple sclerosis is another neurological disease of unknown etiology where the treatment is inadequate and the prognosis is unpredictable, and in an effort to understand the natural history of the condition, many investigators have turned to epidemiology. Data on the distribution of the disease and on the risks of acquiring the disease on migration between high and low risk areas suggest that exposure to an environmental, possibly transmissible factor during late childhood or adolescence may be critical to the subsequent development of the disease in later life — possibly some 15 to 20 years later (for a review see Kurtzke, 1980). This in itself suggests that there may be a long incubation period, possibly involving persistent infection. If this is indeed the case, then a more direct link with an earlier critical episode could perhaps be established by retrospective analysis of the life styles and other characteristics of MS patients and their environments. Many such surveys have been carried out, possibly the most painstaking being those by Poskanzer and his colleagues who analyzed the MS population in the Orkney and Shetland Islands where some of the highest prevalence rates for the disease can be found. These investigators were not able to uncover any significant factors, either genetical, environmental or microbiological, to account for the presence of the disease in these islands (Poskanzer et al., 1980).

A much more contentious hypothesis has been put forward by Cook and his colleagues based on surveys of the contacts of MS patients with dogs in the 5–10 years previous to the onset of the disease. Cook and Dowling (1977) suggested that one of the factors in the initiation of the disease could be infection by canine distemper virus of individuals in close contact with a dog harbouring the virus. According to this hypothesis, other important factors governing the progress of the infection could be the immune status of the individual and possibly the characteristics of the infecting virus (e.g. virulence). Support for their hypothesis came particularly from investigations in the Faroe Islands — a group of islands in the North Sea very similar in many ways to the Orkneys and Shetlands. On these islands, however, MS has been virtually unknown from 1929 except for a period between 1945 and 1956 when an "epidemic" of about 24 cases were recorded and it was suggested (see Kurtzke, 1980), that the landing of British troops on the islands during the Second World War may have introduced some critical extraneous "agent" into the islands to account for the later appearance of the disease.

Cook et al. (1978) discovered that one of the consequences of the landing of the British troops was the introduction of guard dogs and the parallel acquisition of canine distemper disease by the dogs on the islands. Apparently before the landing of troops importation of dogs to the islands was prohibited and over the next few years a very large proportion of the island's dog population succumbed to the disease and particularly to the more virulent, neurologically associated form known as "hard pad". Thus there was at least a temporal association between the acquisition of the canine disease by the dog population and the appearance of MS in the human population. Parallel enquiries on the Orkneys and Shetlands revealed that canine distemper was rife on these islands. Similar associations were uncovered in Iceland (for review see Cook and Dowling, 1980) and on the island of Akiva off the coast of Alaska (personal communication). It is interesting in the light of this hypothesis to learn that the dog population on the Faroe Islands is still not vaccinated against CDV and a serological survey of the canine population has shown the complete absence of CDV neutralizing antibodies (unpublished data). Moreover, multiple sclerosis incidence on the Faroes is still very considerably less than on the nearby Orkney and Shetland Islands although there is considerable movement of the Faroese population to and from Denmark. The hypothesis has aroused considerable controversy, particularly since even the suggestion of an association with pets immediately provides ammunition for the "anti-dog" lobby and in turn provokes an impassioned backlash from the dog lovers. In the wake of this controversy a number of epidemiological studies have been carried out, seeking a significant dog relationship with individual MS patients, and with some exceptions these have not confirmed the original findings of Cook and Dowling in New Jersey (e.g. Hughes et al., 1980). The main difference appears to be that the very high dog contact in the control populations under study made it very difficult to achieve any significance in the corresponding associated MS populations. Attempts have also been made to relate MS incidence in a given area to the incidence of canine distemper encephalitis, but this has failed to show any relationship (Vandevelde and Meier, 1980).

These studies have therefore yielded very inconclusive results and at best can be only considered as indicative of the inadequacy of our understanding of persistent infections and the difficulties in retrospective surveys. The possible relationship of MS to infection via a canine vector is certainly not ruled out, but other avenues will need to be explored before a more definitive and convincing explanation can be established.

SEROLOGICAL POINTERS TO VIRUS INVOLVEMENT IN MS

Surveys of antibody titers to viruses in MS have been extensive and have certainly confirmed the original observations of Adams and Imagawa (1962) of elevated measles antibodies in MS patients. Raised antibody levels against other viruses have been found in MS patients, although far less consistently than against measles, and it is not clear whether the elevated antibody levels merely reflect a hyperactive immune system or are indicative of a specific immune reaction against a measles-related antigen (for a review see Cook and Dowling, 1980). Increased measles antibody levels, however, are not specific to MS patients since similar levels have been obtained in rheumatoid arthritis patients (Shivodaria et al., 1979). It is interesting that elevations of neutralizing antibodies against canine distemper virus have also been found in MS patients (Cook et al., 1979; Hughes et al., 1980; Madden et al., 1981; Appel et al., 1981); there has, however, been one report of no elevation (Krakowka and Koestner, 1978), but only 10 patients were studied in this case. Other methods of assessment of antibody titers using radioimmune assays, complement fixation and analysis of cell-mediated immunity have failed to show a specific association with CDV (Arnadottir, 1980).

These observations, in turn, raise the question of the significance of the levels of CDV neutralizing antibody levels found in human sera. In general, there is a correlation between the titres of CDV and MV in individual sera (cf. Cook et al., 1979; Madden et al., 1981) although there are very significant and consistent differences between the levels of these antibodies in some sera. Thus some human sera contain an apparently higher CDV neutralizing antibody titer than MV, in the absence of any apparent disease and with no apparent abnormal canine contacts, whereas others have very low CDV titres (Fig. 2). The possibility that CDV can

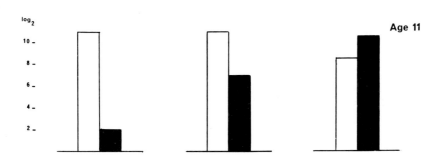

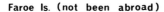

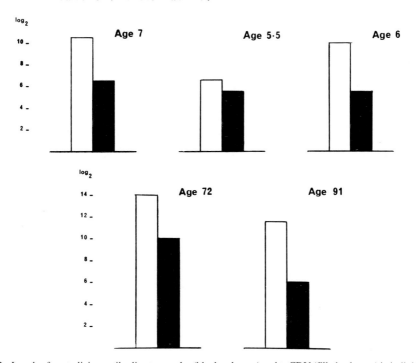

Fig. 2. Levels of neutralizing antibodies to measles (blank columns) and to CDV (filled columns) in individual human sera. The Faroese samples were obtained in 1979 (the last known case of canine distemper in dogs being diagnosed in 1955). Neutralizing antibodies were determined by a micromethod in microtiter plates (Cook et al., 1979).

118

infect humans has been considered on a number of occasions (Bryan, 1928; Adams, 1953), and although there is certainly no clinical evidence of infection, it cannot be ruled out that CDV could gain entry to some human tissues and institute a persistent infection. The available serological evidence, however, indicates that the CDV titers found in human sera are not necessarily related to contact with CDV-infected dogs. Thus analyses of the sera of individuals in the Faroe Islands who have never left the islands, and who have never been in contact with CDV-infected dogs, show that very similar levels of CDV neutralizing antibodies can be achieved in their sera to those who have had the opportunity of being in direct contact with CDV infected dogs (Fig. 2). This is in line with earlier evidence based on the analysis of less well-defined sera (Hopper, 1959) and it also seems that, at least in some cases, the CDV antibody can be adsorbed out by adsorption with measles-infected cells (Appel et al., 1981; Arnadottir, 1980). Nevertheless, it may be of some significance that the relative levels of antibodies against CDV and MV in human sera are in general never achieved in sera obtained from animals either immunized or infected with measles virus (Table I). It is also interesting that the antibody patterns against these two different viruses change significantly as a function of age. Thus, higher antibody levels tend to be found in the student age group and this group also has a much lower ratio of MV to CDV titers than the younger age group (Fig. 3). This suggests a broadening of response as a function of aging — whether this is related to measles vaccination, or to a maturation of the immune system, or perhaps reflects antigen persistence and modulation, cannot be distinguished.

TABLE I

NEUTRALIZATION BY ANIMAL ANTISERA

Neutralizations carried out as described by Cook et al., 1979

| Serum/Virus | CDV | Measles | | |
		Schw.	Edm.	Phil.
Horse anti-CDV	2048	8	64	32
Rabbit anti-measles (Phil)	8	96	1536	512
Rabbit anti-measles (Schw)	16	96	768	192
Rabbit anti-measles (Edm)	16	24	384	96
Bovine anti-PPR	96	8	128	48
Bovine anti-RP	64	16	512	256

The question of possible persistence of measles virus after primary infection has never been satisfactorily resolved, and it is certainly apparent that some individuals can have very high titers of antibody very many years after infection (cf. Fig. 2). The possibility of persistence has also been raised by the claims that thin sections of osteoclasts from bone biopsies of patients with Paget's disease contain 15 mm filaments which can be shown by immunofluorescent and peroxidase methods to be related to measles virus (Rebel et al., 1980) or to respiratory syncytial virus (Mills et al., 1981), this latter virus belonging to the pneumovirus genus of the paramyxoviridae. Since Paget's disease of bone normally presents itself in old age, this suggests a lifetime between initial infection and manifestation of disease. Moreover, a serological survey of measles neutralizing antibody levels has shown that significantly lower levels of antibody are apparent in Paget's disease patients, suggesting that some immunological factor may be associated with the disease onset (unpublished observations). There is also

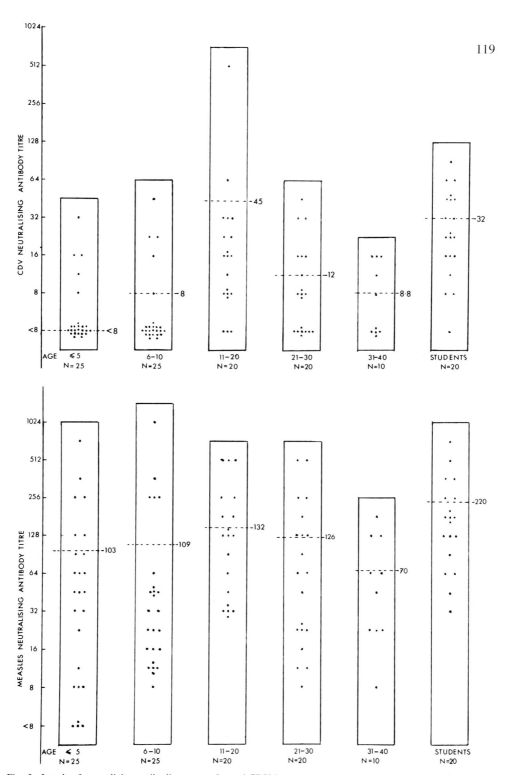

Fig. 3. Levels of neutralizing antibodies to measles and CDV in sera representative of the general population as a function of age. The sera were obtained in 1976 and 1977. The students sera were collected separately in 1976. The dotted lines denote the average titers of a given cohort.

evidence that CDV can persist in infected dogs producing later manifestations of the disease and it has been shown that some strains of CDV can initiate a persistent infection in dogs accompanied by demyelination (Appel and Gillespie, 1972). Where the levels of CDV antibody have been measured, much lower levels are obtained when persistence is the outcome of the infection (Krakowka et al., 1975). From these investigations it is evident that measurements of the levels of virus antibodies of themselves are not necessarily very useful in determining whether there is a persistent infection. In the case of SSPE where there is often quite extensive spread of the virus the immune response can be quite vigorous giving very high yields of measles antibody, but this may not be typical of other syndromes where the virus infection may be closely contained within a very specific location and with minimal expression, which nevertheless may be sufficient to impair normal function in that location.

MORBILLIVIRUS INTERRELATIONSHIPS

The indirect approaches of epidemiology and serology have therefore not been particularly successful in clarifying our understanding of possible persistent infection and its effect on the immune system, and it seems necessary to develop techniques which will detect specifically very small amounts of viral information and to relate this in some defined way to the characteristics of the immune response. The much more complex question of a relationship to disease processes such as demyelination may then be considered more rationally. A prerequisite even to these steps is to characterize in much more detail the antigenic and other relationships between the different viruses within genera. In this way, well-defined molecular probes which are specific to a given virus gene could be constructed and employed in appropriate in situ analyses.

The paramyxoviruses have been relatively poorly characterized, mainly because most of them grow poorly in tissue culture and there are major technical problems in handling viruses and obtaining samples free of contaminating cellular proteins. Most studies of this family have utilized Sendai and NDV and only recently have techniques allowed molecular studies on the more interesting morbillivirus genus.

Initially, attempts were made to analyze the antigenic relatedness between the different morbilliviruses by standard immunological methods. The earliest and most comprehensive was that of Orvell and Norrby (1974) who analyzed cross-reactions using haemagglutinin, haemolysis and neutralization techniques. These authors found that the nucleoprotein antigen of MV, CDV and RV could not be distinguished, and they also concluded that CDV and RV carry an antigen on their envelope which cross-reacts with the MV haemolysin, and that the cross-reaction with the haemagglutinin antigen was not so prominent. However, with the advent of techniques of radioactive labeling and immunoprecipitation, it is now possible to define with considerable clarity the various polypeptide species and to examine their antigenic interrelationships.

On labeling infected cells with [^{35}S]methionine and submitting them to sodium dodecyl sulphate (SDS) polyacrylamide gel electrophoresis (PAGE) followed by autoradiography, it is possible to obtain labeling patterns different to those of uninfected cells. Although in the case of morbillivirus infections there is no dramatic inhibition of background cellular polypeptide synthesis as occurs with other viruses, Fig. 3 shows that cells infected with the Schwartz and Philadelphia strain of measles virus both show differences from the uninfected cell pattern and moreover, differ from each other. The differences can be related to the synthesis of the major virus-specified polypeptides, viz. the G polypeptide (the major envelope glycoprotein), the N

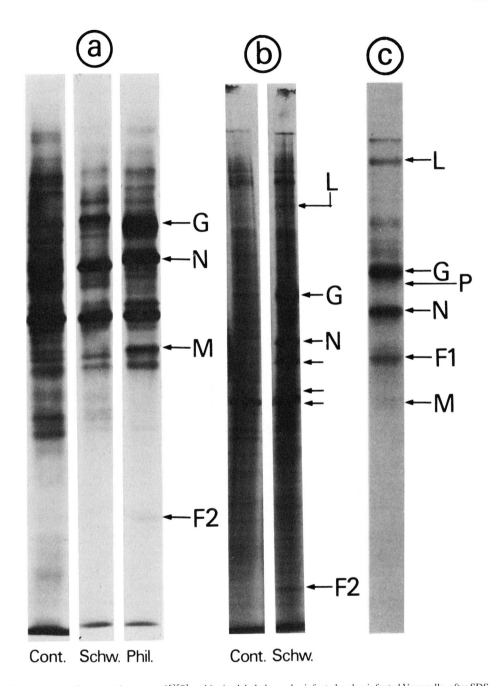

Fig. 4. Autoradiograms of extracts of [³⁵S]methionine labeled measles infected and uninfected Vero cells, after SDS PAGE analysis. Cells were infected or mock-infected (Cont.) with either the Schwartz (Schw.) or Philadelphia/26 (Phil.) strain of measles virus and were labeled for 3 h when the cells were showing initial signs of cytopathic effect. Labeled polypeptides characteristic of the major structural proteins are shown. Other labeled bands, (possibly breakdown products) not seen in control cells are denoted by arrows. Slot C is an autoradiogram of partially purified [³⁵S]methionine labeled measles virus. Cells were extracted and analyzed as described by Russell et al. (1981).

122

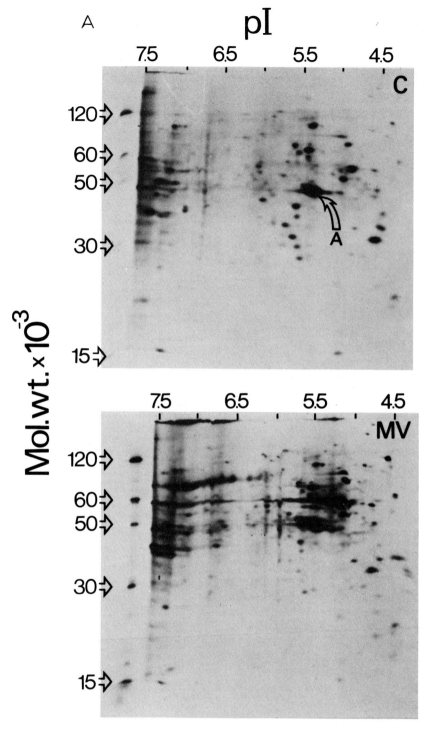

Fig. 5. A: autoradiograms of two-dimensional gels of extracts of [35S]methionine labeled cells infected with the Edmonston strain of measles virus (MV) or mock-infected (C) as described in legend to Fig. 4. Extracts were separated by isoelectric focusing in the first dimension to give a pH gradient as shown. The second dimension was carried out in SDS PAGE along with iodinated adenovirus as a marker giving molecular weight standards as indicated. Methods of 2D gel analysis have been described previously (Boulanger et al., 1979).

polypeptide (nucleocapsid closely associated with the virion RNA), and M the matrix poly-peptide (associated with the virus envelope). It is interesting that these differences in mobilities of the two virus strains are apparent in all 3 of these polypeptides. A more detailed analysis of the differences between the labeling patterns can be obtained by using two-dimensional gel electrophoresis as shown in Fig. 5A.

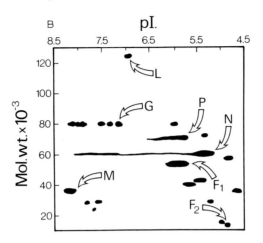

Fig. 5. B: schematic diagram indicating major differences between two-dimensional gels of ^{35}S-labeled measles infected and uninfected cell extracts. The results are based on a series of gels utilizing both 'equilibrium' and 'non-equilibrium' gel systems (O'Farrell et al., 1977). The positions of the virus structural proteins are indicated.

By examination of a number of these patterns, using different conditions, one can construct a two-dimensional differential pattern of the viral-induced polypeptides, and this is shown schematically in Fig. 5B. It will be seen that the labeled polypeptides noted in the one-dimensional gels can be recognized in the two-dimensional gel. However in the case of the G polypeptide, at least 6 different species can be resolved — presumably reflecting differing degrees of glycosylation or other modifications. This is particularly interesting since this surface polypeptide, by analogy with other enveloped viruses, is one which will play a key role in interacting with other biological systems, e.g. in the induction of neutralizing antibodies. The nucleoprotein N (and to a lesser extent the P polypeptide) similarly appear to be indicative of a polypeptide of variable charge, suggesting a multistep modification. At the mobilities corresponding to the M polypeptide there appear to be two species of polypeptides of greatly differing charge, one at a pH of approximately 4.5 and the other about 8.5 or greater. Whether these species represent the same unmodified and modified polypeptide cannot be determined from this pattern. A number of other polypeptides were consistently seen, but it is not clear whether all or only some of them are derived from proteolysis of some larger polypeptide, since this can occur in these labeled extracts.

From these studies, nevertheless, it is apparent that there is considerable scope for antigenic variation within the measles virus structure. Thus there are clear differences in polypeptide mobilities between strains, and the glycoprotein G shows at least 6 different species, possibly indicative of varying conformations and hence of antigenicities. However, it should be noted that the present standard techniques for diagnosing measles virus infection (by HI, CF and neutralization tests) are not capable of detecting these differences and it has always therefore been accepted that measles virus is antigenically stable.

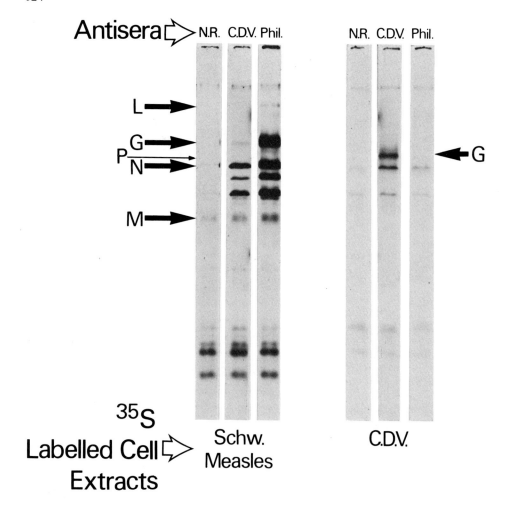

Fig. 6. Autoradiograms of immunoprecipitates derived from interaction of extracts of ^{35}S-labeled Vero cells infected with measles (Schwartz) or with CDV with antisera against C.D.V. and measles (Philadelphia) virus (Phil.) and with normal rabbit serum (N.R.). The immunoprecipitation was facilitated by the addition of staphylococcus protein A as described in Russell et al. (1981).

To determine the antigenic relationships between the various measles strains and canine distemper virus, labeled uninfected and infected cell extracts were incubated with antisera against the different viruses and the washed immune precipitates obtained after addition of staphylococcus protein A were analyzed by SDS PAGE followed by autoradiography. Fig. 6 shows the pattern of polypeptides obtained after incubation of Schwartz measles-infected cell extracts with a rabbit antiserum against the Philadelphia strain and a dog antiserum against canine distemper virus, along with the appropriate controls. Results show that at least 5 polypeptides are specifically precipitated by measles antibody with the measles-infected cells, and that 4 of these are also precipitated with the CDV antiserum, i.e. there is a very close antigenic relationship between measles and CDV, the major difference being in the glyco-protein. Indeed, in some experiments there is some precipitation of the glycoprotein of measles

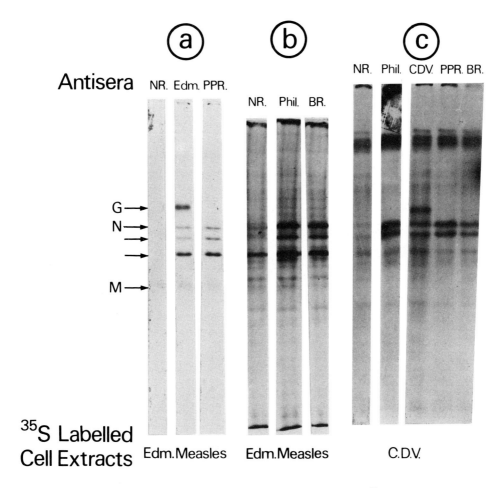

Fig. 7. Autoradiograms of immunoprecipitates derived from interaction of extracts of ^{35}S-labeled cells infected with measles or with CDV with antisera against measles (Edm., Phil.), against CDV, against bovine rinderpest (BR) and peste de petits ruminants (PPR) and normal rabbit serum (NR). Techniques as described in legend to Fig. 6.

by CDV antiserum. Similar results have been obtained by Orvell and Norrby (1980) Hall et al. (1980), Campbell et al. (1980) and Stephenson and ter Meulen (1979).

In CDV-infected cells there is precipitation of the G polypeptide by the CDV antiserum, and in this experiment it has a distinctly faster electrophoretic mobility than the G polypeptide of measles. On carrying out similar cross-reactions with measles and CDV-infected labeled cells and antiserum against measles, CDV, BR and PPR, there was further evidence of very close antigenic relationships, the major difference being once again in the G polypeptide. It is interesting that there is the same kind of relationship observed between different strains of influenza A viruses, i.e. the H2 containing virus only precipitates the haemagglutinin of the homologous virus and not the HI-labeled virus haemagglutinin (see Fig. 8).

The antigenic relationships between all these viruses was also examined by carrying out neutralization with the sera used in the immunoprecipitation tests. The results shown in Table I indicate that the neutralization test appeared to be specific for the homologous virus and the 3

126

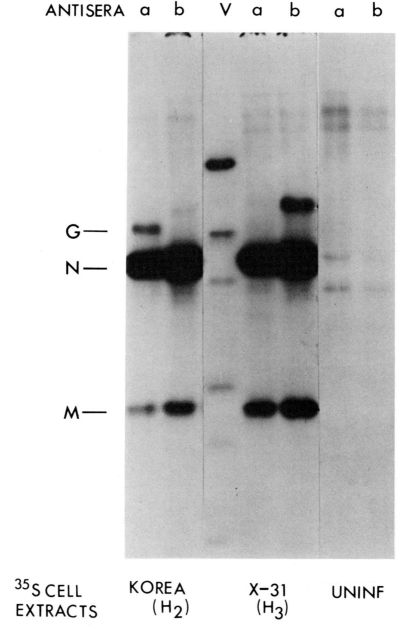

ANTISERA a b V a b a b

G—
N—

M—

^{35}S CELL EXTRACTS KOREA (H$_2$) X-31 (H$_3$) UNINF

Fig. 8. Autoradiogram of immunoprecipitates derived from interaction of extracts of ^{35}S-labeled extracts of chick cells infected by an H2 strain of influenza A (Korea/69) by an H3 strain (×31) and uninfected cell extract with antisera directed against the H2 (Korea) virus (a) and the H3 virus (×31) (b). The haemagglutinin, nucleoprotein and matrix polypeptides are designated by G, N and M respectively. Iodinated adenovirus (Rekosh et al., 1977) is used as a molecular weight marker. Techniques as described in legend to Fig. 6.

rabbit antisera against the different measles virus strains showed a fairly similar pattern of neutralization, although the homologous strain was neutralized relatively more efficiently. It was also notable that the bovine anti-PPR antiserum neutralized CDV significantly better than any of the measles or rinderpest sera which suggested that this virus might be closer to CDV than measles. On the basis of a series of neutralization tests, an indication of the degree of interactions between the 4 members of the morbillivirus genus was obtained and this is shown schematically in Fig. 9.

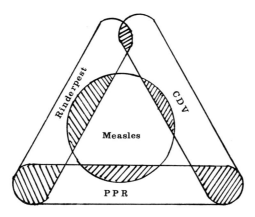

Fig. 9. Schematic diagram illustrating the relative antigenic relationships between the different members of the morbillivirus genus as derived by a series of neutralization tests.

APPLICATION OF IMMUNOPRECIPITATION TECHNIQUES TO PROBLEMS OF NEUROLOGICAL DISEASE

The above results therefore give some indication of the close antigenic relationships between the various members of the morbillivirus genus and offer one other means of analyzing human sera and CSF for the presence of precipitating antibodies to morbillivirus polypeptides. Immunoprecipitation of labeled MV and CDV polypeptides by sera and CSF from MS patients followed by analysis by SDS PAGE has been carried out by a number of investigators to ascertain if there is any specificity in the antigenic response of MS patients (Hayes et al., 1980); (Stephenson et al., 1980). Antibodies against all the measles virus polypeptides (except M) were demonstrated in both the patient and control samples. In the case of CDV polypeptides only the N and F polypeptides appeared to be precipitated by the human sera and CSF, and on the basis of these results it was concluded (Stephenson et al., 1980) that MS could develop without a previous CDV infection. The assumptions behind this conclusion were that the cross-reacting F glycoprotein was the component responsible for cross-neutralization, and that MS patients' sera would be capable of precipitating the more type-specific CDV G polypeptide if they had been infected by that virus. In turn, this presupposed that the techniques would be sensitive enough to detect the antibodies, but more importantly, that the antibody response to a persistent infection would necessarily be mounted against the G polypeptide.

It is relevant to point out that there is now good evidence that antibodies against the measles matrix polypeptide present in convalescent sera, rapidly diminish, are not detected in most adult human sera and are not evident in SSPE sera and CSF in spite of the presence of high

128

levels of antibody against the other measles proteins (Machamer et al., 1980; Hall et al., 1979b). Indeed, a recent study has shown that measles virus proteins, but not the matrix polypeptide, can be detected directly in brain tissue of SSPE patients by protein blotting methods (Hall and Choppin, 1981). These results then, suggest that some of the virological features of SSPE can be explained by the inability of the infected brain cells to synthesize the matrix polypeptide which plays a major role in the assembly of the virus particle at the cell plasma membrane. It has been postulated (Choppin et al., 1981) on this supposition that SSPE can arise as a result of the degree and extent of the original measles infection, and that the virus can infect a specific subset of brain cells which then restrict the replication of virus to intracellular events not susceptible to normal immunological surveillance. An experimental hamster model of SSPE does indeed show a selective disappearance of the measles virus matrix protein from the central nervous system consistent with the above hypothesis (Johnson et al., 1981), although in the case of old dog encephalitis all the CDV polypeptides are precipitated by sera from encephalitic dogs (Hall et al., 1979a). A related hypothesis (Fujinami and Oldstone, 1980) suggests that antibody can modulate the expression of measles virus polypeptides in the infected cell such that synthesis of a specific set of polypeptides (F1, P and M) is decreased, and that this can lead to a persistent and aberrant infection. A corollary to these speculations is that the relatively poor antibody responses to matrix antigen seen in normal individuals may also be the result of a similar persistent and aberrant infection, but without any demonstrable clinical sequelae.

CURRENT DEVELOPMENTS

Standard virological techniques for isolating viruses, either directly or by co-cultivation from diseased tissues, have been utilized by many investigators, particularly in cases of MS, ALS, SSPE, PML (progressive multifocal leucoencephalopathy) and schizophrenia. However, reproducible isolations have only been obtained from SSPE and PML. It is, nevertheless, interesting that members of the paramyxovirus family have been isolated on a number of occasions from MS associated tissues (for a review see Cook and Dowling, 1980; cf. Goswami and Russell, 1981), and it may be that these isolations reflect the ubiquity of the viruses in tissues and in tissue cultures, rather than any direct involvement in the etiology of the disease itself. Furthermore, if one assumes that any of the diseases such as MS are related to a persistent virus infection, as suggested above for SSPE, but limited to a specific loci and expressed only to a limited extent, then the chances of detecting the virus information by these procedures are very slim indeed. Fortunately, recent developments in techniques, particularly in terms of highly specific and sensitive radiolabeled probes and in the use of monoclonal antibodies, offer further, possibly more fruitful, routes to examine these conjectures.

In situ hybridization with labeled nucleic acid probes has been used extensively, particularly to explore the possibility of herpesvirus involvement in cervical carcinoma (e.g. Jones et al., 1978). Similar techniques are now being applied to neurological tissue using cDNA probes from reverse transcripts of measles virion RNA (Haase et al., 1981a, b), and these authors have claimed specific hybridization of measles probe to brain tissue for one out of four MS autopsies and for all SSPE cases examined. The reliability of these results will be greatly improved when better characterized DNA copies of the measles genome become available in the near future. Genetic cloning techniques obviously provide the best means of tackling these problems and several laboratories (e.g. Gorecki and Rosenblatt, 1980) are vigorously pursuing this course.

Monoclonal antibodies against measles virus components have been obtained in a number of laboratories (Birrer et al., 1981a; Togashi et al., 1981; Girauden and Wild, 1981), and it is clear that the supposition that measles virus is antigenically stable is no longer tenable (Birrer et al., 1981b) since neutralizing antibodies against specific epitopes of the G polypeptide of one strain can be obtained which will not neutralize other strains. Whether mutation of the measles virus genome and concomitant antigenic variation can be related to persistent infection and to neurological disease has still to be tested, but the appropriate tools now seem to be available.

It is pertinent at this point to consider the current situation with respect to variation in the influenza viruses. Fine structure analysis (Wiley et al., 1981) has shown that the influenza haemagglutinin has an essentially stable structure consisting of two distinct regions, a peripheral globular region containing the receptor binding site, and antigenic determinants positioned on top of a fibrous stem extending from the membrane. Available data have shown that there are 4 antigenic sites on the globular region, and that at least one amino acid substitution in each of the 4 sites seems to be necessary for the production of new epidemic strains. Thus single site mutations at a few critical sites can influence the biological properties of the haemagglutinin, and it seems not unlikely that a similar situation can exist with measles virus glycoproteins.

The availability of hybridomas should also allow a more discriminating analysis of the other virus polypeptides which show various degrees of antigenic relationships within the morbillivirus genus. Thus, although the nucleoprotein appears to cross-react between CDV and MV, of the hybridomas against the measles nucleoprotein isolated and characterized so far, two only react with measles and not with CDV (Birrer et al., 1981a), and one with both (Russell and Patel, unpublished observations). Similar results can be anticipated with other antigens and it should be possible to build up a series of very specific reagents which can detect either epitopes which are shared between members of the morbilliviruses, or those which are highly specific to a given virus strain. Using these probes it should be possible to analyze in a more meaningful fashion the role of persistent infection and its possible relationship to neurological disease.

CONCLUSIONS

It has been well established that morbilliviruses can initiate persistent infections in tissue culture and that persistence in vivo plays a key role in diseases such as SSPE and the later manifestations of canine distemper. There is, moreover, some suggestion that measles virus persistence under surveillance of the immune system may be operating in the normal healthy individual. While there are interesting pointers to possible involvement of morbilliviruses based on epidemiological and serological studies, much further work will be required to substantiate any of the hypotheses which have been advanced. The new techniques of gene cloning and in situ hybridization, together with the development of appropriate hybridomas, offer potentially interesting novel molecular approaches to this problem of the role of persistent paramyxovirus infection in disease.

ACKNOWLEDGEMENTS

I am indebted to Hilary Bulman, Gunvanti Patel and Marion Hall-Smith for expert technical asistance. I am also grateful to a number of colleagues who supplied sera, viz. Dr. Joan Edwards of the Virus Reference Laboratory, Colindale who made available student sera and

130

the sera of the age cohorts derived originally from the Cross-Infection Laboratories for antistreptolysin titration; Dr. J. Röin and Mr. J. Olsen from Torshaven, Faroe Islands who supplied human and dog sera respectively; Dr. Hamish Inglis, City Hospital, Edinburgh who supplied sera from cases of atypical measles; Dr. B. Underwood, of the Animal Virus Research Institute who supplied bovine sera against rinderpest and peste de petits ruminants viruses; and to Dr. Stuart Cook, Newark, NJ., U.S.A., who supplied information prior to publication.

REFERENCES

Adams, J.M. (1953) Comparative study of canine distemper and a respiratory disease of man. *Pediatrics*, 11 : 15–27.

Adams, J.M., Brown, W.J., Snow, H.D., Lincoln, S.D., Sears, A.W. Jr., Bonefus, M., Holliday, T.A., Cremer, N.E. and Lennette, E.H. (1975) Old dog encephalitis and demyelinating diseases in man. *Vet. Path.*, 12 : 220–226.

Adams, J.M. and Imagawa, D.T. (1962) Measles antibodies in multiple sclerosis. *Proc. Soc. exp. Biol. (N.Y.)*, 3 : 562–566.

Agnarsdottir, G. (1977) In A.P. Waterson (Ed.), *Recent Advances in Clinical Virology*, Churchill Livingstone, London, pp. 21–49.

Appel, M.J.G. and Gillespie, J.H. (1972) Canine Distemper Virus. In *Virology Monographs, Vol. 11*, Springer, New York, pp. 1–96.

Appel, M.J., Glickman, C.T., Raine, C.S. and Tourtellotte, W.W. (1981) Canine viruses and multiple sclerosis. *Neurology*, 31 : 944–949.

Arnadottir, T. (1980) Measles and canine distemper virus. Antibodies in patients with multiple sclerosis determined by radioimmune assay. *Acta neurol. scand.*, 62 : 81–89.

Birrer, M.J., Bloom, B.R. and Udem, S. (1981a) Characterisation of measles polypeptides by monoclonal antibodies. *Virology*, 108 : 381.

Birrer, M.J. Udem, S., Nathanson, S. and Bloom, B.R. (1981b) Antigenic variants of measles virus. *Nature (Lond.)*, 293 : 67–69.

Boulanger, P., Lemay, P., Blair, E.G. and Russell, W.C. (1979) Characterisation of adenovirus protein IX. *J. gen. Virol.*, 44 : 783–800.

Bryan, A.H. (1928) Is canine distemper a danger to children? *Vet. Med.*, 23 : 496–497.

Campbell, J., Cosby, S.L., Scott, B.K., Rima, B.K., Mortin, S.J. and Appel, M. (1980) A comparison of measles and canine distemper virus polypeptides. *J. gen. Virol.*, 48 : 149–159.

Choppin, P.W., Richardson, C.D., Merz, D.C., Hall, W.W. and Scheid, A. (1981) The functions and inhibition of the membrane glycoproteins of paramyxoviruses and myxoviruses and the role of the measles virus M protein in subacute sclerosing paraencephalitis. *J. infect. Dis.*, 143 : 352–363.

Cook, S.D. and Dowling, P.C. (1977) A possible association between house pets and multiple sclerosis. *Lancet*, 1 : 980–982.

Cook, S.D., Dowling, P.C. and Russell, W.C. (1978) Multiple sclerosis and canine distemper. *Lancet*, 1 : 605–606.

Cook, S.D., Dowling, P.C. and Russell, W.C. (1979) Neutralising antibodies to canine distemper and measles virus in multiple sclerosis. *J. Neurol. Sci.*, 41 : 61–70.

Cook, S.D. and Dowling, P.C. (1980) Multiple sclerosis and viruses: an overview. *Neurology*, 30 : 80-91.

Fujinami, R.S. and Oldstone, M.B.A. (1980) Alterations in expression of measles virus polypeptides by antibody: molecular events in antibody-induced antigenic modulation. *J. Immunol.*, 125 : 78–85.

Giraudon, P. and Wild, T.F. (1981) Monoclonal antibodies against measles virus. *J. gen. Virol.*, 54 : 325–332.

Gorecki, M. and Rosenblatt, S. (1980) Cloning of DNA complementary to the measles virus in RNA encoding nucleocapsid protein. *Proc. nat. Acad. Sci. U.S.A.*, 77 : 3686–3890.

Goswami, K.K. and Russell, W.C. (1981) A comparison of paramyxoviruses by immunoprecipitation. J. gen. Virol., 60 : 177–183.

Gross, P.Q., Green, R.H. and McCrea-Curnin, M.G. (1973) Persistent infection with parainfluenza type 3 virus in man. *Amer. Rev. respirat. Dis.*, 108 : 894–898.

Haase, A.T., Ventura, P., Gibbs, C.J. Jr. and Tourtellotte, W.W. (1981a) Measles virus nucleotide sequences: detection by hybridisation in situ. *Science*, 212 : 672–675.

Haase, A.T., Swoveland, P., Stowring, L., Ventura, P., Johnson, K.P., Norrby, E. and Gibbs, C.J., Jr. (1981b) Measles virus genome in infections of the central nervous system. *J. infect. Dis.*, 144 : 154–160.

Hall, W.W., Imagawa, D.T. and Choppin, P.W. (1979a) Immunological evidence for the synthesis of all canine distemper virus polypeptides in chronic neurological diseases in dogs. Chronic distemper and old dog encephalitis differ from SSPE in man. *Virology*, 98 : 283–287.

Hall, W.W., Lamb, R.A. and Choppin, P.W. (1979b) Measles and subacute sclerosing panencephalitis virus proteins: lack of antibodies to the M protein in patients with subacute sclerosing panencephalitis. *Proc. nat. Acad. Sci. U.S.A.*, 76: 2047–2051.

Hall, W.W., Lamb, R.A. and Choppin, P.W. (1980) The polypeptides of canine distemper virus: synthesis in infected cells and relatedness to the polypeptides of other morbilliviruses. *Virology*, 100: 433–449.

Hall, W.W. and Choppin, P.W. (1981) Measles virus proteins in the brain tissue of patients with SSPE – absence of the matrix protein. *New Engl. J. Med.*, 304: 1152–1154.

Hayes, E.C., Gollobin, S.D., Machamer, C.E., Westfall, L.K. and Sweerink, H.J. (1980) Measles-specific antibodies in sera and cerebrospinal fluids of patients with multiple sclerosis. *Infect. Immun.*, 27: 1033–1037.

Hopper, P.K. (1959) Investigations on neutralising antibody to canine distemper virus in human serum from different countries. *Acta Paediat.*, 48: 43–49.

Hughes, R.C., Russell, W.C., Froude, J.R.L. and Jarrett, R.J. (1980) Pet ownership, distemper antibodies and multiple sclerosis. *J. Neurol. Sci.*, 47: 429–432.

Johnson, K.P., Norrby, E., Swoveland, P. and Carrigan, D.R. (1981) Experimental SSPE: selective disappearance of the measles virus matrix protein from the CNS. *J. Infect. Dis.*, 144: 161–165.

Jones, K.W., Fenoglio, C.M., Shevchuck-Chaban, M., Maitland, N.J. and McDougall, J.K. (1978) Detection of herpes virus-2 mRNA in human cervical biopsies by in situ cytological hybridisation. In G. de The, M.A. Epstein and H. Zur Hausen (Eds.), *Oncogenesis and Herpes Viruses*, Vol. 3, part 2, International Agency for Research on Cancer, Lyon, pp. 917–925.

Juergens, S.M., Kurland, L.T., Okazaki, H. and Mulder, D.W. (1980) ALS in Rochester, Minnesota 1925–1977. *Neurology*, 30: 463–470.

Kingsbury, D.W., Bratt, M.A., Choppin, P.W., Hanson, R.P., Hosaka, Y., ter Meulen, V., Norrby, E., Plowright, W., Rott, R. and Wunner, W.H. (1978) Paramyxoviridae. *Intervirology*, 10: 137–152.

Krakowka, S., Olsen, R., Confer, A., Koestner, A. and McCullough, B. (1975) Serologic response to canine distemper viral antigens in gnotobiotic dogs infected with canine distemper virus. *J. infect. Dis.*, 132: 384–392.

Krakowka, S. and Koestner, A. (1978) Canine distemper virus and multiple sclerosis. *Lancet*, 1: 1127–1128.

Kurtzke, J.F. (1980) Epidemiologic contributions to multiple sclerosis. An overview, *Neurology*, 30: 61–79.

Kurtzke, J.F. and Beebe, G.W. (1980) Epidemiology of amyotrophic lateral sclerosis. I. A case-control comparison based on ALS deaths. *Neurology*, 30: 453–462.

Machamer, C.E., Hayes, E.C., Gollobin, S.D., Westfall, L.K. and Zweerink, H.J. (1980) Antibodies against the measles matrix polypeptide after clinical infection and vaccination. *Infect. Immun.*, 27: 817–825.

Madden, D.L., Wallen, W.C., Hauff, S.A., Shekarcki, I.C., Reinikki, P.O., Castellano, G.A. and Sever, J.L. (1981) Measles and canine distemper antibody. Presence in sera from parents with multiple sclerosis and matched control subjects. *Arch. Neurol.*, 38: 13–15.

McCullough, B., Krakowka, S. and Koestner, A. (1974) Experimental canine distemper virus induced demyelination. *Lab. Invest.*, 31: 216–222.

Mills, B.G., Singer, F.R., Weiner, L.P. and Holst, P.A. (1981) Immunohistological demonstration of respiratory syncytial virus antigens in Paget's disease of bone. *Proc. nat. Acad. Sci. U.S.A.*, 78: 1209–1213.

O'Farrell, P.Z., Goodman, H.M. and O'Farrell, P.H. (1977) High resolution two dimensional electrophoresis of basic as well as acidic proteins. *Cell*, 12: 1133–1142.

Orvell, C. and Norrby, E. (1974) Further studies on the immunologic relationships among measles, distemper and rinderpest viruses. *J. Immunol.*, 113: 1850–1858.

Orvell, G. and Norrby, E. (1980) Immunological relationships between homologous structural polypeptides of measles and canine distemper virus. *J. gen. Virol.*, 50: 231–245.

Parkinson, A.J., Muchmore, H.G., McConnell, T.A., Scott, L.V. and Miles, J.A.R. (1980) Serologic evidence for parainfluenza virus infection during isolation at South Pole Station, Antartica. *Amer. J. Epidem.*, 112: 334–340.

Poskanzer, D.C., Prenney, L.B. Sheridan, J.L. and Kondy, J.Y. (1980) Multiple sclerosis in the Orkney and Shetland Islands. I. Epidemiology, clinical factors and methodology. *J. Epid. Comm. Health.*, 34: 229–239.

Rebel, A., Basle, M., Pouplard, A., Kouyoumajian, S., Filmon, R. and Lepatezaur, A. (1980) Viral antigens in osteoclasts from Paget's disease of bone. *Lancet*, 2: 344–346.

Rekosh, D.M.K., Russell, W.C., Bellett, A.J.D. and Robinson, A.J. (1977) Identification of a protein linked to the ends of adenovirus DNA. *Cell*, 11: 283–295.

Risk, W.C. and Haddad, F.S. (1979) The variable natural history of subacute sclerosing panencephalitis. *Arch. Neurol.*, 36: 610–614.

Russell, W.C., Patel, G., Precious, B., Sharp, I. and Gardner, P.S. (1981) Monoclonal antibodies against adenovirus type 5: preparation and preliminary characterisation. *J. gen. Virol.*, 56: 393–408.

Shivodaria, P.V., Fraser, K.B., Armstrong, M. and Roberts, S.D. (1979) Measles virus-specific antibodies and immunoglobulin M antiglobulin in sera from multiple sclerosis and rheumatoid arthritis patients. *Infect. Immun.*, 25: 408–416.

Stephenson, J.R. and ter Meulen, V. (1979) Antigenic relationships between measles and canine distemper viruses: comparison of immune response in animals and humans to individual virus-specific polypeptides. *Proc. nat. Acad. Sci. U.S.A.*, 76: 6601–6605.

Stephenson, J.R., ter Meulen, V. and Kiessling, W. (1980) Search for canine distemper virus antibodies on multiple sclerosis. *Lancet*, ii: 772–775.

Stevens, J.G., Nakamura, R.M., Cook, M.L. and Wilczynski, S.P. (1976) Newcastle disease as a model for paramyxovirus-induced neurological syndromes: pathogenesis of the respiratory disease and preliminary characterisation of the ensuing encephalitis. *Infect. Immun.*, 13: 590–599.

Ter Meulen, V., Hall, W.W. and Kreth, H.W. (1978) Persistent viruses. In J.G. Stevens, G.J. Todaro and C.F. Fox (Eds.), Academic Press, New York, pp. 615–634.

Togashi, T., Orvell, C., Vantdal, F. and Norrby, E. (1981) Production of antibodies against measles virus by use of the mouse hybridoma technique. *Arch. Virol.*, 67: 149–157.

Vandervelde, M. and Meier, C. (1980) Multiple sclerosis and canine distemper encephalitis. *J. Neurol. Sci.*, 47: 255–260.

Wiley, D.C., Wilson, I.A. and Skehel, J.J. (1981) Structural identification of the antibody binding sites of the Hong Kong influenza haemagglutinin and their involvement in antigenic variation. *Nature (Lond.)*, 289: 373–377.

Immunology of Nervous System Infections, Progress in Brain Research, Vol. 59, edited by P.O. Behan, V. ter Meulen and F. Clifford Rose

Immune Response in the CSF in Viral Infections

HARTMUT SIEMES and MARTIN SIEGERT

Westfälische Landeskinderklinik-Universitätsklinik, Alexandrinenstr. 5, 4630 Bochum, and Kinderklinik der Freien Universität, Berlin (F.R.G.)

INTRODUCTION

The local humoral immune response in inflammatory diseases of the central nervous system (CNS) is reflected by an increase in gamma-globulin in the cerebrospinal fluid (CSF) and, more significantly, by the occurrence of oligoclonal gamma-banding. In the detection of local immunoglobulin synthesis, the possibility of changes in the serum gamma-globulin and increased permeability of the blood–CSF barrier to proteins has to be taken into consideration. The purpose of the present study was to evaluate the gamma-globulin reaction in various acute, prolonged, and chronic CNS-infections of viral or presumed viral origin. In addition, the degree of the concomitant blood–CSF barrier disturbance has been determined.

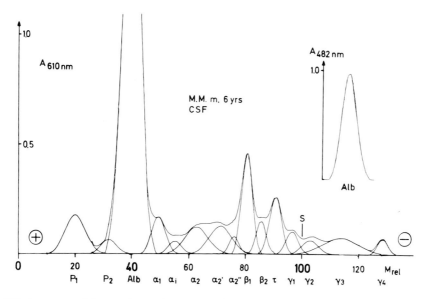

Fig. 1. CSF-phoretrogram (photometric scanning curve and the computer-generated contributing protein fractions) in a 6-year-old boy without CNS disease. A, absorption, scanning of albumin (Alb) at 482 nm, of prealbumins (P1, P2) and globulins at 610 nm; M rel, relative electrophoretic mobility; reference points: Alb (40) and application slot S (100)

134

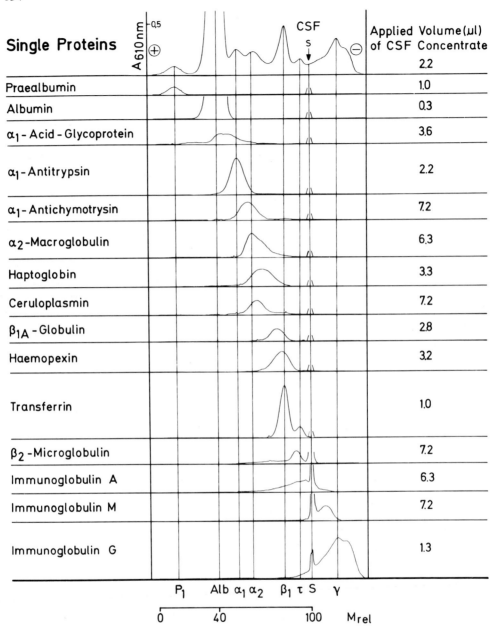

Fig. 2. Identification of the main single plasma proteins of the CSF-phoretrogram by means of immunofixation following electrophoresis. The electrophoretic fractions are designated according to Fig. 1. Immunoglobulin A is located anodically, immunoglobulin M cathodically close to the application slot, gamma 3 is built up by immunoglobulin G, and gamma 4 represents a microglobulin and should not erroneously considered a monoclonal IgG band.

MATERIALS AND METHODS

CSF-proteins were analyzed by quantitative electrophoresis in agarose gel (Siegert and Siemes, 1977). CSF was concentrated by ultrafiltration in collodion tubes and then applied to agarose for electrophoresis followed by fixation and staining. After photometric scanning the phoretograms were evaluated by means of an analogue computer (Du Pont Curve resolver 310) (see Fig. 1). Gaussian curves were adjusted to the single protein fractions. The relative concentration of each fraction was calculated by referring the integral value of its Gaussian to the sum of all Gaussians. The largest gamma-fraction (γ_3) represents immunoglobulin G as demonstrated by the technique of immunofixation electrophoresis (Cawley et al., 1976) (see Fig. 2).

CSF-electrophoresis has been performed in a total of 321 children between 3 months and 15 years of age, of whom 134 served as normal controls. These children had been evaluated for fever, and lumbar puncture was performed to exclude meningitis.

RESULTS

By stereotyped changes of the CSF-protein spectrum, two pathologic reactions can be defined: the pattern of local immune response, and the pattern of blood–CSF barrier disturbance (Fig. 3). The local immune response leads to increase of gamma$_3$-globulin and/or synthesis of oligoclonal gamma-fractions. The elevation of gamma$_3$, including all oligoclonal fractions, has been scored according to Table I.

TABLE I

REPRESENTATION OF ABNORMAL GAMMAGLOBULIN INCREASE (γ_3-FRACTION)

All oligoclonal fractions are included in γ_3; $\underline{X}$, mean; S.D., standard deviation of the mean.

Normal range increase	Points
$\underline{X} + 2$ S.D.	0
2 S.D.–3 S.D.	1
3 S.D.–4 S.D.	2
4 S.D.–5 S.D.	3
and so on	

In the case of a lesion of the CNS barriers, plasma proteins leak into the CSF. Albumin increases, prealbumin (P$_1$), β_1-, τ- and γ_4-globulin decline. For a quantitative estimate of the degree of blood–CSF barrier disturbance the changes of these 5 protein fractions have been scored (see Table II). For evaluation of the blood–CSF barrier disturbance a disproportionate elevation of gamma$_3$-globulin has been corrected. In those patients in whom gamma$_3$, or gamma$_3$ plus the sum of all oligoclonal fractions exceeded the gamma$_3$-values $\underline{X} + 3$ S.D. (mean + 3 S.D.) of the corresponding control group, we reduced their gamma-values to $\underline{X} + 3$ S.D. of the control group; the remaining fractions increased accordingly.

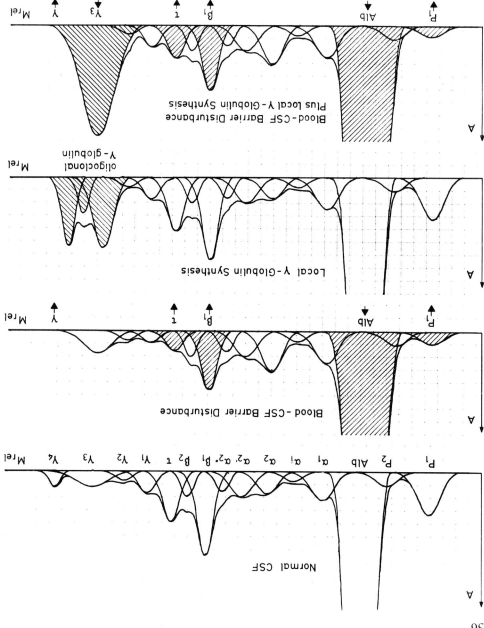

Fig. 3. Illustration of blood–CSF barrier disturbance and local immunoglobulin G production in the CSF. For explanation of the symbols see Fig. 1.; increase or decrease from normal range of relative concentration is indicated by ↑ or ↓.

TABLE II

REPRESENTATION OF THE DEGREE OF BLOOD–CSF BARRIER DISTURBANCE BY CHANGES IN CSF–PROTEIN PATTERN

Maximum possible sum of points: 19. $\bar{X}$, mean, S.D., standard deviation of the mean.

Protein fractions (%)	Normal range	Points						
		1	2	3	4	5	6	7
Prealbumin	$\bar{X} - 2$ S.D.	2–3 S.D.	3–4 S.D.	4–5 S.D.	5–6 S.D.			
Albumin	$\bar{X} + 2$ S.D.	2–3 S.D.	3–4 S.D.	4–5 S.D.	5–6 S.D.			
β_1-globulin	$\bar{X} - 2$ S.D.	2–3 S.D.	3–4 S.D.	4–5 S.D.	5–6 S.D.			
τ-globulin	$\bar{X} - 2$ S.D.	2–3 S.D.	3–4 S.D.	4–5 S.D.		6–7 S.D.	7–8 S.D.	
γ_4-globulin	$\bar{X} - 2$ S.D.	2–3 S.D.	3–4 S.D.	4–5 S.D.				8–9 S.D.

Apart from local production in the CNS, elevation of gamma-globulin may be caused by a lesion of the CNS barrier, resulting in leakage of protein; however, to our present knowledge only one point on our gamma-globulin scale can be reached by maximal increase of barrier permeability.

Age-dependency of normal reference values has been taken into consideration (Siemes et al., 1975). All data have been computed and analyzed by means of the SPSS program.

Aseptic meningitis

Cell count and total protein in 91 children with acute aseptic meningitis are demonstrated in Table III. The known causative agents were mumps virus in 19 of these children, Coxsackie viruses in 6, and ECHO viruses in 3 patients. In the uncomplicated course of the disease both parameters declined to normal levels during the second or third week. The electrophoretic findings of these children are shown in Fig. 4. The protein pattern was characterized by minimal or no increases in gamma-globulin, in association with a slight to moderate blood–CSF barrier disturbance. Mild elevation of the gamma-values may persist for 2–3 weeks. No oligoclonal gamma-globulin could be recognized.

TABLE III

CSF-FINDINGS IN ACUTE UNCOMPLICATED ASEPTIC MENINGITIS (91 CHILDREN)

Mean values, range in parentheses.

Time (days)	Patients (n)	Cell count (per mm³)	Total protein (mg/l)
1	84	320 (21–1680)	432 (145–1060)
4–7	6	157 (10–600)	450 (190–910)
6–18	6	8 (0–23)	311 (253–400)

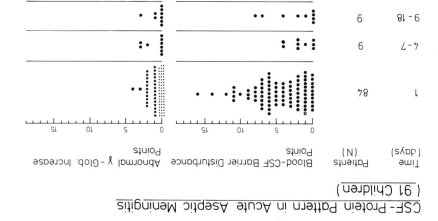

CSF- Protein Pattern in Acute Aseptic Meningitis
(91 Children)

Time (days)	Patients (N)	Abnormal γ-Glob. Increase Points	Blood-CSF Barrier Disturbance Points
1	84		
4-7	9		
6-18	9		

Fig. 4. CSF–protein pattern in acute aseptic meningitis; Time, time since onset of disease; N, number of patients; for explanation of the scales see Tables I and II.

Prolonged aseptic meningitis

In 16 children with a more protracted course of aseptic meningitis, two different CSF reactions occurred (Table IV). One reaction showed a further increase in total protein during the third to sixth week. This group comprised 7 children, 4 of whom had mumps meningitis and one Coxsackie B virus meningitis. A second reaction was an increase in cell count with or without concomitant rise of total protein concentration. In this group of 9 children there were 5 cases of mumps meningitis and one meningitis caused by an enterovirus infection. Electrophoretic protein analysis revealed that increase of total protein only was due to moderate to severe blood–CSF barrier disturbance without changes in gamma-globulin (Fig. 5). In most of the children with rising cell counts, however, oligoclonal gamma-globulin was formed; in addition, signs of an ongoing blood–CSF barrier disturbance were seen.

TABLE IV

CSF-FINDINGS IN PROLONGED ASEPTIC MENINGITIS (GROUP A AND B, 8 CHILDREN EACH)

Mean values, range in parentheses.

Time (days)	Patient (n)	Cell count (per mm³)	Total protein (mg/l)
Group A (with increase of total protein only)			
17–39	7	38 (3–100)	1380 (1030–1910)
50–360	4	5 (2–14)	480 (330–520)
Group B (with increase of total protein and/or cell count)			
15–28	6	229 (68–430)	1043 (230–1950)
41–58	5	103 (11–170)	688 (430–1200)

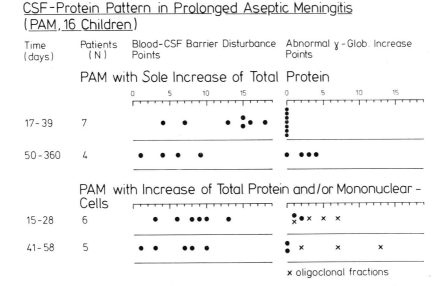

Fig. 5. CSF–protein pattern in prolonged aseptic meningitis.

Acute encephalitis

CSF was analyzed in 60 children with acute para- or post-infectious encephalitis. Identified infectious agents included the following: rubeola virus in 14 cases; Coxsackie virus in 5 cases; adenovirus and rubella virus in 3 cases each; and influenza and parainfluenza viruses in 2 cases each. There were also two children with postvaccinial encephalitis. Cell count and total protein declined slowly over a period of weeks or months (Table V). There was a marked blood–CSF

TABLE V

CSF-FINDINGS IN ACUTE PARA- AND POSTINFECTIOUS ENCEPHALITIS (60 CHILDREN)

Mean values, range in parentheses.

Time (days)	Patients (n)	Cell count (per mm³)	Total protein (mg/l)
1	31	82 (0–650)	541 (220–2000)
4–13	18	46 (0–207)	572 (179–862)
18–44	18	30 (0–165)	430 (190–960)
59–90	11	14 (0–92)	372 (180–770)

barrier disturbance which was observed, not only during the initial stage, but also during the following weeks (Fig. 6). In the majority of these patients, an increase in gamma-globulin was seen. It appeared either initially or at some point during the course of the disease. During the third to the seventh week, oligoclonal gamma-banding was demonstrated in 4 of 18 children, although there were neither clinical complications nor rises in cell count or total protein.

CSF-Protein Pattern in Acute Encephalitis (HSV-Encephalitis Exluded, 60 Children)

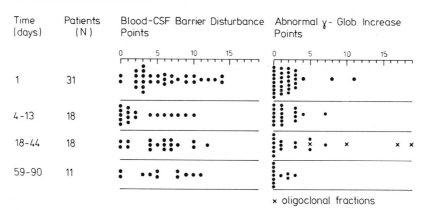

Fig. 6. CSF–protein pattern in acute para- and postinfectious encephalitis.

Herpes simplex virus encephalitis

Herpes simplex virus encephalitis, as an example of primary encephalitis, was characterized by an intense blood–CSF barrier disturbance and normal gamma-globulin values at the beginning of the illness (Fig. 7). Whereas the children improved clinically, there was an excessive local humoral immune response which lasted for many months. Oligoclonal gamma-globulin was noticed in one child.

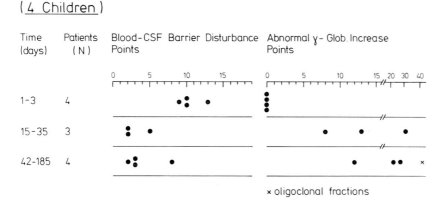

Fig. 7. CSF–protein pattern in herpes simplex virus encephalitis.

Prolonged encephalitis

In 7 children with prolonged para- of postinfectious encephalitis, cell count and total protein remained high for weeks or months or even transiently increased during this period (Table VI).

TABLE VI

CSF-FINDINGS IN PROLONGED ENCEPHALITIS (7 PATIENTS)

Mean values, range in parentheses.

Patients (n)	Time (days)	Cell count (per mm³)	Total protein (mg/l)
6	18–35	164 (10–370)	1522 (720–2240)
6	47–91	139 (53–292)	1002 (570–1770)
4	104–360	10 (0–15)	370 (240–470)

Etiology was unknown except in two cases in which a varicella zoster virus and a Coxsackie B virus were identified. All these children displayed oligoclonal gamma-fractions, the rise in gamma-globulin being remarkable in some of these patients (Fig. 8). Blood–CSF barrier disturbance seemed to resolve slowly.

142

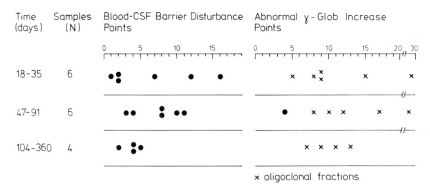

Fig. 8. CSF–protein pattern in prolonged para- or postinfectious encephalitis.

Chronic progressive encephalitis

In only 3 of 9 children with chronic progressive encephalitis were the causative agents identified. Rubella virus and varicella zoster virus caused encephalitis in one child during maintenance therapy for acute lymphoblastic leukaemia, and rubeola virus produced encephalitis in a child with nephrosis treated with corticosteroids. These children showed consistently elevated cell counts as well as total protein persisting for months or years, the mean value of the latter parameter revealing a rising tendency (Table VII). In association with the active blood–CSF barrier disturbance, a marked oligoclonal gamma-reaction was displayed (Fig. 9).

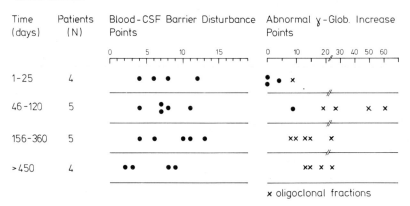

Fig. 9. CSF–protein pattern in chronic progressive encephalitis.

TABLE VII

CSF-FINDINGS IN CHRONIC PROGRESSIVE ENCEPHALITIS (9 PATIENTS)

Mean values, range in parentheses.

Time (days)	Patients (n)	Cell count (per mm³)	Total protein (mg/l)
1–25	4	48 (3–160)	535 (120–1120)
46–120	5	207 (5–365)	672 (370–1390)
156–360	5	241 (32–403)	848 (470–1370)
>450	4	184 (83–244)	942 (610–1200)

SUMMARY AND CONCLUSIONS

In acute aseptic meningitis, minimal or no abnormal gamma-globulin increases were observed. In acute para- and postinfectious encephalitis, however, a marked local humoral immune response may occur. The most striking increases in gamma-globulin can be noticed in herpes simplex virus encephalitis during phases of clinical improvement. In many cases of prolonged meningitis and in all cases of prolonged para- and postinfectious encephalitis, an intense local humoral immune response was recognized. The most constant finding of chronic progressive encephalitis was an increase in gamma-globulin and the presence of oligoclonal gamma-fractions. Table VIII lists the pathological conditions which have been found to be associated with oligoclonal gamma-globulin. This list is compiled from examination of about 2000 children with a broad spectrum of CNS disorders. In the present study, detection of CSF oligoclonal gamma-globulin in conventional agarose gel electrophoresis was usually associated with prolonged or chronic CNS infections of various etiologies. This phenomenon appeared nearly always in connection with a pleocytosis. It occurred to some extent under conditions of immunologic immaturity or immunosuppression, which could mean that total elimination of infectious agents was impeded. In the CNS infections of known etiology studied

TABLE VIII

CNS DISEASES ASSOCIATED WITH OCCURRENCE OF OLIGOCLONAL GAMMA-GLOBULIN IN THE CSF

	Viral origin	Non-viral or unknown origin
Newborn period, infancy	Congenital infections: cytomegalovirus, rubella virus	Congenital infection: toxoplasmosis. Bacterial meningitis, especially: (1) after corticosteroid therapy; (2) associated with subdural effusions
(Pre-)school age, adolescence	(Acute), prolonged or chronic meningitis, encephalitis	
	Progressive encephalitis following immunosuppressive therapy	Bacterial or fungal meningitis following immunosuppressive therapy, leukemia, medulloblastoma, multiple sclerosis
	Subacute sclerosing panencephalitis	

144

so far, oligoclonal gamma-globulin revealed antibody activity directed against components of the causal agent (Vandvik and Norrby, 1973; Sköldenberg et al., 1976; Porter et al., 1977; Iwashita, 1978; Vandvik et al., 1978). One might suppose that a prolonged or continuous local antigenic stimulation would lead to proliferation of clones of lymphocytes, which release antibodies into the CSF.

ACKNOWLEDGEMENTS

The authors particularly thank Mrs. C. Weigel for data processing. This work was supported in part by the Deutsche Forschungsgemeinschaft (Si 289/1-1).

REFERENCES

Cawley, L.P., Minard, B.J., Tourtelotte, W.W., Ma, B.J. and Chelle, C. (1976) Immunofixation electrophoretic techniques applied to identification of proteins in cerebrospinal fluid. *Clin. Chem.*, 22: 1262–1268.

Iwashita, H., Araki, K., Kuroiwa, Y. and Matsumoto, T. (1978) Occurrence of Candida-specific oligoclonal IgG antibodies in the CSF with Candida meningoencephalitis. *Ann. Neurol.*, 4: 579–581.

Porter, K.G., Sinnamon, D.G. and Gillies, R.R. (1977) Croptococcus neoformans-specific oligoclonal immunoglobulins in cerebrospinal fluid in cryptococcal meningitis. *Lancet*, i: 1262.

Siegert, M. and Siemes, H. (1977) Agarose gel electrophoresis of cerebrospinal fluid proteins and analysis of the pherogram profiles by analogue computer. *J. clin. Chem. clin. Biochem.*, 15: 635–644.

Siemes, H., Siegert, M. and Rating, D. (1975) Das Liquorproteinprofil normaler Kinder und seine Abhängigkeit vom Lebensalter. *Neuropädiatrie*, 6: 383–397.

Sköldenberg, B., Carlström, A., Forsgren, M. and Norrby, E. (1976) Transient appearance of oligoclonal immunoglobulins and measles virus antibodies in the cerebrospinal fluid in a case of acute measles encephalitis. *Clin. exp. Immunol.*, 23: 421–425.

Vandvik, B. and Norrby, E. (1973) Oligoclonal IgG antibody response in the central nervous system to different measles virus antigens in subacute sclerosing panencephalitis. *Proc. nat. Acad. Sci. U.S.A.*, 70: 1060–1063.

Vandvik, B., Norrby, E., Steen-Johnsen, J. and Stensvold K. (1978) Mumps meningitis: prolonged pleocytosis and occurrence of mumps virus-specific oligoclonal IgG antibodies in the cerebrospinal fluid. *Europ. Neurol.*, 17: 13–22.

Immunology of Nervous System Infections, Progress in Brain Research, Vol. 59, edited by P.O. Behan, V. ter Meulen and F. Clifford Rose

Immune Complexes in Subacute Sclerosing Panencephalitis

ALEXANDER M. ABDELNOOR[1], SUHAYL S. DHIB-JALBUT[2],
HANIA K. TAMER[1] and FUAD S. HADDAD[3]

[1]*Department of Microbiology,* [2]*Medicine, and* [3]*Surgery, Faculty of Medicine, American University of Beirut, Beirut*
(Lebanon)

INTRODUCTION

In a previous study we demonstrated that patients with SSPE responded normally to skin test antigens, had normal isohemagglutinin titers, elevated serum IgG, IgA, and IgM levels, elevated CSF IgG levels and elevated serum and CSF measles antibody titers (MAT). It was also observed that both serum and CSF IgG levels increased with progression of the disease, while the specific measles antibody titers remained at the same level (Dhib-Jalbut et al., 1981). This finding suggested to us that antigenic stimuli other than the measles virus may be involved in the disease. We later reported the possible involvement of parainfluenza type I virus, in addition to the measles virus, in the pathogenesis of SSPE (Abdelnoor et al., 1982).

During the course of our investigations, it was noted that a certain number of sera obtained from patients with SSPE had an altered complement profile. This led us to search for circulating immune complexes in patients with SSPE. This chapter reports our findings.

MATERIALS AND METHODS

Patients

Twenty-seven patients with SSPE were included in this study. They consisted of two stage I, 11 stage II, 11 stage III, and 3 stage IV patients. The diagnosis and clinical stage of the disease were established on clinical, electroencephalographic and serological grounds (Haddad et al., 1977).

Specimens

Blood was drawn from patients. Sera from these specimens were obtained and after complement levels and activity were determined, the remaining sera were stored at $-20°C$ until used.

C_{3C}, C_4 and C activity determinations

C_{3C} and C_4 levels were determined by radial immunodiffusion (Mancini et al., 1965). Normal values for C_{3C} and C_4 ranged between 55 and 120 mg/dl (mean = 82 mg/dl) and 20–50 mg/dl (mean = 30 mg/dl) respectively. Complement activity was determined by the method described by Lachmann et al. (1973). The diameter of the zone of hemolysis in normal subjects ranged between 5 and 5.5 mm. Values less than 5 mm, obtained when patients' sera were analyzed, was considered as low.

Detection of circulating immune complexes (IC)

Circulating IC were detected by testing the ability of serum specimens to aggregate platelets. One-tenth of a ml of serum was added to platelet-rich plasma (PRP) at 37°C. Any aggregation that occurred was detected using a chronolog aggregometer. Adenosine diphosphate (2×10^{-5} M) and serum from normal healthy individuals were used as positive and negative controls respectively.

RESULTS

Complement profile

The mean and range of C_{3C}, C_4 and C activity obtained in SSPE patients are presented in Table I. Although the mean values of SSPE patients were not significantly different from the normal controls, C_{3C}, C_4, and/or C activity were altered in 14 patients (3 had high C_{3C} and C_4 and low complement activity; 1 had high C_{3C}; 2 had high C_4; 2 had low C_4; 1 had high C_{3C} and

TABLE I

COMPLEMENT PROFILE IN SSPE PATIENTS

Number of SSPE patients studied	C_{3C} mg/dl		C_4 mg/dl		C activity (mm)		Remarks
	Mean	Range	Mean	Range	Mean	Range	
27	96.1	47–214	36.6	16–64	4.8	3–5.4	14/27 patients had an altered complement profile
	S.D. ±34		S.D. ±14.3		S.D. ±0.77		

TABLE II

COMPLEMENT PROFILE IN RELATION TO CLINICAL STAGE

Clinical stage	Number of patients	C_{3C}		C_4		C activity		Number of patients having altered complement profile
		Mean	Range	Mean	Range	Mean	Range	
I	2	84.7	84–85.4	27.7	27.4–28	5	5–5	0
		S.D. ±1		S.D. ±0.42				
II	11	100.7	47–160	42.6	19–64	4.8	3–5.5	9
		S.D. ±30.6		S.D. ±14.2		S.D. ±0.8		
III	11	99.7	58–214	36.9	16–64	4.7	3–5.4	5
		S.D. ±28		S.D. ±16.1		S.D. ±0.94		
IV	3	101	95–105	30	25–35	5.1	5–5.2	0
		S.D. ±5.5		S.D. ±5		S.D. ±0.1		

C_4; 1 had low C_{3C} and C_4; 1 had high C_{3C} and low complement activity; 1 had high C_4 and low complement activity, and two had low complement activity). It was observed that in stages I and IV, complement profiles were normal while 9 in stage II and 5 in stage III had altered complement profiles (Table II).

Circulating immune complexes

Fifteen patients had detectable circulating IC, 5 of which also had an altered complement profile. Three of the 5 patients were in stage II and the other 2 were in stage III (Table III). IC was not detected in 9 patients with an altered complement profile.

TABLE III

IMMUNE COMPLEXES AND COMPLEMENT PROFILE IN RELATION TO CLINICAL STAGE

Clinical stage	Number of patients	Number of patients with IC	Number of patients with IC and altered complement profile
I	2	1	0
II	11	5	3
III	11	7	2
IV	3	2	0

DISCUSSION

Dayan and Stokes (1972), Philips (1972), Oldstone et al. (1975) and Derakhshan et al. (1981) demonstrated or suggested the presence of IC in the circulation of patients suffering from SSPE, but did not correlate the presence or absence of these complexes with the complement profile of the patients. Ahmed et al. (1974) has demonstrated the presence of a specific blocking factor in the sera and CSF of SSPE patients. It is conceivable that this factor is IC since it was precipitated by antibodies against IgG and C_3. Furthermore, one of the sites at which IC can be deposited is the choroid plexus (Oldstone, 1975). This makes the supposition of the involvement of IC in the pathogenesis of SSPE more probable. If such is the case, our findings suggest that complement-dependent and complement-independent mechanisms are involved, since 5 IC-positive patients had an altered complement profile and the other 10 had normal complement profiles. The number of patients in stages I and IV is too small to be able to make a meaningful correlation between IC, complement and the severity of the disease.

Furthermore, the finding in 9 patients of an altered complement profile, in the absence of IC, suggests that factors other than IC may be activating complement, possibly by the alternate pathway; or IC, although present, were not detected by the method used.

Further studies are being conducted to elucidate the role of IC in the pathogenesis of SSPE.

ACKNOWLEDGEMENTS

We gratefully acknowledge the assistance of Dr. Riad Khalifeh and Dr. Adnan Cherif for referring SSPE patients to the Registry. Miss Seta Keuroghlian assisted in the typing of the

148

manuscript. This study was supported in part by Grant 38-5723 from the Lebanese National Research Council and by a grant from the Research Committee of the American University of Beirut.

REFERENCES

Abdelnoor, A.M., Dhib-Jalbut, S.S. and Haddad, F.S. (1982) Different virus antibodies in serum and cerebrospinal fluid of patients suffering from SSPE. *J. Neuroimmunol.*, 2: 27–34.

Ahmed, A., Strong, D.N., Sell, K.W., Thurman, G.B., Knudsen, R.C., Wistar, R. Jr. and Grace, W.R. (1974) Demonstration of a blocking factor in the plasma and spinal fluid of patients with SSPE. *J. exp. Med.*, 139: 902–924.

Dayan, A.D. and Stokes, M.I. (1972) Immune complexes and visceral deposits of measles antigens in SSPE. *Br. Med. J.*, 2: 374–376.

Derakhshan, I., Massoud, A., Foroozanfar, N. et al. (1981) SSPE: clinical and immunologic study of 23 patients. *Neurology*, 31: 177–178.

Dhib-Jalbut, S.S., Abdelnoor, A.M. and Haddad, F.S. (1981) Cellular and humoral immunity in SSPE, *Infect. Immun.* 33: 34–42.

Haddad, F.S., Risk, W.S. and Jabbour, J.T. (1977) SSPE in the Middle East, report of 99 cases. *Ann. Neurol.*, 3: 211–217.

Lachmann, P.J., Hobart, M.J. and Aston, W.P. (1973) Complement. In D.M. Weir (Ed.), *Handbook of Experimental Immunology*, 2nd Ed., Blackwell Scientific Publications, Oxford.

Mancini, G.A., Carbonara, O. and Heremans, J.F. (1965) Immunochemical quantitation of antigens by single radial immunodiffusion. *Immunochemistry*, 2: 235–254.

Oldstone, M.B.A. (1975) Virus neutralization and virus-induced immune complex disease. Virus-antibody union resulting in immunoprotection or immunologic injury — two sides of the same coin. *Progr. Med. Virol.*, 19: 84–119.

Oldstone, M.B.A., Bokish, V.A., Dixon, F.J., Barbosa, L.H., Fucillo, D. and Sever, J.L. (1975) SSPE: destruction of human brain cells by antibody and complement in an autologous system. *Clin. Immunol. Immunopathol.*, 4: 52.

Philips, P.E. (1972) Immune complexes in SSPE. *New Engl. J. Med.*, 286: 949.

Immunology of Nervous System Infections, Progress in Brain Research, Vol. 59, edited by P.O. Behan, V. ter Meulen and F. Clifford Rose

Immunological Abnormalities and Immunotherapeutic Attempts in Subacute Sclerosing Panencephalitis

P.O. BEHAN and WILHELMINA M.H. BEHAN

Departments of Neurology and Pathology, Glasgow University, Glasgow, Scotland (U.K.)

INTRODUCTION

Subacute sclerosing panencephalitis (SSPE) is a rare encephalitis associated with persistent measles virus infection. It affects primarily children and has been known for half a century. Measles virus was first isolated from brain tissue by Horta-Barbosa et al. (1969) and since then has been recovered from both autopsy and biopsy nervous tissue and from the lymph nodes of affected children (Horta-Barbosa et al., 1971). The pathogenesis of the disease is an enigma since we have no idea why the measles virus persists in the central nervous system (CNS) in these cases. One attractive hypothesis is that a defect in the normal immune mechanisms underlies the continuing infection. Some support for this is provided by the fact that SSPE occurs more frequently in children who have had measles before the age of two years, when the virus may have been introduced into the body at a time when the immune system was immature. Patients with impaired immunity may develop an SSPE-like syndrome (Aicardi et al., 1977; Wolinsky et al., 1977), but in spite of the virological and pathological similarities, this appears to be a different disease.

Burnet (1968) proposed originally that the illness occurred in patients with disorders of immunoregulation and several reports suggest that this may be true. Gerson and Haslam (1971) studied 4 boys with SSPE and noted that skin test responses to 6 common antigens were impaired, skin grafts were rejected more slowly than normal, and contact sensitivity to dinitrochlorobenzene (DNCB) could not be induced. In addition, 3 of the children had low serum concentrations of immunoglobulin A (IgA) while germinal centers and plasma cells were deficient in their lymph nodes, suggesting a reduction in humoral immunity. Kolar (1968) had already reported that SSPE patients were negative on skin testing to purified protein derivative (PPD). This impairment of cutaneous reactivity to ubiquitous antigens does seem to be a genuine feature of SSPE, reported also by several other workers (Kreth et al., 1974; Valdimarsson et al., 1974; Livni et al., 1976; Swick et al., 1976). The anergy bears no relationship to the age, sex or stage of the disease. Unlike Gerson and Haslam (1971), Kreth et al. (1974) were able to sensitize their patients to DNCB.

Cell-mediated skin test reactions to measles virus have been reported consistently as negative (Kolar, 1968; Jabbour et al., 1969; Gerson and Haslam, 1971; Valdimarsson et al., 1974), but such studies are meaningless because no standard measles antigen is available for skin testing (Nelson et al., 1966; Lennon et al., 1967).

In vitro examination of lymphocytes from cases of SSPE at first revealed defective responses to measles virus (Moulias et al., 1971; Vandvik, 1970; Lischner et al., 1972), but later investigations have given conflicting results, e.g. some workers (Saunders et al., 1969; Thurman et al., 1973) found increased blastogenesis but others (Klajman et al., 1973; Valdimarsson et al., 1974; Ruckdeschel et al., 1975; Matthew et al., 1975) detected no effect. Using a different technique, lymphokine production (macrophage-inhibiting factor) by lymphocytes from cases of SSPE exposed to measles virus was documented by certain investigators (Mizutani et al., 1971; Ahmed et al., 1974; Sheremata et al., 1978) but this finding could not be confirmed by others (Moulias et al., 1971; Klajman et al., 1973; Valdimarsson et al., 1974; Livni et al., 1976). In addition, it has been shown that lymphocytes from both normal healthy controls and from patients with SSPE, when used in cell-mediated cytotoxicity tests, give similar results (Kreth et al., 1975a; Steele et al., 1976; Yamanaka et al., 1977; Perrin et al., 1977; Ewan and Lachmann, 1977).

The picture is complicated even more by reports that blocking factors which affect cell-mediated responses in SSPE are present. Allen et al. (1973) and Swick et al. (1976) found that lymphocyte transformation to phytohaemagglutinin (PHA) was impaired if plasma from patients with SSPE was incorporated into the test system. Ahmed et al. (1974) found specific blocking factors in these subjects and they suggested that the blocking was due to the immune complexes which they detected in both serum and CSF. Once again controversy exists, however, because certain investigators (Steele et al., 1976; Ewan and Lachmann, 1977) confirmed the findings of Ahmed and co-workers, while Kreth and ter Meulen (1977) and Perrin et al. (1977) were unable to do so and reported also that cell-mediated cytotoxicity to measles virus was increased.

Finally, in contrast to the early studies, recent investigations of general cellular immunity have revealed no abnormalities. Thymus-derived (T) lymphocytes are present in normal numbers, as determined by rosetting techniques (Valdimarsson et al., 1974; Blaese and Hofstrand, 1975; Kreth et al., 1979) and in vitro lymphocyte responses to ubiquitous antigens have also been reported as normal (Sharma et al., 1971; Klajman et al., 1973; Valdimarsson et al., 1974; Kreth et al., 1974; Blaese and Hofstrand, 1975; Livni et al., 1976).

We report here our experience with a large group (13 cases) of patients with SSPE, the results of detailed immunological studies carried out, and the outcome of several different attempts at immunotherapy.

PATIENTS

A total of 13 patients were studied, although it was not possible to carry out the same immunological tests in all cases. All the children had undisputed SSPE, with the diagnosis based on clinical, electrophysiological, virological and immunological features. There were 7 boys and 6 girls and their ages at presentation ranged from 5 to 14 years. Nine of the 13 had had measles before the age of two years.

Atypical features included the appearance of spider naevi in 4 of the girls during the course of the disease: all 4 had at least one naevus on the face, chest and arm. Bilateral papilloedema, which resolved rapidly, was the presenting sign in one of these girls.

One patient was remarkable because, when first seen complaining of a disturbance in sleep rhythm and nightmares, there was no increased anti-measles antibody in her serum and her EEG was normal. Six months later, the serum titer had risen to 1/4096 and specific anti-measles antibody was detected in the CSF at a titer of 1/64. The characteristic EEG abnormalities were now present on hyperventilation. A curious feature was that when first seen, she had no detectable serum IgA, but normal concentrations were present when the disease became evident clinically, and remained during the rest of her 6 month course.

IMMUNOLOGICAL METHODS

Histocompatibility (HLA) typing

HLA typing was carried out in 6 patients (cases 1, 2, 4, 6, 8, 10), using peripheral blood lymphocytes and a battery of 120 antisera to define the antigens in a microcytotoxicity technique (Kissmeyer-Nielsen and Dick, 1979). The control population consisted of 342 random (unrelated) healthy subjects from the same geographical region, i.e. the west of Scotland.

Estimation of lymphocyte subpopulations

Mononuclear cells were isolated from heparinized blood samples obtained from cases 1 (stage I disease), case 4 (stage 2) and case 8 (stage 3). Ficoll-Hypaque (Pharmacia) gradient density centrifugation was used. Cells were stained with Ortho-mune monoclonal antibodies (OK) T3, T4, T8 and Ia 1 (Ortho Diagnostic Systems, Buckinghamshire, U.K.), followed by fluorescein-conjugated anti-mouse IgG (sheep F (ab)2 anti-mouse Ig fluorescein-conjugated, New England Nuclear, Boston, MA, U.S.A.) according to the method of Reinherz et al. (1979). Analysis of the lymphocytes was performed on a fluorescence-activated cell sorter (FACS IV, Becton Dickinson, Mountain View, CA, U.S.A.) using logarithmic amplification of the fluorescence signal (Ledbetter et al., 1980) and 90° scatter to eliminate all contaminating monocytes (Richie et al., 1983). The Ia 1 percentage obtained was therefore considered to represent B-cells and activated T-cells only. The T3 antibody labeled all peripheral blood T-lymphocytes while the T4 identified the helper/inducer subpopulation and the T8, the cytotoxic/suppressor cells.

Skin tests

Eleven patients (all cases except numbers 11 and 12) were skin tested by injecting 0.1 ml of each of the test antigens intradermally into the cleaned, volar aspect of the left arm. The antigens used were streptokinase/streptodornase, 10 units (SK/SD, Varidase, Lederle Laboratories) candida albicans 0.5 % (Hollister-Steier Laboratories), Old Tuberculin, 5 units, and measles antigen (Mevilin-L measles vaccine, live attenuated), 0.1 ml of 1 in 2 dilution of stock solution (Duncan, Flockhart, London, U.K.). The tests were read at 6, 24 and 48 h: any area of induration was then noted and the product of its two maximum diameters measured.

Peripheral blood leucocyte protein synthesis

The in vitro technique, using whole blood, as described by Pauly et al. (1973) was employed in 5 patients (cases 1, 2, 6, 7 and 8). The uptake of tritiated leucine by peripheral blood lymphocytes following phytohaemagglutinin (PHA, Burroughs Wellcome) stimulation, was measured over a 22-h period. A dose–response curve for a range of concentrations of PHA (0.65 μg/ml–8.33 μg/ml) was plotted and compared to that obtained using 30 normal healthy controls of the same age.

Inhibition of leucocyte migration

The leucocyte migration inhibition assay of Soborg and Bendixen (1967) was used in 6 patients (cases 2, 3, 4, 5, 6, 8). The results were expressed as:

$$\text{index of inhibition} = \frac{\text{surface area in presence of antigen}}{\text{surface area in absence of antigen}} \times 100.$$

Each result was the average of at least 4 capillary measurements and unless the measurements were all within 15% of one another, the result was discarded. An inhibition index of more than 70% was considered significant.

The same antigens as used in the skin tests were employed, at the final concentrations indicated. These were measles antigen (Mevilin-L, 1/5 dilution of stock solution), candida albicans (0.1 ml/ml), purified protein derivative (200 units/ml) and SK/SD (50 units/ml). If transfer factor therapy was given, the tests were done before and after this therapy.

Search for serum-blocking factors

The peripheral blood lymphocyte protein assay described above was used as follows:

Healthy donor lymphocytes and pooled serum from SSPE cases

Sixty milliliters of venous blood from healthy donors was collected. The cells obtained were washed 3 times in tissue culture fluid RPMI 1640 and a lymphocyte count was done. The cell suspension was then divided into 4 aliquots and tissue culture medium was added to each to give a final concentration of 1×10^6 lymphocytes/3 ml. The medium was supplemented with one of the following: (I) 10% autologous serum; (II) 10% foetal calf serum; (III) 10% serum pooled from 13 cases of SSPE; (IV) 10% serum pooled from patients with other chronic neurological diseases.

The cells were cultured for 48 h at 37°C and tritiated leucine was added and the material divided into 3 ml aliquots. Protein synthesis over the following 22 h, on stimulation by the range of PHA concentrations indicated above, was then measured.

Repeated washing of lymphocytes from the patients to remove putative blocking factors

Lymphocytes from cases 6, 8, 9, 10, 11, 13 were washed carefully 3 times in large volumes of RPMI 1640. They were then resuspended in tissue culture fluid supplemented with autologous or foetal calf serum and protein synthesis to PHA stimulation over a 22-h period was measured as described, in each case.

Immunoglobulins

Serum immunoglobulin concentrations of IgG, IgM and IgA were measured by single radial immunodiffusion, using commercially obtained monospecific antisera (Oxford Laboratories, Diffu-gen reagents), in all 13 patients.

Complement studies

The following cases were examined: 1, 2, 3, 4, 6, 7, 8, 10. The functioning efficiency of the complement system was assayed in terms of the total haemolytic complement activity (CH50 units). The concentrations of C1q, C3, C4 and factor B in EDTA plasma were determined by radial immunodiffusion, and evidence of C3 and factor B breakdown products were sought. Commercially available antisera were used. Standard methods were used (Kent and Fife, 1963; Laurel, 1965).

Immune complex assays

These were done in all 13 patients.

Solid phase C1q assay. This was performed as described by Hay et al. (1976) using radiolabeled anti-human IgG antibodies. The assay detects as low as 16 μg/ml of aggregated IgG in serum.

Staphylococcus aureus binding assay (Barkas, 1981). Complexes were precipitated from serum using polyethylene glycol 6000 at a final concentration of 5%. The precipitates were washed and redissolved in phosphate-buffered saline, then incubated with a 1% (v/v) suspension of staphylococcus aureus. After washing, bound complexes were detected using radiolabeled protein A. The lower limit of sensitivity of the assay is 3–6 μg/ml of aggregated IgG in the serum. In both these assays an equal number of age and sex matched controls were processed simultaneously. The control population consisted of normal volunteers. Samples classed as positive were those yielding values greater than the mean and two standard deviations of the control results.

Anticomplementary assay. Serum anticomplementary assays were also carried out (Mayer, 1961).

RESULTS

HLA typing

The HLA haplotypes of the 6 cases are shown in Table I. No significant association with any particular haplotype was detected.

TABLE I

HLA TYPING IN 6 CASES OF SSPE

Case no.	A series	B series	C series
1	2, 24	27, 35	W4
2	1, 28	8, W27/AJ	
4	1, 9	8, 14	? W2, W6
6	2	12, 21	
8	1	8 W22	W3
10	2, 3	21, 18	W6

TABLE II

LYMPHOCYTE SUBSETS IN 3 CASES OF SSPE

Results are expressed as the mean ± S.E.M.

Subjects	% Reactivity with monoclonal antibodies				T4/T8 ratio (number of patients)
	T3	T4	T8	Ia 1	
Case no. 4 (stage 1)	78	52	20	10	2. 6:1
Case no. 1 (stage 2)	70	55	20	20	2. 8:1
Case no. 8 (stage 2)	76	54	23	9	2. 3:1
Other neurological diseases (n = 15)	70 ± 3	45 ± 2	24 ± 1	19 ± 1	< 4:1 (15)
Normal subjects (n = 20)	75 ± 2	49 ± 2	25 ± 2	12 ± 1	< 4:1 (20)

154

In Table II, the results in the 3 cases are shown, compared to a group of patients with other neurological diseases, and a group of healthy controls. No significant deviations from the normal were noted: in particular there was no loss of suppressor/cytotoxic cells.

Skin tests

The results are summarized in Table III. Five children were in stage 1 of the disease; they were otherwise healthy. Two had impaired responses to SK/SD and candida antigens. They did show a positive reaction to PPD but, in this group of children, a negative response to PPD could not be evaluated properly because none of them had had BCG immunization. Of the 3 children with stage 2 disease, two showed similarly defective responses to SK/SD and candida while one of the 3 children at stage 3, reacted in the same way. Thus, impaired responses to common antigens were detectable at all stages of disease activity, but nonetheless children with advanced disease did show perfectly normal reactions. Measles antigen produced no skin reactions in any of the children.

TABLE III

SKIN TESTS IN 11 CHILDREN WITH SSPE

Case no.	Clinical stage	SK/SD	Candida	Old Tuberculin	Measles
1	2	−	−	−	−
2	1	−	−	−	−
3	1	+	+	−	−
4	1	−	−	−	−
5	3	−	−	+	−
6	1	+	+	+	−
7	3	+	+	−	−
8	3	+	+	−	−
9	1	+	−	+	−
10	2	−	−	+	−
13	2	+	+	−	−

Peripheral blood lymphocyte protein synthesis

Of the 5 children tested, two (cases 6 and 8) shared a highly significant impairment of lymphocyte response (Fig. 1). Both had stage 3 disease at this time. One of them had shown a normal response on several previous occasions while in stage 2. The other 3 children, one of whom was also in stage 3, were normal to testing.

Inhibition of leucocyte migration

The inhibition indices to stimulation with the different antigens are shown in Table IV.

Search for serum-blocking factors

These results were entirely negative. No evidence of serum-blocking factors was detected.

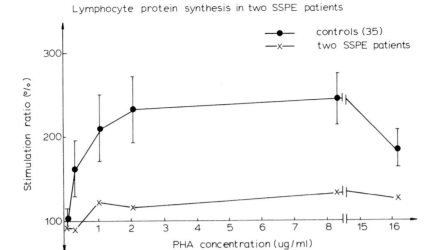

Fig. 1. Peripheral blood lymphocyte protein synthesis in two patients with SSPE, compared to that in normal healthy controls.

TABLE IV

LEUCOCYTE INHIBITION INDEX TO COMMON ANTIGENS IN 6 PATIENTS WITH SSPE

An inhibition index of more than 30% was considered positive.

Case no.	SK/SD	Candida	PPD	Measles
2	10	19	28	12
3	92	88	12	0
4	22	56	28	8
5	36	7	62	4
6	69	25	58	6
8	70	85	30	0

Serum immunoglobulins

In the main these were normal, but in 4 cases there was a mild increase in IgG, up to 14.8 g/l. The serum IgM concentrations were all within the normal range, as were the IgA levels, except in one patient (case 3) whose serum IgA was undetectable when first seen, but returned to normal 6 months later and remained so during the rest of her course. The normal ranges were: IgG = 4.5–13.8 g/l; IgM = 0.32–1.5 g/l; IgA = 0.5–2.6 g/l.

Complement studies

Of the 8 patients investigated, marginal increases in the serum CH50 units and the C3 concentrations were detected in 6, and reductions in the C4 component in 5. Two of these latter children had evidence of C3 conversion (10% and 15%; normal range 0–5%). It was considered that there was evidence of complement activation, possibly due to circulating immune complexes, in 4 cases.

Immune complex assays

The staphylococcus aureus assay was positive in all cases tested, while the C1q and anticomplementary assays were each positive in one-third of the samples tested. The results of the latter two assays correlated poorly. These results indicated that a range of immune complexes from very small ones, present in antigen excess, to larger complement-fixing aggregates, were present at all stages of the disease.

Immunotherapy

Use of transfer factor (TF)

Preparation of material. Donors were family members and healthy subjects, each of whom gave one pint of blood. All subjects were negative for syphilis and hepatitis antigen. Blood was obtained by venepuncture or by the use of a cell separator. The leucocytes were separated, washed twice in phosphate-buffered saline (PBS) and then lysed by freezing and thawing 5 times. The lysate was then dialyzed against distilled water. The dialyzate was lyophilized and sealed in glass vacuum containers until use. All samples were tested for pyrogenicity and sterility and were passed through a millipore filter. Each dose of TF consisted of the material obtained from $4.5–10 \times 10^8$ lymphocytes. As therapy, each of the patients received s.c. and i.m. injections of TF obtained from 5 donors, over a period of one week.

A total of 5 children were treated as indicated: cases 2 and 11, stage 1; case 12, stage 2; cases 5 and 7, stage 3. There were no adverse effects, but no evidence of improvement, clinically, electrophysiologically or by estimation of the anti-measles antibody titers in the serum or CSF, was noted. In 3 of the cases, detailed immunological studies, including skin tests, were carried out before and after the therapy. Apart from one possible skin conversion from PPD-negative to positive, no changes were found.

Thymectomy

Thymectomy was carried out in 6 children: cases 1, 4, 6, stage 1; cases 8, 9 and 10, stage 3. Of the 3 patients treated in stage 1, two are now dead but one is still alive, ambulant, but with all the features of SSPE, 3 years after the operation. In one boy the disease continued to progress slowly for 4 years until, within a few months, he passed rapidly from stage 1 to stage 3 and died. The other child's course showed no response at all to thymectomy. As regards the children treated in stage 3, two are now dead, having shown no detectable response to the operation, and although the last boy is still alive, this is almost certainly entirely due to excellent nursing care.

The thymuses were all histologically normal. The material is being studied at present in Professor ter Meulen's laboratory. In addition, 6 dogs were injected intracerebrally with the thymic tissue and studied over the ensuing year. No clinical, electrophysiological or immunological abnormalities were detected in these animals.

Interferon therapy

The children treated were cases 2, 8 and 9. Case 2 was a girl of 13, still in stage 1 but with neurological signs developing. Cases 8 and 9 were boys of 6 and 7 years, in stage 2. All 3 had already had thymectomies and the girl had also had three 2-liter plasma exchanges.

Human leucocyte interferon (IFN α-type P-IF-A) was purchased from a Danish laboratory. It had been produced by in vitro induction in human buffy coat leucocytes, using Sendai virus. The activity of the semi-purified product was 3×10^6 IU/ml, assayed by plaque reduction of vesicular stomatitis virus in human amniotic cells.

Case 8 was given 25 daily i.m. injections of 1.0 ml. Case 9 had 90 similar i.m. injections, while case 2 received 20 doses. The first boy deteriorated rapidly and died after the last injection, showing no clinical or laboratory evidence of improvement. The second boy showed a continuing increase in serum anti-measles antibody titer, which reached 1/8096, and no clinical benefit at all was observed. His EEG findings also remained unchanged. The third child was given an additional 12×10^6 IU of interferon intrathecally, over a period of 3 days. This led to a sterile meningitis (7000 leucocytes/ml CSF) accompanied by fever, but again, no clinical benefit. Mild temperature rises were associated with the i.m. injections in all children, occurring usually 3–4 h after the injections. No other side-effects were observed. Samples of CSF from these 3 cases, other patients with SSPE, and subjects with multiple sclerosis, were coded and analyzed for interferon activity: none was detected except in one specimen of CSF which contained 10 IU/ml. This was from the child who had had 90 i.m. injections. We concluded that partially purified human leucocyte interferon was of no value in these cases.

Plasma exchange

Five children (cases 1 and 6, stage 1; cases 8, 9 and 10, stage 3) were treated. In each case, 16 liters of plasma were exchanged on continuous flow cell separators, over a period of a week. Replacement fluid consisted of Plasma Protein Fraction.

No clinical change was seen in any of the children and their EEGs remained the same. Their serum anti-measles antibody titers fell rapidly during the exchanges but reached their original values within the following three weeks.

DISCUSSION

All 13 of these patients had undisputed SSPE, fulfilling the clinical, virological, electrophysiological and immunological criteria for diagnosis of the disease. With regard to the clinical features, it is worth commenting on the presence of spider naevi in 4 patients. Simpson (1961) observed similar lesions in SSPE. He thought that the disease might be associated with infective hepatitis because he had obtained a history of a previous attack of jaundice in 3 of his patients. Liver function tests in our patients were all entirely normal, so that the presence of the spider naevi may have been coincidental.

One of our patients was first seen before her serum anti-measles antibody titer was increased and when no other features of the disease were present except very mild cerebral involvement which had given rise to persistent nightmares. Six months later a high titer of anti-measles antibody was detected, together with EEG abnormalities. This case contrasts with the only similar one reported in the literature (ter Meulen et al., 1982). This was a child who developed SSPE and from whom a serum specimen had been fortuitously obtained one year previously when there were no clinical signs. A high titer of anti-measles antibody was already detectable in the early specimen.

We were unable to show any association between SSPE and a specific HLA haplotype in our 13 children. Kurent et al. (1975) have suggested a possible linkage with HLA W29, but other workers have not been able to find any other HLA associations (Kreth et al., 1975b). Reports that the disease has occurred in only one of identical twins, militate against such a genetic association (Chao, 1962; Whittaker et al., 1972; D'Onghia et al., 1974; Houff et al., 1979).

The ability to study such a large group of patients with SSPE gave us a unique opportunity to see whether or not we could find unequivocal evidence of disordered immune mechanisms. We were able to study lymphocyte subpopulations in only 3 patients, but our finding of normal values for these subsets, adds support to previous reports that T-lymphocytes are normal when measured by other techniques (Valdimarsson et al., 1974; Blaese and Hofstrand, 1975; Kreth and Pabst, 1979). We can confirm that a variable amount of hyposensitization as demonstrated by cutaneous reactivity to common antigens, exists in the patients. This has been a common finding by investigators (Gerson and Haslam, 1971; Valdimarsson et al., 1974; Kreth et al., 1974; Livni et al., 1976; Swick et al., 1976). We found no correlation between the stage of the disease and the loss of cutaneous reactivity and we did not try to induce sensitization to DNCB.

Using the technique of peripheral blood lymphocyte protein synthesis, we detected a subtle but definite lymphocyte abnormality in some of these children. A similar abnormality has been previously reported in a wide variety of illnesses, including malignancy (Levy and Kaplan, 1974; Thomas et al., 1975), autoimmune disease (Simpson et al., 1976) and adverse drug reactions (Behan et al., 1976). The same lesion has been found by this test in patients with motor neuron disease (Behan, 1979) where other in vitro investigations by other workers have confirmed the presence of the abnormality. Similar impairment of PHA-induced responses occurs in acute viral infections (Mellman and Wetton, 1963).

The mechanism which produces the defect is unknown: serum-blocking factors, intrinsic lymphocyte abnormalities or defective PHA receptors could all give this picture, which indeed may be nonspecific and not immunologically-related. A serum factor which depresses lymphocyte function has been reported in infections (Levene et al., 1969) and more particularly, in SSPE (Ahmed et al., 1974). We could not confirm that such a blocking factor was present in our patients. The PHA receptors on the lymphocytes are probably normal in these cases, because the PHA response measured by the uptake of titrated thymidine over 3 days (instead of 22 h) was normal.

Zweiman's work (1972) is pertinent to our findings. He observed that the addition of autoclaved, noninfectious measles virus preparations imapired significantly the lymphocyte proliferation induced by nonspecific mitogens and tuberculin. He and his colleagues (Zweiman et al., 1971) had demonstrated previously that there was a similar depression of reactivity in lymphocytes from patients who had received measles vaccine. Thus the most likely explanation for the defective response in the peripheral blood lymphocyte protein synthesis assay, and for the variable responses on skin testing, must be that they are due to the effect of persistent measles virus.

By means of the leucocyte inhibition assay we were able to show that although the patients had impaired lymphocyte function as detected in the protein synthesis assay, nevertheless, lymphokines were produced in response to common antigens. The literature on cell-mediated immunity in SSPE, using in vitro techniques of investigation, is confusing. The discrepancies between the results of various assays have already been outlined in the Introduction. It would seem that, as regards ubiquitous antigens, there is a consensus of opinion that immune responses in these patients are normal. As far as measles antigen goes, however, the evidence is more difficult to interpret. We have already listed the workers who claim to have found sensitization to measles virus in SSPE subjects and those who have not.

Graziano et al. (1975) reported that they had produced a reliable in vitro system for demonstrating cellular hypersensitivity to measles. They claimed that the recognition of viral antigen by sensitized lymphocytes in patients with SSPE, depended on the antigen being bound to, or associated with, a cell membrane. We used a similar measles antigen preparation in our studies, but were quite unable to obtain reproducible evidence of positive lymphokine production. The data in this area are so conflicting that no firm conclusions can be drawn at this time.

Reports of a blocking factor present in the serum and CSF of patients with SSPE, add to the present confusion (Ahmed et al., 1974). The blocking factor reported was heat-labile and neutralized by rheumatoid factor; it did not stop the production of leucocyte-inhibiting factor by stimulated PPD-sensitive lymphocytes, and was 10 times more potent when obtained from CSF compared to serum. The factor was though to consist of immune complexes. We were unable to demonstrate any serum-blocking factors in our cases, but we did not use the same antigen (SSPE-virus preparation) as Sell et al. (1973). It seems likely that although no nonspecific blocking factors are seen, a specific blocking factor for SSPE virus may be present. Such a specific blocking factor is assumed to consist of immune complexes (Ahmed et al., 1974). Certain workers have confirmed the presence of blocking effects (Valdimarsson et al., 1974; Steele et al., 1976; Ewan and Lachmann, 1977) while others have reported that cell-mediated cytotoxicity is enhanced rather than depressed by the addition of SSPE serum (Kreth and ter Meulen, 1977; Perrin et al., 1977).

Serum IgA was undetectable in one of our cases when she was first seen. IgA production is related to intact thymic function and abnormalities in IgA metabolism can be correlated with impaired immunity (Shakir et al., 1978). How a transient deficiency in IgA might arise is unknown, but we have observed a similar phenomenon in a young girl who developed transverse myelopathy after a nonspecific viral infection.

There is compelling evidence that humoral immunity is abnormal in SSPE. The presence of immune complexes in these patients is discussed elsewhere in this book by Abdelnoor and colleagues. Dayan and Stokes (1972) demonstrated by immunofluorescence that immune complexes were present in renal glomeruli in these cases and that measles antigens can be found in spleen, liver and lymph nodes. Antibody and complement have been detected in nervous tissue in SSPE patients (Philips, 1972; Oldstone et al., 1975). We found circulating immune complexes and evidence of complement activation in the patients we studied here. Derakhshan et al. (1981) have postulated that the complexes are pathogenetic. But whether or not tissue damage is due to these deposits cannot be stated without further investigation. Certainly, attempted removal of the aggregates by plasma exchange produced no benefit in our cases of SSPE.

There has been a report of the possible benefit of thymectomy in this disorder (Kolar et al., 1967), but we found no evidence of amelioration of the disease in patients in stage 3, although in two patients who were in stage 1, there was a suggestion that the thymectomy might have modified and prolonged the clinical course. Because of the variable picture that occurs in SSPE, however, this observation would need to be tested in a much larger group of subjects. There were no histological abnormalities in the thymuses removed.

Transfer factor therapy was quite without any effect. The claims that this treatment has a role in immunologically-mediated disorders are highly controversial and not now generally accepted. Critical analysis of the many reports of the use of this substance in SSPE, reveal that it is of no benefit (Reinhert et al., 1975; Vandvik, 1973; Kackell et al., 1975; ter Meulen et al., 1975; Blaese et al., 1975; Valdimarsson et al., 1975).

Human leucocyte interferon (IFN α-type P-IF-A) was without benefit in these cases of SSPE. Interferon inducers (Leavitt et al., 1971) have also been reported as ineffective in this disorder. Plasma exchange was used empirically, in an attempt to manipulate the patients' immune systems and to remove the putative pathogenetic immune complexes. This therapy proved of no value, similarly to previous reports of plasmapheresis or of exchanging the CSF (Sell et al., 1975).

Our experience in the 13 cases reported here suggests that, although it is possible that immune factors are involved in the pathogenesis of SSPE, present techniques are inadequate for their demonstration and the immunotherapies currently available are of no benefit to the patients.

ACKNOWLEDGEMENTS

We wish to thank Drs I.T. Draper, I.D. Melville and S. Currie for providing some of the patients studied here. This work was supported by the Andrew Noble Fund.

REFERENCES

Ahmed, A., Strong, D.M., Sell, K.W., Thurman, G.B., Knudsen, R.C., Wistar, R. and Grace, W.R. (1974) Demonstration of a blocking factor in the plasma and spinal fluid of patients with subacute sclerosing panencephalitis. *J. exp. Med.,* 139: 902–924.

Aicardi, J., Goutieres, F., Arsenio-Nunes, M. and Lebon, P. (1977) Acute measles encephalitis in children with immunosuppression. *Paediatrics,* 59: 232–239.

Allen, J., Oppenheim, J., Brody, J.A. and Miller, J. (1973) Labile inhibitor of lymphocyte transformation in plasma from a patient with subacute sclerosing panencephalitis. *Infect. Immun.,* 8: 80–82.

Barkas, T. (1981) A rapid simple sensitive assay for immune complexes using Staphylococcus immuno-absorbent. *J. Clin. lab. Immunol.,* 5: 59–65.

Behan, P.O., Behan, W.M.H., Zacharias, F.J. and Nichols, J.T. (1976) Immunological abnormalities in patients who had the oculomucocutaneous syndrome associated with practolol therapy. *Lancet,* ii: 984–987.

Behan, P.O. (1979) Cell-mediated immunity in motor neurone disease and poliomyelitis. In F.C. Rose (Ed.), *Clinical Neuroimmunology,* Blackwell Scientific Publications, Oxford, pp. 259–272.

Blaese, R.M. and Hofstrand, H. (1975) Immunocompetence in patients with SSPE. *Arch. Neurol.,* 32: 494–495.

Blaese, R.M., Hofstrand, H., Krebs, H. and Sever, J. (1975) Evaluation of transfer factor in the therapy of SSPE. *Arch. Neurol.,* 32: 505.

Burnet, F.M. (1968) Measles as an index of immunological function. *Lancet,* 2: 610–613.

Chao, D. (1962) Subacute inclusion body encephalitis. Report of three cases. *Paediatrics,* 61: 501–510.

Dayan, A.D. and Stokes, M.I. (1972) Immune complexes and visceral deposits of measles antigens in SSPE. *Brit. Med. J.,* 2: 374–376.

Derakhshan, I., Massoud, A., Foroozanfar, N. (1981) SSPE: clinical and immunologic study of 23 patients. *Neurology,* 31: 177–178.

D'Onghia, C.A., Lefevre, A.B., Canelas, H.M., Grossmann, R.M., Salles-Gomes, L.F. and Saldanha, P.H. (1974) Subacute sclerosing panencephalitis in only one member of a monozygotic twin pair. *J. neurol. Sci.,* 21: 323–333.

Ewan, P.W. and Lachmann, P.J. (1977) Demonstration of T-cell and K-cell cytotoxicity against measles-infected cells in normal subjects, multiple sclerosis and subacute sclerosing panencephalitis. *Clin. exp. Immunol.,* 30: 22–31.

Gerson, K.L. and Haslam, R.H.A. (1971) Subtle immunologic abnormalities in four boys with subacute sclerosing panencephalitis. *New Engl. J. Med.,* 285: 78–81.

Graziano, K.D., Ruckdeschel, J.S. and Mardiney, M.R. (1975) Cell-associated immunity to measles (Rubeola). The demonstration of in vitro lymphocyte tritiated thymidine incorporation in response to measles complement fixation antigen. *Cell Immunol.,* 15: 347–359.

Hay, F.C., Nineham, L.J. and Roitt, I.M. (1976) Routine assay for the detection of immune complexes of known immunoglobulin class using solid phase C1q. *Clin. exp. Immunol.,* 24: 396–400.

Horta-Barbosa, L., Fuccillo, D.A., Sever, J.L. and Zeman, W. (1969) Subacute sclerosing panencephalitis: isolation of measles virus from a brain biopsy. *(Nature (Lond.),* 221: 974.

Horta-Barbosa, L., Hamilton, R., Wittig, B., Fuccillo, D.A., Sever, J.I. and Vernon, M.L. (1971) Subacute sclerosing panencephalitis: isolation of suppressed measles virus from lymph node biopsy. *Science,* 173: 840–841.

Houff, S.A., Madden, D.L. and Sever, J.L. (1979) Subacute sclerosing panencephalitis in only one of identical twins. *Arch. Neurol.,* 36: 854–856.

Jabbour, J.T., Roane, J.A. and Sever, J.L. (1969) Studies of delayed dermal hypersensitivity in patients with subacute sclerosing panencephalitis. *Neurology,* 19: 929–931.

Kackell, Y.M., Grob, P.J., Kreth, H.W., Kibler, R. and ter Meulen, V. (1975) Transfer factor therapy in patients with subacute sclerosing panencephalitis. *J. Neurol.,* 211: 39–49.

Kent, J.F. and Fife, E.H., Jr. (1963) Precise standardization of reagents for complement fixation. *Amer. J. Trop. Med. Hyg.,* 12: 103–116.

Kissmeyer-Nielsen, H. and Dick, H.M. (1979) Lymphocytotoxicity testing. In Heather M. Dick and F. Kissmeyer-Nielsen (Eds.), *Histocompatibility Techniques,* Elsevier/North-Holland, Amsterdam, pp. 9–37.

Klajman, A., Sternbach, M., Ranon, L., Drucker, M., Geminder, D. and Sadan, M. (1973) Impaired delayed hypersensitivity in subacute sclerosing panencephalitis. *Acta paediat. scand.*, 62: 523–526.

Koch, F., Becker, W. and Schwick, H.G. (1970) Leichte ketten der immunoglobuline im liquor cerebrospinalis bei patienten mit panenzephalitis. *Dtsch. Med. Wochenschr.*, 95: 391–393.

Kolar, O. (1968) Measles and subacute sclerosing panencephalitis. *Lancet*, ii: 1242.

Kolar, O., Obrucnik, M., Behounkova, L., Musil, J. and Penickova, V. (1967) Thymectomy in subacute sclerosing panencephalitis. *Brit. med. J.*, 111: 22–24.

Kreth, H.W. and ter Meulen, V. (1977) Cell-mediated cytotoxicity against measles virus in SSPE. I. Enhancement by antibody. *J. Immunol.*, 118: 291–295.

Kreth, H.W. and Pabst, F. (1979) Recent findings on cell-mediated immune reactions in acute measles and SSPE. In D.A.J. Tyrrell (Ed.), *Aspects of Slow and Persistent Virus Infections. 2. New Perspectives in Clinical Microbiology*, Martinus Nijhoff, The Hague, pp. 553–559.

Kreth, H.W., Kackell, Y.M. and ter Meulen, V. (1974) Cellular immunity in SSPE patients. *Med. Microbiol. Immunol.*, 160: 191–199.

Kreth, H.W., Kackell, Y.M. and ter Meulen, V. (1975a) Demonstration of in vitro lymphocyte-mediated cytotoxicity against measles virus in SSPE. *J. Immunol.*, 114: 1042–1046.

Kreth, H.W., ter Meulen, V. and Eckert, G. (1975b) HL-A and subacute sclerosing panencephalitis. *Lancet*, ii: 415–416.

Kreth, H.W., Ahmed, A. and ter Meulen, V. (1979) B lymphocyte function in SSPE: is there lack of suppressor cells? In D. Karcher, A. Lowenthal and A.D. Strosberg (Eds.), *Humoral Immunity in Neurological Diseases*, Plenum, New York, pp. 553–559.

Kurent, J.E., Sever, J.L. and Terasaki, P.I. (1975) HA-AW29 and subacute sclerosing panencephalitis. *Lancet*, i: 927–928.

Laurel, C.-B. (1965) Antigen-antibody crossed electrophoresis. *Analyt. Biochem.*, 10: 358–361.

Leavitt, T.J., Merigan, T.C. and Freeman, J.M. (1971) Hemolytic-uremic-like syndrome following polycarboxylate interferon induction. *Amer. J. Dis. Child.*, 121: 43–47.

Ledbetter, J.A., Rouse, R.V., Micklem, H.S. and Herzenberg, L.A. (1980) T-cell subsets defined by expression of Lyt-1, 2, 3 and Thy-1 antigens. *J. exp. Med.*, 152: 280–295.

Lennon, R.G., Isacson, P., Rosales, T., Elsea, W.R., Karzon, D.T. and Wilkelstein, W. (1967) Skin tests with measles and poliomyelitis vaccines in recipients of inactivated measles virus vaccine. *JAMA*, 200: 99–104.

Levene, G.M., Turk, J.L., Wright, D.J.M. and Grimble, A.G.S. (1969) Reduced lymphocyte transformation due to a plasma factor in patients with active syphilis. *Lancet*, ii: 246–247.

Levy, R. and Kaplan, H.S. (1974) Impaired lymphocyte function in untreated Hodgkin's disease. *New Engl. J. Med.*, 290: 181–186.

Lishner, H.W., Sharma, M.K. and Grover, W.D. (1972) Immunologic abnormalities in subacute sclerosing panencephalitis. *New Engl. J. Med.*, 286: 786–787.

Livni, E., Kott, E., Danon, Y., Kuritzky, A. and Joshua, H. (1976) Cell-mediated immunity in subacute sclerosing panencephalitis. *Israel J. Med. Sci.*, 12: 1183–1188.

Matthew, E.B., Krasny, M., Fuccillo, D.A. and Sever, J.L. (1975) Lymphocyte blastogenesis to viral antigens in SSPE. *Arch. Neurol.*, 32: 497–498.

Mayer, M.M. (1961) Complement and complement fixation. In E.A. Kabat and M.M. Mayer (Eds.), *Experimental Immunochemistry*, 2nd Edn., Charles C. Thomas, Springfield, IL, pp. 133–240.

Mellman, W.J. and Wetton, R. (1963) Depression of the tuberculin reaction by attenuated measles vaccine. *J. Lab. clin. Med.*, 61: 453–458.

Mizutani, H., Mizutani, H., Saito, S., Nihei, K. and Izuchi, T. (1971) Cellular hypersensitivity in subacute sclerosing panencephalitis. *JAMA*, 216: 1201–1202.

Moulias, R.L., Reinert, P. and Goust, J.M. (1971) Immunologic abnormalities in subacute sclerosing panencephalitis. *New Engl. J. Med.*, 285: 1090.

Nelson, J.D., Sandusky, G. and Peck, F.B. (1966) Measles skin test and serologic response to intradermal measles antigen. *JAMA*, 198: 185–186.

Oldstone, M.B.A., Bokish, V.A., Dixon, F.J., Barbosa, L.H., Fuccillo, D. and Sever, J.L. (1975) Subacute sclerosing panencephalitis: destruction of human brain cells by antibody and complement in an autologous system. *Clin. Immunol. Immunopathol.*, 4: 52.

Pauly, J.L., Sokal, J.E. and Han, T. (1973) Whole-blood culture technique for functional studies of lymphocyte reactivity to mitogens, antigens and homologous lymphocytes. *J. lab. Clin. Med.*, 82: 500–512.

Perrin, L.H., Tishon, A. and Oldstone, M.B.A. (1977) Immunologic injury in measles virus infection. III. Presence and characterization of human cytotoxic lymphocytes. *J. Immunol.*, 118: 282–290.

Philips, P.E. (1972) Immune complexes in SSPE. *New Engl. J. Med.*, 286: 949.

Reinert, P., Goust, J.M., Moulias, R. and Teman, G. (1975) Immunotherapy in SSPE. *Arch. Neurol.*, 32: 502.

162

Reinherz, E.L., Kung, P.C., Goldstein, G. and Schlossman, S.F. (1979) A monoclonal antibody with selective reactivity with functionally mature human thymocytes and all peripheral human T cells. *J. Immunol.,* 123: 1312–1317.

Richie, A.W.S., Gray, R.A. and Micklem, H.S. (1983) Right angle light scatter: a necessary parameter in flow cytofluorimetric analysis of human peripheral blood mononuclear cells, *J. immunol. Meth.,* in press.

Ruckdeschel, J.C., Dunmire, C. and Mardiney, M.R. Jr. (1975) Cell-associated immunity to measles in SSPE: evidence for impaired lymphocyte transformation in response to measles antigen. *Arch. Neurol.,* 32: 497.

Saunders, M., Knowles, M., Chambers, M.E., Caspary, E.A., Gardner-Medwin, D. and Walker, P. (1969) Cellular and humoral responses to measles in subacute sclerosing panencephalitis. *Lancet,* i: 72–74.

Sell, K.W., Thurman, G.B., Ahmed, A. and Strong, D.M. (1973) Plasma and spinal-fluid blocking factor in SSPE. *New Engl. J. Med.,* 288: 215–216.

Sell, K.W., Ahmed, A. and Bailey, D.W. (1975) Attempts to remove an inhibitor of cellular immunity found in plasma and spinal fluid in patients with SSPE. *Arch. Neurol.,* 32: 502–503.

Shakir, R.A., Behan, P.O., Dick, H. and Lambie, D.G. (1978) Metabolism of immunoglobulin A, lymphocyte function and histocompatibility antigens in patients on anticonvulsants. *J. Neurol. Neurosurg.* Psychiat., 41: 307–311.

Sharma, M.K., Grover, W.D., Huff, D.S., Baird, H.W. and Lischner, H.W. (1971) Studies of immunologic competence in subacute sclerosing panencephalitis (SSPE). *Clin. Res.,* 19: 730.

Sheremata, W., Sazant, A. and Watters, G. (1978) Subacute sclerosing panencephalitis and multiple sclerosis: in vitro measles immunity and sensitization to myelin basic protein. *Canad. Med. Assoc.,* 118: 509–513.

Simpson, J.A. (1961) Subacute inclusion-body encephalitis: a possible association with infective hepatitis. *Lancet,* ii: 685–687.

Simpson, J.A., Behan, P.O. and Dick, H.M. (1976) Studies on the nature of autoimmunity in myasthenia gravis. Evidence for an immunodeficiency type. *Ann. N.Y. Acad. Sci.,* 274: 382–389.

Soborg, M. and Bendixen, G. (1967) Human lymphocyte migration as a parameter of hypersensitivity. *Acta med. scand.,* 181: 247–256.

Steele, R.W., Fuccillo, D.A., Hensen, S.A., Vincent, M.M. and Bellanti, J.A. (1976) Specific inhibitory factors of cellular immunity in children with subacute sclerosing panencephalitis. *J. Pediat.,* 88: 56–62.

Swick, H.M., Brooks, W.H., Roszman, T.L. and Caldwell, D. (1976) A heat-stable blocking factor in the plasma of patients with subacute sclerosing panencephalitis. *Neurology,* 26: 84–88.

Ter Meulen, V., Grob, P.J., Kreth, H.W., Kackell, Y.M. and Kibler, R. (1975) Transfer factor therapy in patients with SSPE. *Arch. Neurol.,* 32: 501.

Ter Meulen, V., Stephenson, J.R. and Kreth, H.W. (1982) Subacute sclerosing panencephalitis. In *Comprehensive Virology, Vol. 18,* in press.

Thomas, D.G.T., Lanigan, C.B. and Behan, P.O. (1975) Impaired cell-mediated immunity in bain tumours. *Lancet,* i: 1389–1390.

Thurman, G.B., Ahmed, A.A., Strong, D.M., Knudsen, R.C., Grace, W.R. and Sell, K.W. (1973) Lymphocyte reactivity of patients infected with subacute sclerosing panencephalitis virus or cytomegalovirus: in vitro stimulation in response to viral-infected cell lines. *J. exp. Med.,* 138: 839–846.

Valdimarsson, H., Agnarsdottir, G. and Lachmann, P.J. (1974) Cellular immunity in subacute sclerosing panencephalitis. *Proc. roy. Soc. Med.,* 67: 1125–1129.

Valdimarsson, H., Agnarsdottir, G. and Lachmann, P.J. (1975) The treatment of SSPE with transfer factor. *Arch. Neurol.,* 32: 503.

Vandvik, B. (1970) Immunological studies in subacute sclerosing panencephalitis. *Acta neurol. scand.,* 46, Suppl. 43: 232.

Vandvik, B. (1973) Immunopathological aspects in the pathogenesis of subacute sclerosing panencephalitis, with special reference to the significance of the immune response in the central nervous system. *Ann. Clin. Res.,* 5: 308–315.

Whitaker, J.N., Sever, J.L. and Engel, W.K. (1972) Subacute sclerosing panencephalitis in only one of identical twins. *New Engl. J. Med.,* 287: 364–366.

Wolinsky, J.S., Swoveland, P., Johnson, K.P. and Baringer, J.R. (1977) Subacute measles complicating Hodgkin's disease in an adult. *Ann. Neurol.,* 1: 452–457.

Yamanaka, T., Chiba, S., Nakao, T., Okabe, N., Takahashi, N., Saito, S., Kitayama, T., Mishima, H., Konno, K. and Fujiwara, K. (1977) Cell-mediated immunity to measles virus in subacute sclerosing panencephalitis. *Tohoku J. exp. Med.,* 122: 175–181.

Zweiman, B., Pappagianis, D., Maibach, H. and Hildreth, E.A. (1971) Effect of measles immunisation on tuberculin hypersensitivity and in vitro lymphocyte reactivity. *Int. Arch. Allergy,* 40: 834–841.

Zweiman, B. (1972) Effect of viable and non-viable measles virus on proliferating human lymphocytes. *Int. Arch. Allergy,* 43: 600–607.

Immunology of Nervous System Infections, Progress in Brain Research, Vol. 59, edited by P.O. Behan, V. ter Meulen and F. Clifford Rose
© *1983 Elsevier Science Publishers B.V.*

Subacute Sclerosing Panencephalitis: Are Antigenic Changes Involved in Measles Virus Persistence?

MICHAEL J. CARTER and V. TER MEULEN

Institute for Virology and Immunobiology, University of Würzburg, Versbacher Str. 7, D-8700 Würzburg (F.R.G.)

INTRODUCTION

Subacute sclerosing panencephalitis (SSPE) is a rare, fatal complication of measles virus infection arising years after acute measles. During this chronic disease process, characteristic measles virus inclusions are present in the cells of the central nervous system (CNS) (Freeman et al., 1967; Connolly et al., 1967; ter Meulen et al., 1967, 1969), and the patients display an elevated serum antibody titer to all measles virus polypeptides. This response does not include anti-matrix protein (M) activity (Hall and Choppin, 1979; Wechsler et al., 1979; Stephenson and ter Meulen, 1979). Where this response can be detected, it is consistent with antibody remaining from the previous acute infection (Hall and Choppin, 1979). A similar pattern is observed in the CSF, where antibodies produced also lack an anti-matrix protein activity. In the CNS, however, the immunoglobulins synthesized are oligoclonally restricted and probably, therefore, secreted from lymphocyte clones which have invaded this compartment. The epidemiology, immunology and current knowledge of the measles virus involved have recently been reviewed (ter Meulen et al., 1983). During SSPE, infectious virus is not present either in the CNS or other tissues, but it has proved possible, in some cases, to rescue a measles-like virus by cocultivation techniques (reviewed by Agnarsdottir, 1977). These viruses may differ from measles virus, and from each other, but no single, stable property differentiates them. In fact, differences between various strains of measles virus are of a similar magnitude to those observed between SSPE and measles viruses (Agnarsdottir, 1977; Fraser and Martin, 1978). In the experiments reported here, we have attempted to differentiate these agents further using monoclonal antibodies raised against purified measles virus Edmonston. In no case is an isolate of measles virus available from the acute phase of infection preceding the develoment of SSPE by the same patient. We have attempted to model this event in vitro by using a tissue culture of Vero cells persistently infected with an SSPE virus "Lec", and to compare this system to other carrier cultures. These in vitro persistent infections differ from any in vivo persistence since they are maintained in the absence of an immune response and may therefore provide an insight into the importance of that phenomenon in the development of SSPE.

MATERIALS AND METHODS

Measles virus Edmonston was grown in Vero or CV-1 cells as described in the text. The Lec SSPE virus was isolated by cocultivation techniques from the brain of a child with SSPE

164

(Barbanti-Brodano et al., 1970), and a persistent infection (Lec PI) was established in Vero cells as described (ter Meulen et al., 1981). This persistent infection has now been maintained in our laboratory for over two years.

Immune precipitation of infected cell polypeptides was performed using cell [^{35}S]methionine-labeled lysates prepared at 16 h p.i. (Edmonston), 24 h p.i. (Lec lytic) or 16 h after cell passage (Lec PI). Lysate preparation and immunoprecipitation were carried out in RIPA buffer (10 mM Tris-HCl, pH 7.4, 0.15 M NaCl containing 0.1 % SDS, 1 % Triton X-100 and 1 % sodium deoxycholate as described by Lamb et al. (1978). Immunoprecipitated proteins were analyzed on 10 % polyacrylamide gels using the method of Laemmli (1970) and visualized by fluorography (Bonner and Laskey, 1974). Messenger RNA was isolated from cellular cytoplasmic fractions and selected by oligo dT chromatography (Barrett et al., 1979). mRNA was translated in a reticulocyte lysate system kindly provided by Dr. S. Siddell. This was prepared as described by Pelham and Jackson (1976) with modifications described by Siddell et al. (1980). The preparation of monoclonal antibodies and the radioimmuno-binding assay has already been described (ter Meulen et al., 1983). Serological assays, haemagglutination inhibition (HAI), neutralization (NT) and haemolysin inhibition (HLI) tests were carried out as described (Norrby and Gollmar, 1975).

RESULTS

In our laboratory we have prepared some 75 hybridoma antibodies. Of these, 21 were found to immunoprecipitate the H-polypeptide, 1 the nucleocapsid, and 2 the matrix protein of measles virus Edmonston. The remainder were not positive by this technique, even though all bound to high titers in a radioimmunoassay. The biological properties of the anti-H-hybridomas have been tested, and on this basis, these antibodies were divided into 5 groups (ter Meulen et al., 1981). These groups are summarized below (Table I). This type of analysis has

TABLE I

PROPERTIES OF MEASLES HYBRIDOMA MYELOMA ANTIBODIES

All hybridoma failed to inhibit the haemolysin reaction. No antibodies were obtained with high neutralization titers (NT) but undetectable haemagglutination inhibition (HI) titers.

Group	Example	Properties
1	173	No detectable HI or NT
2	298	HI-positive, no detectable NT
3	585, 26	HI and NT activities similar
4	323	HI > NT. Both activities easily detectable
5	155	HI < NT. Both activities easily detectable

provided the first evidence that a given antigenic determinant on the H-polypeptide could be altered in functional significance between measles and SSPE virus strains. That is, the site for a given antibody may still be present, but the antibody–antigen combination no longer produces the same biological effect (ter Meulen et al., 1981). Preliminary data from direct competitive

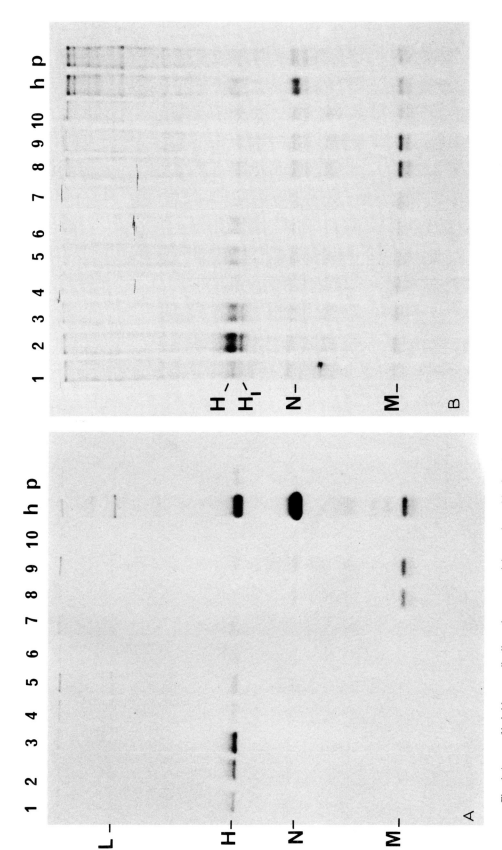

Fig. 1. A: use of hybridoma-antibodies to immunoprecipitate polypeptides from Lec virus-infected Vero cells. Immunoprecipitation was performed in 50 μl vols. at 4°C using 1 μl of undiluted rabbit serum or 5 μl of ascites fluid diluted 1 : 10. Immune complexes were precipitated after 30 min, using staphylococcal protein A coupled to sepharose beads and armed with rabbit anti-mouse immunoglobulins (Dako). h, rabbit hyperimmune serum, raised against purified SSPE virus Lec; p, preimmune rabbit serum; lanes 1–6, anti-H hybridoma antibodies, (nos. 173, 155, 585, 298, 32a, 26); lane 7, anti-N hybridoma antibody (no. 2273); lanes 8 and 9, anti-M hybridoma antibody (no. 128 and 263); lane 10, non measles-virus directed hybridoma antibody. B : proteins immunoprecipitated from Lec PI cell lysates. Method and hybridoma antibody used as in A.

binding experiments indicate that these 5 groups occupy at least 3 partially overlapping sites on the H-protein molecule. The two anti-matrix protein monoclonals (263 and 128) appear to bind at distinct sites on this protein and their binding is not mutually exclusive. Further characterization of the N-polypeptide awaits the isolation of more monoclonal antibodies. This panel of antibodies was used in a comparison of Lec PI cells and Vero cells lytically infected with Lec virus by immunoprecipitation (Fig. 1).

Both anti-M-antibodies were found to immunoprecipitate M-protein from lytic Lec infections. This protein was immunoprecipitated as a double band and this was also observed in some measles virus Edmonston infections. It seems, therefore, that M-protein may exist in two related forms. Recently, Rima et al. (1981) have provided evidence that a cleavage product of the measles virus P-protein also runs in this area. These two hybridoma antibodies also precipitated M protein from Lec PI cell lysates. Owing to the lower level of virus polypeptide expression in this cell line, a much higher background was obtained, but reference to the control monoclonal antibody, raised against a totally unrelated antigen, shows this precipitation to be clearly specific. The anti-nucleocapsid antibody did not react with N protein of the parent Lec virus, nor with that formed in persistence, so that we are unable to draw any conclusions regarding this protein. The anti-haemagglutinin hybridoma antibodies revealed an interesting effect. Only 4 of the 6 antibodies used were clearly positive in the immune precipitation reaction: 173, 155, 585 and 32, when tested with antigens produced in lytic Lec virus infection. These same antibodies also precipitated H protein from Lec PI cell lysates. In this case, however, the monospecific antibodies precipitated the H polypeptide as a double band, H and H_1. Currently, peptide mapping studies are underway to clearly establish the relationship between these polypeptides. Other hybridoma antibodies, namely 298 and 26, were borderline in this technique. In view of the high background, it is difficult to be definitive on this point. Monoclonal antibodies which failed to definitively immunoprecipitate this protein from Lec virus-infected cell lysates, were used in immunofluorescence tests. This provided firm evidence for antigenic change during persistency, since 2 antibodies, 131 and 132, failed to bind to Lec PI cells whilst still combining well with antigens present in cells lytically infected with the Lec parent virus (Table II). This test is more sensitive than immunoprecipitation because a firm antibody–antigen combination is not required.

TABLE II

ANTIGENIC VARIATION IN MEASLES H-POLYPEPTIDE DURING PERSISTENT INFECTION

Immunofluorescence assay using infected tissue culture cells.

Clone number	Edmonston	Lytic Lec	Lec PI
585	+	+	+
131	+	+	−
152	+	+	−
SSPE serum	+	+	+

Thus it may be concluded that antigenic changes have arisen in the course of a persistent infection. These may be related to the double band observed in the specific immunoprecipitation of H-polypeptide from Lec PI cells. Whether this latter effect was due to differences in polypeptide synthesis, modification or turnover was unclear. For this reason, and also in an attempt to decrease the non-specifically precipitating background, this phenomenon was examined by immunoprecipitation of polypeptides formed in vitro. mRNA was extracted from Lec PI cells or from Vero cells lytically infected with Lec virus. In addition, mRNA was prepared from uninfected cells and from two other measles virus carrier cell lines. The N-1 cell line was produced by the cocultivation technique from SSPE brain material (Doi et al., 1972). The agent carried in these cells is exclusively cell-associated and infectious virus has never been detected. The carrier Lu106 cell line was originally established by Norrby (1967) and does shed infectious virus. The polypeptides detected by this procedure are shown in Fig. 2.

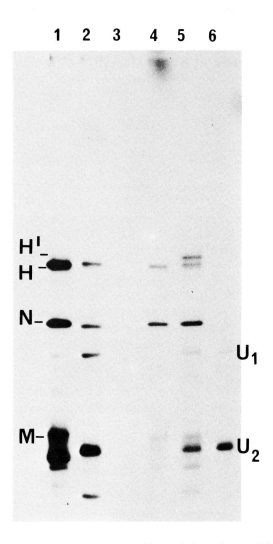

Fig. 2. In vitro translation of mRNA. mRNA was translated in a reticulocyte lysate cell-free system and immunoprecipitated using hyperimmune rabbit serum raised against SSPE virus Lec. The two prominent bands U_1 and U_2 in lane 6 presumably reflect contaminating host-cell polypeptides in this virus preparation. mRNA from: lane 1, carrier Lu cells; lane 2, N-1 cells (SSPE agent); lane 3, no mRNA added; lane 4, Lec PI cells; lane 5, Vero cells lytically infected with SSPE virus Lec; lane 6, uninfected cells. Bands were assigned by reference to a hyperimmune serum precipitation of an infected cell lysate.

Two polypeptides are immunoprecipitated specifically from the translation products of uninfected cells (Fig. 2, track 1) U_1 and U_2. The translation system itself has no immunoprecipitating protein product, and in the absence of added mRNA no products are detected (Fig. 2, track 4). A comparison of proteins formed by the Lec P1 and lytic Lec infected cell mRNA shows that 2 bands are detectable in the H protein region (H and H^1), when mRNA from a lytic infection is used but not when Lec PI cell mRNA is translated. H protein precipitated from Lec virus-infected cell lysates was observed to comigrate with the larger component of the H peptide doublet detected in Lec PI cells (H in Fig. 1). The in vitro translation product of mRNA from Lec PI cells co-migrated with the lower band (H) formed by mRNA extracted from Vero cells lytically infected with SSPE virus Lec. This band may therefore represent the precursor of the fully modified H protein observed in Fig. 1. Since no smaller product was detected amongst the in vitro translation products of Lec PI cells, the split H band (H and H_1) in Fig. 1, may represent post-translational modification of polypeptide H in Fig. 2. This modification either does not occur in lytically infected cells, or cannot be detected in extracts prepared under these conditions.

The higher molecular weight protein H^1 in Fig. 2 is at present not understood. It is possible that this product is normally rapidly degraded or modified so that it migrates in a different position. The absence of such a protein in the translation products of mRNA from Lec PI cells, however, is surprising, and suggests a difference in virus expression between the lytic and persistent infections examined. This might be due to the phase of virus replication in which the Lec PI cells are fixed. If this stage is normally short-lived in a lytic infection, then it may be difficult to detect by translation of total cellular mRNA, or by prolonged labeling of cellular proteins. The relevance of these apparent differences in virus expression to antigenic differences between lytic and persistent infections observed in Table II is at present unclear.

Analysis of the M-protein is more difficult since the host band U2 runs close to virus M. The position of M was determined from a lytically infected Vero cell extract. This protein was readily detected among the translation products of virus-releasing carrier Lu cell mRNA. It was present also in the Lec PI protein product, but no protein can be detected in this position in the non-virus yielding N-1 cell line. In a previous communication, we were unable to detect Lec virus M protein in Lec PI cells, but noted this product among the proteins formed in vitro. It would seem that this result can be explained by the high background observed in Fig. 1B, a problem which has now been overcome by the use of anti-M-monoclonal antibodies. Consequently, there is no reason to postulate translational control of M protein in the Lec PI cell system. We are currently searching for mRNA for this protein in the N-1 cell line, using a cloned cDNA copy of the Edmonston M-protein message, and for the protein itself using monoclonal antibodies. The other small bands detected in Fig. 2 are thought to be breakdown products from the nucelocapsid protein.

DISCUSSION

In this report we have observed the occurrence of antigenic change during SSPE virus persistence. This was observed as the loss of ability to bind 2 monoclonal antibodies, and evidence for an alteration in virus expression has been gathered. It seems clear that a rapid mutational drift may occur during virus-persistence in vitro. Holland et al. (1979) reported that a continual evolution in virus-specific RNA was demonstrable during vesicular stomatitis virus persistence. Most of these changes were manifested in the production of small plaque, temperature-sensitive mutants. This is to be expected since it may be supposed that the effect of most amino acid substitutions would be to destabilize a particular protein, and relatively few would lead to complete loss of function. A similar situation presumably exists during morbilli-virus persistence. We have demonstrated changes in H-protein antigenicity during SSPE virus persistence in the absence of antibody selection. Furthermore, the production of small plaque, or ts mutants during measles virus persistence is already well documented (ter Meulen et al., 1973; Haspel et al., 1973; Gould and Linton, 1975; Ju et al., 1978). Moreover, the ts mutants fail to complement each other, and ts (+) revertants retain their small plaque phenotype (Haspel et al., 1973). This suggests each virus had accumulated a number of different mutations. The observation that the measles virus released may alter with time of persistence further supports this concept (Rustigian et al. 1966; Wechsler et al., 1979; Wild et al., 1981).

During measles virus persistence in vivo it is possible that a competent host immune response might drive this mutation such that the virus remained "one-step ahead" of the host. Viruses are able to mutate easily in response to monoclonal antibodies: this is true of influenza (Laver et al., 1979), rabies (Wiktor and Koprowski, 1980), and also of measles virus (Birrer et al., 1981). It is clearly not quite so easy, however, to evade a polyvalent immune response such as encountered in vivo. It is important in this context to emphasize that SSPE viruses are neutralized by circulating antibodies, even if they are not quite so sensitive as measles viruses (Payne and Baublis, 1973). This could lead to conditions of partial neutralization and it is conceivable that a mutant virus might then be able to establish persistence more easily.

A second role of antibody could be modulation of antigen expression. Antibody has been shown to directly influence virus antigen expression, both at the cell surface and intracellularly (Joseph and Oldstone, 1975; Gould and Almeida, 1977; Fujinami and Oldstone, 1979). One of the first casualties of this process seems to be the expression of virus M-protein. Some evidence favours this event in vivo. It had been observed that after hamsters were inoculated with SSPE virus, infectious virus could at first be recovered, but gradually became more cell-associated. The time required for this process could be lengthened by inoculation of anti-lymphocyte serum or thymectomy (Byington and Johnson, 1975; Johnson et al., 1975). Following intracerebral inoculation of hamsters, the expression of M protein was found to gradually decrease, whilst that of N remained high (Johnson et al., 1981). Finally, SSPE patients display a low or absent immune response to M protein, suggesting that this protein is no longer available to the immune system as an antigen.

No M protein can be detected in the SSPE N-1 cell line and it is impossible to rescue virus from this cell line or from a similar line isolated by Thormar et al. (1978). In many other cases attempts to isolate a virus from SSPE autopsy material have failed, whereas in other instances co-cultivation techniques have led to M-protein production and virus release. Thus it is possible that the mechanism of measles virus persistence may differ from one individual to another, or within different areas of the same brain.

SUMMARY

SSPE virus "Lec" was used to establish a persistent infection in Vero cells. Late passages of this culture (225), which shed no detectable infectious virus, were compared to lytic "Lec" virus infections, using monoclonal antibodies in immune precipitation and immune fluorescence reactions. The data indicate that the haemagglutinin molecule (H) has undergone antigenic change during virus persistence in vitro. Antigenic change in the matrix (M) protein was not detected. The Lec persistent infection was compared to carrier cultures of measles virus (Carrier Lu 106 cells), and an SSPE agent (N-1), by in vitro translation of the extracted mRNA. The relevance of these observations to the mechanism of virus persistence and SSPE is discussed.

ACKNOWLEDGEMENTS

This work is supported by Deutsche Forschungsgemeinschaft and Volkswagenstiftung. We thank Margaret Willcocks and Sieglinde Löffler for valuable technical assistance and Helga Kriesinger for typing the manuscript.

REFERENCES

Agnarsdottir, G. (1977) Subacute sclerosing panencephalitis. In Waterson, A.P. (Ed.), *Recent Advances in Clinical Virology*, Churchill Livingstone, Edinburgh, pp. 21–49.

Barbanti-Brodano, G., Oyanagi, S., Katz, M. and Koprowski, H. (1970) Presence of two different viral agents in brain cells of patients with subacute sclerosing panencephalitis. *Proc. Soc. exp. Biol. (N.Y.),* 134: 230–236.

Barret, T., Wolstenholme, A.J. and Mahy, B.W.J. (1979) Transcription and replication of influenza virus RNA. *Virology*, 98: 211–225.

Birrer, M.J., Udem, S., Nathenson, S. and Bloom, B.R. (1981) Antigenic variants of measles virus. *Nature (Lond.),* 293: 67–69.

Bonner, W.M. and Laskey, R.A. (1974) A film detection method for tritium labelled proteins and nucleic acids in polyacrylamide gels. *Europ. J. Biochem.*, 46: 83–88.

Byington, D.P. and Johnson, K.P. (1975) Subacute sclerosing panencephalitis virus in immunosuppressed adult hamsters. *Lab. Invest.*, 32: 91–97.

Connolly, J.H., Allen, I.V., Hurwitz, L.J. and Miller, J.H.D. (1967). Measles-virus antibody and antigen in subacute sclerosing panencephalitis. *Lancet*, 1: 542–544.

Doi, Y., Samse, T., Nakajima, M., Okawa, S., Katoh, T., Itoh, H., Sato, T., Oguchi, K., Kumanishi, T. and Tsubaki, T. (1972) Properties of a cytopathic agent isolated from a patient with subacute sclerosing panencephalitis in Japan. *Jap. J. Med. Sci. Biol.*, 25: 321–333.

Fraser, K.B. and Martin, S.J. (1978) *Measles Virus and its Biology.* Academic Press, London.

Freeman, J.M., Magoffin, R.L., Lennette, E.H. and Herndon, R.M. (1967) Additional evidence of the relations between subacute inclusion-body encephalitis and measles virus. *Lancet*, 2: 129–131.

Fujinami, R.S. and Oldstone, M.B.A. (1979) Antiviral antibody reacting on the plasma membrane alters measles virus expression inside the cell. *Nature (Lond.)*, 279: 529–530.

Gould, E.A. and Linton, P.E. (1975) The production of a temperature-sensitive persistent measles virus infection. *J. gen. Virol.*, 28: 21–28.

Gould, J.J. and Almeida, J.D. (1977) Antibody modification of measles in vitro infection. *J. med. Virol.*, 1: 111–118.

Hall, W.W. and Choppin, P.W. (1979) Evidence for the lack of synthesis of the M polypeptide of measles virus in brain cells from SSPE. *Virology*, 99: 443–447.

Haspel, M.V., Knight, P.R., Duff, R.G. and Rapp, F. (1973) Activation of a latent measles virus infection in hamster cells. *J. Virol.*, 12: 690–695.

Holland, J.J., Grabau, E.A., Jones, C.L. and Sember, B.L. (1979) Evolution of multiple genome mutations during long-term persistent infection by vesicular stomatitis virus. *Cell*, 16: 495–504.

Johnson, K.P., Feldman, E.G. and Byington, D.P. (1975) Effect of neonatal thymectomy on experimental subacute sclerosing panencephalitis in adult hamsters. *Infect. Immun.*, 12: 1464–1469.

Johnson, K.P., Norrby, E., Swoveland, P. and Carrigan, D.R. (1981) Experimental subacute sclerosing panencephalitis. Selective disappearance of measles virus matrix protein from the central nervous system. *J. infect. Dis.*, 144: 161–168.

Joseph, B.S. and Oldstone, M.B.A. (1975) Immunologic injury in measles virus infection. II. Suppression of immune injury through antigenic modulation. *J. exp. Med.*, 142: 864–876.

Ju, G., Udem, S., Razer-Zisman, B. and Bloom, B. (1978) Isolation of a heterogenous population of temperature sensitive mutants of measles virus from persistently infected human lymphoblastoid cell lines. *J. exp. Med.*, 147: 1637–1652.

Laemmli, U.K. (1970) Cleavage of structural proteins during the assembly of the head of bacteriophage T4. *Nature (Lond.)*, 227: 680–685.

Lamb, R.A., Etkind, P.R. and Choppin, P.W. (1978) Evidence for a ninth influenza viral polypeptide. *Virology*, 91: 60–78.

Laver, W.G., Air, G.M., Webster, R.G., Gerhard, W., Ward, C.W. and Dopheide, T.A.A. (1979) Antigenic drift in type A influenza virus: sequence differences in the hemagglutinin of Hong Kong (H3N2) variants selected with monoclonal hybridoma antibodies. *Virology*, 98: 226–237.

Norrby, E. (1967) A carrier cell line of measles virus in Lu 106 cells. *Arch. ges. Virusforsch.*, 20: 15–224.

Norrby, E. and Gollmar, Y. (1975) Identification of measles virus-specific hemolysis-inhibiting antibodies separate from hemagglutination-inhibiting antibodies. *Infect. Immun.*, 11: 231–239.

Payne, F.E. and Baublis, J.V. (1973) Decreased reactivity of SSPE strains of measles virus with antibody. *J. infect. Dis.*, 127: 505–511.

Pelham, H.R.B. and Jackson, R.J. (1976) An efficient mRNA dependent translation system from reticulocyte lysates. *Europ. J. Biochem.*, 67: 247–256.

Rima, B.K., Lappin, S.A., Roberts, M.W. and Martin, S.J. (1981) A study of phosphorylation of the measles membrane protein. *J. gen. Virol.*, 56: 447–450.

Rustigian, R. (1966) Persistent infection of cells in culture by measles virus. I. Development and characteristics of Hela sublines persistently infected with complete virus. *J. Bacteriol.*, 92: 1792–1804.

Siddell, S.G., Wege, H., Barthel, A. and ter Meulen, V. (1980) Coronavirus JHM: cell-free synthesis of structural protein p60. *J. Virol.*, 17: 10–17.

Stephenson, J.R. and ter Meulen, V. (1979) Antigenic relationships between measles and canine distemper virus. Comparison of immune response in animals and humans to individual virus-specific polypeptides. *Proc. nat. Acad. Sci. U.S.A.*, 76: 6601–6605.

Stephenson, J.R., Siddell, S.G. and ter Meulen, V. (1981) Persistent and lytic infections with SSPE virus; a comparison of the synthesis of virus-specific polypeptides. *J. gen. Virol.*, 57: 191–197.

Ter Meulen, V., Müller, D. and Joppich, C. (1967) Fluorescence microscopy studies of brain tissue from a case of subacute progressive panencephalitis. *Germ. Med. Mth.*, 12: 438–441.

Ter Meulen, V., Enders-Ruckle, G., Müller, D. and Joppich, G. (1969) Immunhistological, microscopical and neurochemical studies on encephalitides. III. Subacute progressive panencephalitis. Virological and immuno-histological studies. *Acta Neuropath.*, 12: 244–259.

Ter Meulen, V., Katz, M. and Käckell, Y.M. (1973) Properties of SSPE virus; tissue culture and animal studies. *Ann. Clin. Res.*, 5: 293–297.

Ter Meulen, V., Löffler, S., Carter, M.J. and Stephenson, J.R. (1981) Antigenic characterization of measles and SSPE virus haemagglutinin by monoclonal antibodies. *J. gen. Virol.*, 57: 357–364.

Ter Meulen, V., Stephenson, J.R. and Kreth, H.W. (1983) Subacute sclerosing panencephalitis. In H. Fraenkel-Conrat and R.R. Wagner (Eds.). *Comprehensive Virology, Vol. 18*, Plenum Press, in press.

Thormar, H., Mehta, P.D. and Brown, H.R. (1978) Comparison of wild-type and subacute sclerosing panencephalitis strains of measles virus. Neurovirulence in ferrets and biological properties in cell cultures. *J. exp. Med.*, 148: 674.

Wechsler, S.L., Rustigian, R., Stallcup, K.C., Byers, K.B., Winston, S.H. and Fields, B.N. (1979) Measles virus-specific polypeptide synthesis in 2 persistently infected Hela cell lines. *J. Virol.*, 31: 677–684.

Wechsler, S.L., Weiner, H.L. and Fields, B.N. (1979) Immune response in subacute sclerosing panencephalitis: reduced antibody response to the matrix protein of measles virus. *J. Immunol.*, 123: 884–889.

Wiktor, T.J. and Koprowski, H. (1980) Antigenic variants of rabies virus. *J. exp. Med.*, 152: 99–112.

Wild, T.F., Bernard, A. and Greenland, T. (1981) Measles virus: evolution of a persistent infection in BGM cells. *Arch. Virol.*, 67: 297–308.

Immunology of Nervous System Infections, Progress in Brain Research, Vol. 59, edited by P.O. Behan, V. ter Meulen and F. Clifford Rose

Latency and other Consequences of Infection of the Nervous System with Herpes Simplex Virus

T.J. HILL, W.A. BLYTH, D.A. HARBOUR, E.L. BERRIE and A.B. TULLO

Department of Microbiology, University of Bristol, Bristol (U.K.)

THE SIGNIFICANCE OF THE NEUROTROPISM OF HERPES SIMPLEX VIRUS

The production of encephalitis by herpes simplex virus (HSV) in laboratory animals was one consequence of infection with the virus that came to light early in the history of virology (e.g. Goodpasture and Teague, 1923). In man, however, the virus's natural host, such severe destructive disease occurs only extremely rarely (Longson, 1977) in comparison with the establishment of the much more subtle and long-lasting state of latency in the tissues of the host's nervous sytem (Stevens and Cook, 1973; Baringer, 1975). Hence the phenomenon of neurotropism, first noted in laboratory animals, may reflect the requirement of the virus to reach the nervous system in order to establish latency. In such animals it seems that the controls which direct the virus into the latent state are less effective than in man and thereby the likelihood of a destructive infection of the central nervous system is greater. As a result of this different balance a considerable proportion of experimentally infected animals suffer a productive infection of the peripheral nervous system (PNS) and central nervous system (CNS) during primary infection and recover, though carrying a latent infection. The consequences of both active and latent infection can therefore be studied. Consequences of the former include pathological changes such as demyelination in the CNS while recurrent disease can result from activation of virus from the latent infection.

Spread of active infection through the nervous sytem will first be considered; demyelination resulting from this spread will then be discussed. Following this, some of the consequences of latent infection and its reactivation will be described.

SPREAD OF HSV TO AND WITHIN THE NERVOUS SYSTEM

If laboratory animals are inoculated with HSV at a peripheral site, the virus travels rapidly to the sensory ganglia and CNS via the peripheral nerves (Kristensson et al., 1971; Cook and Stevens, 1973; Baringer, 1975). The speed with which this transport occurs, about 2 mm/h (Kristensson et al., 1971; Field and Hill, 1974) suggests that retrograde axonal transport is involved (Kristensson, 1978). An alternative means of spread would be by infection of contiguous glial cells, but this would be very much slower: 1 mm/day (Narang, 1977; Narang and Codd, 1978). Moreover, in adult animals Schwann cells appear to be relatively resistant to infection with HSV (Cook and Stevens, 1973; Hill and Field, 1973). More direct evidence for intra-axonal transport of virions has come from electron microscopic observations of virions within axons (Hill et al., 1972; Cook and Stevens, 1973; Baringer and Swoveland, 1974; Kristensson et al., 1974).

Recent observations on the mouse ear model (Hill et al., 1975) by Eleanor Berrie in this laboratory, suggest that once the virus has reached the CNS many parts of the brain can become infected (Table I). In particular, it is noteworthy that virus can be isolated from the brainstem of all mice, sometimes at high titer, on the sixth day after infection. However, 60–70% of such animals survive and become clinically normal (except for ear paralysis, see below).

TABLE I

ISOLATION OF INFECTIOUS HSV FROM THE BRAINS OF MICE AFTER INFECTION OF THE RIGHT EAR

Mice were 4 weeks old, female, outbred, inoculated in right ear with 3×10^5 pfu (Hill et al., 1975). Region of the brain: right and left halves homogenized together. Data show virus isolated / total tested.

Region of brain	Days after infection				
	4	5	6	7	8
Olfactory lobe	0/8	0/8	0/13	0/8	0/8
Cerebral hemispheres	1/8	0/8	3/13	6/8	0/8
Cerebellum	0/8	2/8	7/13	5/8	1/8
Brainstem	6/8	4/8	12/13	7/8	3/8

Similar results have also been obtained in our laboratory by Dr. Andrew Tullo after inoculation of the mouse cornea (Table II). Again, although virus can be isolated from the brainstem of all mice on the fourth day after infection, 70% of these animals will survive. Sequential observations on animals infected in the cornea indicate that the virus first reaches the ophthalmic part of the trigeminal ganglion and the ipsilateral brainstem. Two days later the virus reaches the maxillary part of the ganglion, and after a further day, the mandibular branch.

TABLE II

ISOLATION OF HSV FROM THE TRIGEMINAL GANGLION AND BRAINSTEM OF MICE AFTER INFECTION OF THE CORNEA

Mice were 8 weeks old, male, outbred, cornea scarified through suspension containing 0.6×10^5 pfu. All mice showed signs of keratitis and most had lid margin disease. None showed signs of neurological disease.

Days after infection	Trigeminal ganglion (ipsilateral)			Brainstem	
	Ophthalmic I	Maxillary II	Mandibular III	Ipsilateral	Contralateral
1	0/4	0/4	0/4	0/4	0/4
2	2/4	0/4	0/4	1/4	0/4
3	2/4	0/4	0/4	1/4	0/4
4	4/4	1/4	0/4	4/4	0/4
5	3/3	2/3	2/3	3/3	1/3
6	3/3	3/3	1/3	3/3	3/3
7	3/3	2/3	3/3	3/3	3/3
9	0/2	0/2	0/2	2/2	0/2
11	0/3	0/3	0/3	1/3	0/3

These observations suggest that infection of the non-ophthalmic divisions of the ganglion may occur by spread of HSV back into the ganglion from the brainstem. The herpes virus of pseudorabies has also been shown to spread from the CNS to other neural and extraneural tissues (Field and Hill, 1974).

From all these observations it seems clear that, during the primary infection at least in mice, HSV is able to spread to, within and from the CNS.

DEMYELINATION AS A CONSEQUENCE OF INFECTION WITH HSV

As mentioned earlier it seems that the glia of the peripheral nervous system are relatively resistant to infection with HSV. In contrast, the glia of the CNS appear to be susceptible to infection (Townsend and Baringer, 1976; Townsend and Baringer, 1978; Townsend, 1981a). This may in part explain the intriguing demyelinating lesions which have been described in the CNS after inoculation of the mouse eye (Townsend and Baringer, 1976; Townsend and Baringer, 1978; Kristensson, et al., 1978). Such demyelination occurs predominantly in the central part of the trigeminal nerve root and ends abruptly at the junction with the PNS. We have now made similar observations in mice infected in the skin of the ear. At the time this model was first described (Hill et al., 1975), it was noted that paralysis of the ear often occurred within the first 6–10 days after infection. It is clear from recent observations that, at

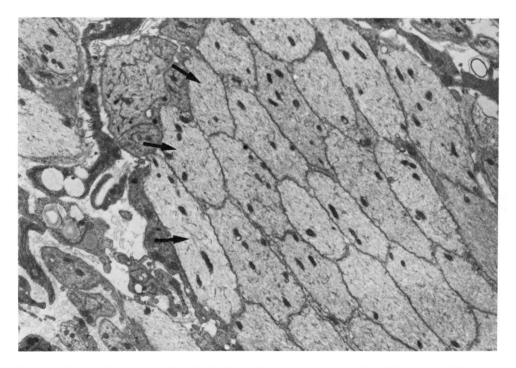

Fig. 1. Brainstem adjacent to root of the right facial nerve from mouse with ear paralysis. The animal was killed on the fourteenth day after infection of the right ear with 3×10^5 pfu HSV. Ear paralysis appeared on the sixth day after infection and therefore the paralysis was likely to have been permanent (Fig. 3). Group of about 20 demyelinated axons (arrows). Magnification: $\times 6700$.

the time ear paralysis develops, there is always demyelination of the central part of the facial nerve root (the facial or VII cranial nerve supplies motor nerves to the muscles of the ear) (Figs. 1 and 2). Animals which do not develop ear paralysis show no such lesions. This model therefore provides a system in which an easily demonstrable clinical sign can be related to a virally-induced demyelinating lesion in the CNS.

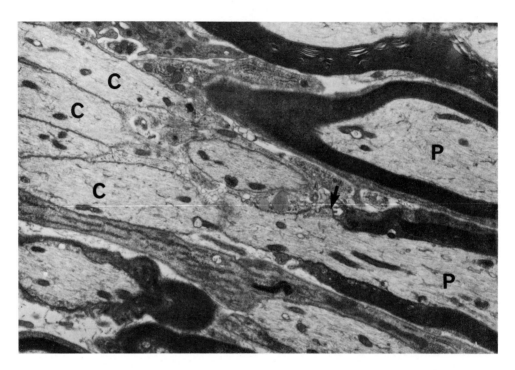

Fig. 2. Root of right facial nerve (same mouse as Fig. 1) at the junction of peripheral and central nervous system (arrow). The myelin of the peripheral axons (P) is intact but the central axons (C) are demyelinated. Magnification: × 9800.

A further advantage of the model is that the time of onset of ear paralysis gives an indication of whether mice are likely to survive or die from the infection. In outbred mice nearly all animals which die show ear paralysis, and the majority of such animals first show paralysis on the fifth day after infection (Fig. 3). By contrast, in animals that eventually survive and which develop ear paralysis, the majority first show paralysis on the sixth day after infection. This difference is not seen in the one inbred strain (NIH) that we have examined in detail (Fig. 4). In this inbred strain, as might be expected, the response is more uniform so that, whether they eventually die or survive, most mice first develop paralysis on the fifth day after infection.

In both outbred mice and the inbred strain NIH, however, it is clear that the recovery from ear paralysis in surviving animals is related to the day on which the paralysis first appears. In such animals, 90 % of those which first show ear paralysis on, or later than the seventh day after infection (outbred) or sixth day (NIH), will recover by the fifteenth day. Hence, in most of these animals the paralysis lasts for only 8–9 days. On the basis of these observations it is possible to select, with some degree of certainty, those in which the paralysis will be transient. Preliminary observations on such animals suggest that the demyelination in the root of the

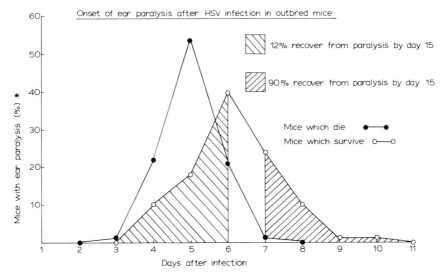

Fig. 3. Onset of ear paralysis after HSV infection in outbred mice. Daily observations were made on 183 four-week-old outbred mice after inoculation of the right ear with 3×10^5 pfu HSV type 1 (Hill et al., 1975); 78 (43 %) mice died and of the survivors 68 % developed ear paralysis.

$$* \ \frac{\text{Number of surviving mice (or mice which die) first showing ear paralysis}}{\text{Total of surviving mice (or mice which die) which develop ear paralysis}} \times 100.$$

facial nerve is limited to the region near the CNS/PNS junction. In contrast, in those animals with permanent ear paralysis (beyond the fifteenth day after infection), the demyelination extends from the outer part of the nerve root deep into the brainstem. Within the brainstem the demyelination is almost entirely limited to the tract of the facial nerve.

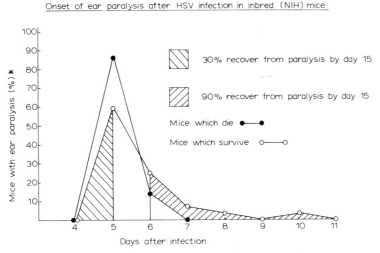

Fig. 4. Onset of ear paralysis after HSV infection in inbred (N1H) mice. Daily observations were made on 60 four-week-old N1H mice after inoculation of the right ear with 6×10^5 pfu (Harbour et al., 1981); 29 (48 %) mice died and of the survivors 90 % developed ear paralysis.

$$* \ \frac{\text{Number of surviving mice (or mice which die) first showing ear paralysis}}{\text{Total of surviving mice (or mice which die) which develop ear paralysis}} \times 100.$$

The production of demyelination by HSV in the CNS may involve direct effects of virus infection on the glia of the CNS (Townsend, 1981a) and also more indirect immunological mechanisms (Townsend and Baringer, 1979; Townsend, 1981b), e.g. the so-called "bystander" effect (Kristensson et al., 1979b). The mechanisms underlying the recovery of animals from ear paralysis have yet to be elucidated, but these could include rewrapping of demyelinated axons by Schwann cells from the periphery (Blakemore, 1976). Evidence for this repair process has been seen in the nerve root even in mice with permanent paralysis. Long-term observations on mice which suffered transient paralysis suggest that paralysis may recur. If these observations are confirmed this model may prove of value in attempts to investigate the involvement of HSV in chronic neurological disease (see below).

LATENT INFECTION

Possible differences between the PNS and CNS

Usually within 10–14 days after primary infection of a laboratory animal such as the mouse, infectious virus can no longer be demonstrated in homogenates of sensory ganglia or CNS (Tables I and II). After this time, latent infection can be demonstrated in the ganglia of the majority (80–90%) of animals. The explantation methods used to detect the latent infection are shown in Fig. 5. Using such methods latency has also been demonstrated in the CNS (Knott et al., 1973; Cabrera et al., 1980) but at a much lower incidence: 5% in one series of experiments (Cabrera et al., 1980). However, the size of this difference in incidence may reflect the difficulty of demonstrating latency in the CNS, more than a real difference in its occurrence (Kastrukoff et al., 1981), since Cabrera et al. (1980) demonstrated viral DNA in the brains of 30% of mice in which the incidence of latent infection in the brain was 5% and in the trigeminal ganglion 95%. From our own experience it is clear that virus reaches the CNS of many animals that will survive (Tables I and II) but as yet we have failed to demonstrate latency in this site.

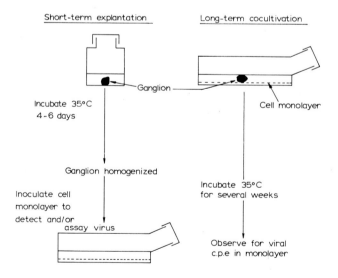

Fig. 5. Methods of culture used to detect latent infection with HSV.

Latency and the immune response

In discussing the possible consequences of latent infection with respect to the immune response, it is important to consider which cells in the nervous system harbour the latent virus and what viral functions are expressed.

Within the sensory ganglion there is now good evidence that the neuron is the site of latent infection (Cook et al., 1974; McClennan and Darby, 1980). Whether this is also true for the CNS remains to be established.

Once latency is established, all reports but one (Schwartz et al., 1978) show the absence of infectious virus in the ganglion. Indeed the weight of evidence is in favour of the "static state" of latency (Roizman, 1965) in which the whole viral genome is present but is extensively repressed (Table III). In such a state the latently infected neuron might express few, if any, viral antigens and they have not been detected during latent infection (Stevens and Cook, 1973). Therefore, no significant immunological response may be provoked unless the infection is reactivated. Support for this suggestion is provided by observations on latently infected mice which have low or undetectable levels of serum neutralizing antibodies (Sekizawa et al., 1980). Such animals develop neutralizing antibodies after a stimulus which is known to cause reactivation of virus in the ganglion.

TABLE III

PRESENCE AND EXPRESSION OF VIRAL FUNCTIONS IN THE LATENTLY INFECTED MOUSE GANGLION

		Expression	Reference
Viral genome	Complete	+	(Stevens and Cook, 1973)
	Complete	+	(human) (Baringer, 1975)
	Defective or non-inducible	+	(human) (Brown et al. 1979)
Viral DNA		+	(Puga et al. 1978)
Viral polypeptides	Antigens	−	(Stevens and Cook, 1973)
Viral mRNA		−	(Puga et al. 1978)
Productive infection		−	(Stevens and Cook, 1973)
		+	(Schwartz et al. 1978)

Reactivation of latency

The processes involved in removal of ganglia from the host and culture of the tissue in vitro clearly cause reactivation of the latent infection. Observations on a number of model systems, particularly in mice (Table IV), show that a variety of procedures can cause reactivation of the latent infection in vivo. They include nerve section, treatment with immunosuppressive drugs, and various kinds of trauma to the peripheral tissue which receives sensory nerves from the ganglion. The mechanisms whereby these stimuli might induce reactivation are discussed elsewhere (Hill, 1981). In the mouse ear model we have now shown that a stimulus (stripping the originally infected skin with cellophane tape) which induces recurrent disease in 30–50% of animals (Hill et al., 1978) also induces reactivation of virus in the ganglion (Fig. 6). Moreover, the application of dimethylsulphoxide (DMSO) to the ear, although inducing a lower incidence of recurrent disease, induces infectious virus in the ganglion and skin as efficiently as does stripping with cellophane tape.

TABLE IV

REACTIVATION OF LATENT INFECTION IN THE GANGLION OF MICE

Site of primary infection	Treatment	Site of reactivation of virus	Reference
Footpad	Section of peripheral nerve	Lumbosacral dorsal root ganglia	Walz et al. (1974)
Footpad	Intratracheal injection of pneumococci or mucin	Lumbosacral dorsal root ganglia	Stevens et al. (1975)
Intraocular	Postganglionic neurectomy	Superior cervical autonomic ganglion	Price and Schmitz (1978)
Cornea	Cyclophosphamide or X-rays	Trigeminal ganglion	Openshaw et al. (1979b)
Cornea	Cyclophosphamide, prednisolone, antithymocyte serum or trauma to ganglion	Trigeminal ganglion	Hill et al. (1981)
Cornea or lip	Dry-ice on lip	Trigeminal ganglion	Openshaw et al. (1979a)
Cornea or lip + passive immunization	Dry-ice on lip	Reactivation shown by seroconversion of "antibody-negative" mice	Sekizawa et al. (1980)
Ear	Cellophane tape stripping, application of xylene, retinoic acid or DMSO to ear	Cervical dorsal root ganglia	Harbour et al. (1983)

The immunological consequences of such reactivation in the ganglion are at present largely unknown. From the work of Sekizawa et al. (1980), cited previously, it is likely that the production of neutralizing antibody is stimulated, but effects on cell-mediated responses have not so far been reported. Baringer and Swoveland (1974) observed an accumulation of mononuclear cells around a few productively infected neurons in latently infected ganglia from rabbits. Furthermore, Kristensson et al., 1979a) noted significant numbers of lymphocytes in latently infected ganglia from mice. Whether such immune cells are present as a response to reactivation of latency, or whether they are concerned with maintenance of latency, remains to be established.

It is also of importance to discover whether peripheral stimuli, such as cellophane tape stripping or application of DMSO to the skin, can induce reactivation of any putative latent infection in the CNS.

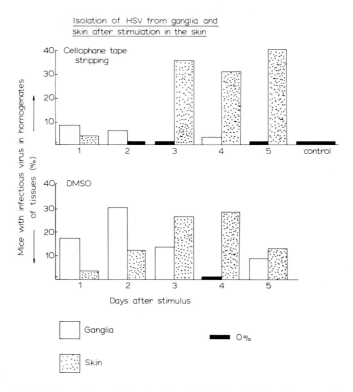

Fig. 6. Isolation of HSV from ganglia and skin after stimulation in the skin. The right ears of latently infected mice were stripped with cellophane tape (Hill et al., 1978) or treated with 50 μl of dimethylsulphoxide (DMSO). The incidence of latent infection in these animals would be about 85 % (Hill et al., 1978). On the first to fifth day after either treatment the second and third cervical ganglia and skin of the right ear of groups of mice (20–30/day for each stimulus) were ground, frozen and thawed and inoculated onto Vero cells to detect infectious virus (Harbour et al., 1983).

Consequences of reactivation for the host

It is assumed, perhaps incorrectly, that while the virus remains in the latent state in the nervous system the host suffers no ill effect. Once the infection has been reactivated a number of proven or hypothetical consequences may follow (Table V). Some of these consequences are discussed elsewhere (Hill and Blyth, 1976; Hill, 1981). With reference to neurological disease, perhaps the most serious and devastating result of reactivation would be the induction of encephalitis. There is no direct evidence that in man this rare disease can result from such reactivation (Longson and Bailey, 1977). However, in latently infected rabbits, encephalitis can be induced by anaphylactic shock (Good and Campbell, 1948) or injection of adrenalin (Schmidt and Rasmussen, 1960) so that a similar sequence of induction of herpetic encephalitis in man cannot be ruled out.

The suggestions that HSV may be associated with disorders of the autonomic nervous system (or tissues receiving an autonomic nerve supply), chronic neurological disease or psychological disorders, are largely speculative. It is true that HSV can establish latency in autonomic ganglia of animals (Price et al., 1975) and man (Warren et al., 1978), but whether, as suggested by Price and Notkins (1977) this is associated with clinical disease has yet to be

TABLE V

EVENTS WHICH MAY RESULT FROM REACTIVATION OF THE LATENT INFECTION

Note that points 4–6 are at present hypothetical.

(1)	Shedding of virus at the periphery without associated clinical disease
(2)	Recurrence of lesions at the periphery
(3)	Encephalitis
(4)	Disorders associated with dysfunction of the autonomic nervous system or recurrence of lesions in tissues innervated by autonomic ganglia?
(5)	Chronic neurological disease?
(6)	Psychological disorders?

demonstrated. A number of studies suggest that patients with some psychological disorders may have increased incidence of antibodies to HSV (Cleobury et al., 1971; Lycke et al., 1974). Similarly, patients with Bell's palsy have a higher incidence and titers of antibodies to HSV than controls (Vahlne et al., 1981). One study (Sequiera et al., 1979) reports that HSV DNA can be detected in brain tissue from psychiatric patients. Clearly it is important to discover to what extent HSV or fragments of its genome can be found in the CNS of the population at large. If such virus is present in the brain, it is also important to determine its association, if any, with neurological and other diseases. The host's immunological response to infection with the virus (see Nash, this volume) will also need to be fitted into the final picture. The availability of a system in which a well-defined neuropathy is associated with HSV infection (the mouse ear paralysis model) may help in answering some of these intriguing questions.

ACKNOWLEDGEMENTS

We are grateful for the excellent technical assistance of Penny Stirling, Peter Standing and Carolyn Shimeld. The work was supported by grants from the MRC and Wellcome Trust (A.B.T.).

REFERENCES

Baringer, J.R. (1975) Herpes simplex virus infection of nervous tissue in animals and man. *Progr. med. Virol.*, 20: 1–26.

Baringer, J.R. and Swoveland, P. (1974) Persistent herpes simplex virus infection in rabbit trigeminal ganglia. *Lab. Invest.*, 30: 230–240.

Blakemore, W.F. (1976) Invasion of Schwann cells into the spinal cord of the rat following local injection of lysolecithin. *Neuropath. appl. Neurobiol.*, 2: 21–39.

Brown, S.M., Subak-Sharpe, J.H., Warren, K.G., Wroblewska, Z. and Koprowski, H. (1979) Detection by complementation of defective or uninducible (herpes simplex type 1) virus genomes latent in human ganglia. *Proc. nat. Acad. Sci. U.S.A.*, 76: 2364–2368.

Cabrera, C.V., Wohlenberg, C., Openshaw, H., Rey-Mendez, M., Puga, A. and Notkins, A.L. (1980) Herpes simplex DNA sequences in the CNS of latently infected mice. *Nature (Lond.)*, 288: 288–290.

Cleobury, J.R., Skinner, G.R.B., Thouless, M.E. and Wildy, P. (1971) Association between psychopathic disorder and serum antibody to herpes simplex virus (type 1). *Brit. Med. J.*, i: 438–439.

Cook, M.L. and Stevens, J.G. (1973) Pathogenesis of herpetic neuritis and ganglionitis in mice: evidence for intraaxonal transport of infection. *Infect. Immun.*, 7: 272–288.

Cook, M.L., Bastone, V.B. and Stevens, J.G. (1974) Evidence that neurons harbour latent herpes simplex virus. *Infect. Immun.*, 9: 946–951.

Field, H.J. and Hill, T.J. (1974) The pathogenesis of pseudorabies in mice following peripheral inoculation. *J. gen. Virol.*, 23: 145–157.

Goodpasture, E.W. and Teague, O. (1923) Experimental production of herpetic lesions in organs and tissues of the rabbit. *J. med. Res.*, 44: 121–133.

Good, R.A. and Campbell, B. (1948) The precipitation of latent herpes simplex encephalitis by anaphylactic shock. *Proc. Soc. exp. Biol. N.Y.*, 68: 82–87.

Harbour, D.A., Hill, T.J. and Blyth, W.A. (1981) Acute and recurrent herpes simplex in several strains of mice. *J. gen. Virol.*, 55: 31–40.

Harbour, D.A., Hill, T.J. and Blyth, W.A. (1983) Recurrent herpes simplex in the mouse: inflammation in the skin and activation of virus in the ganglia following peripheral stimulation. *J. gen. Virol.*, in press.

Hill, T.J. (1981) Mechanisms involved in recurrent herpes simplex. In A.J. Nahmias, W.R. Dowdle and R.F. Schinazi (Eds.), *The Human Herpesviruses*, Elsevier, New York, pp. 241–244.

Hill, T.J., Field, H.J. and Roome, A.P.C. (1972) Intra axonal location of herpes simplex virus particles. *J. gen. Virol.*, 15: 253–255.

Hill, T.J. and Field, H.J. (1973) The interaction of herpes simplex virus with cultures of peripheral nervous tissue: an electron microscopic study. *J. gen. Virol.*, 21: 123–133.

Hill, T.J., Field, H.J. and Blyth, W.A. (1975) Acute and recurrent infection with herpes simplex virus in the mouse: a model for studying latency and recurrent disease. *J. gen. Virol.*, 28: 341–353.

Hill, T.J. and Blyth, W.A. (1976) An alternative theory of herpes simplex recurrence and a possible role for prostaglandins. *Lancet*, i: 397–398.

Hill, T.J., Blyth, W.A. and Harbour, D.A. (1978) Trauma to the skin causes recurrence of herpes simplex in the mouse. *J. gen. Virol.*, 39: 21–28.

Hill, T.J., Ahluwalia, K. and Blyth, W.A. (1981) Infection with herpes simplex virus in the eye and trigeminal ganglia of mice. In R. Sundmacher (Ed.), *Herpetic Eye Diseases*, J.F. Bergmann, Munchen, pp. 37–42.

Kastrukoff, L., Long, C., Doherty, P.C., Wroblewska, Z. and Koprowski, H. (1981) Isolation of virus from brain after immunosuppression of mice with latent herpes simplex *Nature (Lond.)*, 291: 432.

Knott, F.B., Cook, M.L. and Stevens, J.G. (1973) Latent herpes simplex virus in the central nervous system of rabbits and mice. *J. exp. Med.*, 138: 740–744.

Kristensson, K. (1978) Retrograde transport of macromolecules in axons. *Ann. Rev. Pharmacol. Toxicol.*, 18: 97–110.

Kristensson, K., Lycke, E. and Sjöstrand, J. (1971) Spread of herpes simplex virus in peripheral nerves. *Acta neuropath.*, 17: 44–53.

Kristensson, K., Ghetti, B. and Wisniewski, H.M. (1974) Study of the propagation of herpes simplex virus (type 2) into the brain after intraocular infection. *Brain Res.*, 69: 189–201.

Kristensson, K., Vahlne, A., Persson, L.A. and Lycke, E. (1978) Neural spread of herpes simplex types 1 and 2 in mice after corneal or subcutaneous (footpad) inoculation. *J. Neurol. Sci.*, 35: 331–340.

Kristensson, K., Svennerholm, B., Persson, L., Vahlne, A. and Lycke, E. (1979a) Latent herpes simplex virus trigeminal ganglionic infection in mice and demyelination in the central nervous sytem. *J. Neurol. Sci.*, 43: 253–264.

Kristensson, K., Thormar, H. and Wisniewski, H.M. (1979b) Myelin lesions in the rabbit eye model as a bystander effect of herpes simplex and Visna virus sensitisation. *Acta Neuropath.*, 48: 215–217.

Longson, M. and Bailey, A.S. (1977) Herpes encephalitis. In A.P. Waterson (Ed.), *Recent Advances in Clinical Virology, Vol. 1*, Churchill and Livingstone, Edinburgh, pp. 1–19.

Lycke, E., Norby, R. and Roos, B. (1974) A serological study on mentally ill patients. *Brit. J. Psychiat.*, 124: 273–279.

McLennan, J.L. and Darby, G. (1980) Herpes simplex virus latency: the cellular location of virus in dorsal root ganglia and the fate of the infected cell following virus activation. *J. gen. Virol.*, 51: 213–243.

Narang, H. (1977) The pathway into the central nervous system after intraocular infection of herpes simplex (type 1) virus in rabbits. *Neuropath. appl. Neurobiol.*, 3: 490.

Narang, H.K. and Codd, A.A. (1978) The pathogenesis and pathway into the central nervous system after intraocular infection of herpes simplex virus type 1 in rabbits. *Neuropath. applied Neurobiol.*, 4: 137.

Openshaw, H., Puga, A. and Notkins, A.L. (1979a) Herpes simplex virus infection in sensory ganglia, immune control, latency and reactivation. *Fed. Proc.*, 38: 2660.

Openshaw, H., Asher, L.V. Wohlenberg, C., Sekizawa, T. and Notkins, A.L. (1979b) Acute and latent infection in sensory ganglia with herpes simplex virus: immune control and virus reactivation. *J. gen. Virol.*, 44: 205–215.

Price, R.W., Katz, B.J. and Notkins, A.L. (1975) Latent infection of the peripheral autonomic nervous system with herpes simplex virus. *Nature (Lond.)*, 257: 686–688.

Price, R. and Notkins, A.L. (1977) Viral infections of the autonomic nervous system and its target organs: pathogenetic mechanisms. *Med. Hypoth.*, 3: 33.

Price, R.W. and Schmitz, J. (1978) Reactivation of latent herpes simplex virus infection of the autonomic nervous system by postganglionic neurectomy. *Infect. Immun.*, 19: 523–532.

Puga, A., Rosenthal, J.D., Openshaw, H. and Notkins, A.L. (1978) Herpes simplex virus DNA and mRNA sequences in acutely and chronically infected trigeminal ganglia of mice. *Virology*, 89: 102–111.

Roizman, B. (1965) An inquiry into the mechanisms of herpes infections of man. In M. Pollard (Ed.), *Perspectives in Virology, IV*, Hocker, New York, 283.

Schmidt, J.R. and Rasmussen, A.F. (1960) Activation of latent herpes simplex encephalitis by chemical means. *J. infect Dis.*, 106: 154–158.

Schwartz, J., Whetsell, W.O. and Elizan, T.S. (1978) Latent herpes simplex virus infection of mice. Infectious virus in homogenates of latently infected dorsal root ganglia. *J. Neuropath. exp. Neurol.*, 37: 45–55.

Sekizawa, T., Openshaw, H., Wohlenberg, C. and Notkins, A.L. (1980) Latency of herpes simplex virus in absence of neutralizing antibody: a model of reactivation. *Science*, 210: 1026–1028.

Sequiera, L.W., Jennings, L.C., Carrasso, L.H., Lord, M.A., Curry, A. and Sutton, R.N.P. (1979) Detection of herpes virus genome in brain tissue. *Lancet*, ii: 609–612.

Stevens, J.G. and Cook, M.L. (1973) Latent herpes simplex virus in sensory ganglia. *Persp. Virol.*, 8: 171–188.

Stevens, J.G., Cook, M.L. and Jordan, M.C. (1975) Reactivation of latent herpes simplex virus after pneumococcal pneumonia in mice. *Infect. Immun.*, 11: 635.

Townsend, J.J. (1981a) The relationship of astrocytes and macrophages to CNS demyelination after experimental herpes simplex virus infection. *J. Neuropath. exp. Neurol.*, 40: 369–379.

Townsend, J.J. (1981b) The demyelinating effect of corneal HSV infections in normal and nude (athymic) mice. *J. Neurol. Sci.*, 50: 435–441.

Townsend, J.J. and Baringer, J.R. (1976) Comparative vulnerability of peripheral and central nervous tissue to herpes simplex virus. *J. Neuropath. exp. Neurol.*, 35: 100.

Townsend, J.J. and Baringer, J.R. (1978) Central nervous system susceptibility to herpes simplex infection. *J. Neuropath. exp. Neurol.*, 37: 255–262.

Townsend, J.J. and Baringer, J.R. (1979) Morphology of the CNS disease in immunosuppressed mice after peripheral HSV inoculation. *Lab. Invest.*, 40: 178–182.

Vahlne, A., Edström, S., Arstila, P., Beran, M., Ejnall, M., Nylen, O. and Lycke, E. (1981) Bell's palsy and herpes simplex virus. *Arch. Otolaryngol.*, 107: 79–81.

Walz, M.A., Price, R.W. and Notkins, A.L. (1974) Latent ganglionic infection with herpes simplex virus types 1 and 2: viral reactivation in vivo after neurectomy. *Science*, 184: 1185–1187.

Warren, K.G., Brown, S.M., Wroblewska, Z., Gilden, D., Koprowski, H. and Subak-Sharpe, J. (1978) Isolation of latent herpes simplex virus from the superior cervical and vagus ganglions of human beings. *New Engl. J. Med.*, 298: 1068–1069.

Immunology of Nervous System Infections, Progress in Brain Research, Vol. 59, edited by P.O. Behan, V. ter Meulen and F. Clifford Rose

Cell-Mediated Immune Responses in Herpes Simplex Virus-Infected Mice

A.A. NASH

Department of Pathology, University of Cambridge, Tennis Court Road, Cambridge (U.K.)

INTRODUCTION

The importance of cell-mediated immunity in the defense against herpes simplex virus infections is now well documented. However, hitherto, surprisingly little information is available on the particular lymphocyte subsets involved in protection against the primary infection and in immune surveillance against latent and recurrent infections. In order to study the detailed immune response against herpes simplex virus type 1 infection the mouse ear model was used in which the primary, latent and recurrent phases of the disease have been well defined (Hill et al., 1975). Briefly, following the inoculation of herpes into the ear pinna, a local infection is produced in which infective virus titers become maximal on the third day and gradually dwindle to become undetectable after a week. Infectious virus can also be recovered from the dorsal root ganglia during the third to fifth day, but the titers are much lower than those detected in the pinna. After a period of 20 days, about 90 % of the mice are likely to be latently infected, i.e. infective virus can be recovered from the ganglia only after a period of culture in vitro (Field et al., 1979).

CELL-MEDIATED IMMUNITY DURING THE PRIMARY INFECTION

To study cell-mediated immune responses during the primary infection, a functional characterization of the cell types present in the lymph node draining the infected pinna was undertaken. Four days after infection with 10^5 pfu herpes simplex virus type 1 (clone SC16) cytotoxic T-cells are detected, which have maximal activity between days 6 and 8 and dwindle to undetectable levels by day 14 (Nash et al., 1980). These cells are H-2K, D-restricted, and are specific for herpes simplex. During the time when cytotoxic T-cell activity can be detected, the adoptive transfer of delayed hypersensitivity (DH) to normal syngeneic recipients is effective. The DH activity is maximum 48 h after transfer/infection, is mediated by T-cells which are specific for herpes and are H-2$1_A$ region restricted (Nash et al., 1981a). In addition to cytotoxic T-cell and DH-T cell activity, the draining lymph nodes also contain virus-specific T cells which depress infective virus titers in the pinna when adoptively transferred to infected syngeneic recipients. This anti-viral T-cell response is present in the node between days 4 and 12 and is restricted by the H-2K(D) and I_A subregion. This suggests a role for both cytotoxic

T-cells and their helpers or DH-T cells (Nash et al., 1981a). The suggestion that more than one T-cell subset is required for host resistance to herpes simplex, as defined by H-2 mapping experiments, was made by Howes et al. (1979).

CELL-MEDIATED IMMUNITY DURING LATENCY

After 20 days, during the period of virus latency, the draining lymph node contains memory cells for the various populations discussed in the previous section. A general memory response can be detected by the lymphocyte proliferation assay, in which lymph node cells are cultured with herpes virus antigen for 5 days and [^{3}H]thymidine incorporation measured. The cells undergoing proliferation are T cells and persist in the draining lymph node throughout the life of the mouse. These memory cells also appear in the contralateral node and the spleen, but in reduced numbers compared to the draining node. Specific cytotoxic T-cell memory can be demonstrated in the draining node following a re-injection of infective virus at the site of the primary infection. The cytotoxic response generated is effective at low effector to target ratios and the cells appear in the node by day 2 post-challenge (Nash et al., 1980).

Perhaps the most interesting cell type demonstrable at these times is an Ig-positive, Thy 1.2-negative, non-macrophage cell which can suppress an established DH response when transferred into herpes pre-sensitized recipients (Nash and Gell, 1980). Alternatively, this cell type can suppress the adoptive transfer of DH when mixed with DH-positive cell suspensions. The suppressor cells are specific for herpes and interestingly are restricted to the draining node. Although B-suppressor cells are not detected in vaccinia-infected mice, they are found in mice infected with a thymidine kinase-deficient mutant, which does not produce a latent infection. It is considered that these cells act as homeostatic regulators of DH reactions, in which the intensity and duration are controlled. These cells do not affect the induction of DH reactions.

CELL-MEDIATED IMMUNITY DURING RECURRENCES: A MODEL FOR STUDYING SPECIFIC DH UNRESPONSIVENESS

In man, defects in cell-mediated immunity, as measured by a failure to produce lymphokines such as macrophage migration inhibition factor (MIF), have been measured during recurrent herpes infections (Shillitoe et al., 1977). Similar findings have been made in a guinea pig-herpes model (Donnenberg et al., 1980). These observations suggest that the failure to mobilize macrophages (and possibly other cell types) at the site of a herpes infection leads to local virus replication resulting in a clinical disease. How does such a failure occur? The rapid localization of macrophages at sites of antigen deposition is considered to be a property of DH-T cells. It is known that such cells are particularly sensitive to regulation by suppressor cells (e.g. B suppressor cells — previous section). In addition, it is also possible to suppress the induction of DH reactions by injecting herpes simplex virus i.v. (Nash et al., 1981b). In this model, mice simultaneously injected i.v. and s.c. are rendered DH unresponsive. This form of tolerance is rapidly induced, of long duration and specific for the herpes type used in the initial i.v. injection. Part, if not all, of the tolerance mechanism is due to suppressor T-cells (Nash et al., 1981c). Simultaneous to the induction of tolerance of DH, immunity to the virus is also established in the form of neutralizing antibodies and cytotoxic T-cell responses (Nash and Ashford, 1982). Consequently a form of split T-cell tolerance exists following this type of injection protocol.

An important feature of this model is that the draining lymph nodes from DH-tolerized mice do not contain transferable DH cells, neither do they contain cells capable on transfer of reducing infective virus titers in normal recipients, despite the presence of transferable cytotoxic T-cells (Nash and Ashford, 1982). These data argue in favour of a role for DH in rapidly localizing anti-viral cell mechanisms in order that an efficient eradication of virus is produced.

Another feature of this model is that latent infections are established in the cervical dorsal root ganglia, thus allowing an evaluation of the role of DH-T-cells in the immune surveillance against herpes recurrences. Whether or not functional cell defects of this type will predispose the herpes-infected host to a greater incidence of, and/or more severe recrudescenses, is still an open question. At least this model provides an opportunity to test the hypothesis.

ACKNOWLEDGEMENT

This work was supported by the Medical Research Council of Great Britain.

REFERENCES

Donnenberg, A.D., Bell, R.B. and Aurelian, L. (1980) Immunity to herpes simplex virus type 2. Development of virus-specific lymphoproliferative and LIF responses in HSV-2 infected guinea pigs. *Infect. Immun.*, 30: 90–109.

Field, H.J., Bell, S.E., Elion, G.B., Nash, A.A. and Wildy, P. (1979) Effect of acycloguanosine treatment on acute and latent herpes simplex infections in mice. *Antimicrobial Agents and Chemotherapy*, 15: 554–561.

Hill, T.J., Field, H.J. and Blyth, W.A. (1975) Acute and recurrent infection with herpes simplex. *J. gen. Virol.*, 28: 341–353.

Howes, E.L., Taylor, W., Mitchison, N.A. and Simpson, E. (1979) MHC matching shows that at least two T-cell subsets determine resistance to HSV. *Nature (Lond.)*, 277: 67–68.

Nash, A.A. and Gell, P.G.H. (1980) Cell-mediated immunity in herpes simplex virus infected mice: suppression of delayed hypersensitivity by an antigen specific B lymphocyte. *J. gen. Virol.*, 48: 359–364.

Nash, A.A. and Ashford, N.P.N. (1982) Split T-cell tolerance in herpes simplex virus infected mice and its implication for anti-viral immunity. *Immunology*, in press.

Nash, A.A., Quartey-Papafio, R. and Wildy, P. (1980) Cell mediated immunity in herpes simplex virus-infected mice: functional analysis of lymph node cells during periods of acute and latent infection, with reference to cytotoxic and memory cells. *J. gen. Virol.*, 48: 309–317.

Nash, A.A., Phelan, J. and Wildy, P. (1981a) Cell mediated immunity in herpes simplex virus-infected mice: H-2 mapping of the delayed-type hypersensitivity response and antiviral T cell response. *J. Immunol.*, 126: 1260–1262.

Nash, A.A., Gell, P.G.H. and Wildy, P. (1981b) Tolerance and immunity in mice infected with herpes simplex virus: simultaneous induction of protective immunity and tolerance to delayed type hypersensitivity. *Immunology*, 43: 153–159.

Nash, A.A., Phelan, J., Gell, P.G.H. and Wildy, P. (1981c) Tolerance and immunity in mice infected with herpes simplex virus: studies on the mechanism of tolerance to delayed type hypersensitivity. *Immunology*, 43: 363–369.

Shillitoe, E.J., Wilton, J.M.A. and Lehner, T. (1977) Sequential changes in cell-mediated immune responses to herpes simplex virus after recurrent herpetic infections in humans. *Infect. Immun.*, 18: 130–137.

Immunology of Nervous System Infections, Progress in Brain Research, Vol. 59, edited by P.O. Behan, V. ter Meulen and F. Clifford Rose

T-Cell Control of Herpesvirus Infections: Lessons from the Epstein–Barr Virus

A.B.RICKINSON

Department of Pathology, University of Bristol, The Medical School, Bristol BS8 1TD (U.K.)

INTRODUCTION

The historical association of the Epstein–Barr (EB) virus with two human malignancies, Burkitt's lymphoma and nasopharyngeal carcinoma, has rightly provoked enormous interest in the oncogenic potential of this agent (Epstein and Achong, 1979; Klein, 1979) and has tended to set it aside as a rather special member of the human herpesvirus group. Whilst undoubtedly important, this involvement with malignant disease should not be allowed to impose too strongly upon the wider view of EB virus biology from which it is clear that, overall, this agent displays a finely balanced and largely apathogenic relationship with its host species, quite characteristic of that shown by many other herpesvirus.

Thus, in primitive communities, primary EB virus infection occurs naturally during the first few years of life when it is almost always clinically silent. Paradoxically, when infection is delayed until the second decade or later, as happens increasingly in the Western world, it is accompanied in at least a proportion of cases by the clinical symptoms of infectious mononucleosis (IM) (Henle et al., 1968; Henle and Henle, 1979a). Primary infection at whatever age regularly induces permanent seroconversion to EB virus antibody-positivity and establishes a carrier state, whereby the virus persists for life as an apparently non-productive infection in the lymphoid tissues of the serologically immune host (Nilsson et al., 1971). This persistent infection is very largely asymptomatic and periods of renewed virus replication can occur without clinical sequelae, as witnessed by the detection of infectious virus in the throat washings of a proportion of healthy seropositive individuals (Gerber et al., 1972). As with other human herpesviruses, this pattern of "latent" infection interspersed with periodic virus secretion guarantees that EB virus remains endemic even within quite small and isolated host communities (Henle and Henle, 1979b).

IMMUNOLOGICAL CONTROL OF LATENT HERPESVIRUS INFECTIONS

The importance of cell-mediated immune mechanisms in the control of herpesvirus infections has for some time been apparent from clinical observations. Thus immunodeficient children with impaired cellular responses are particularly susceptible to severe infection with these agents (Shore and Feorino, 1981). Moreover, allograft recipients receiving immunosuppressive therapy suffer reactivations of latent herpes simplex (HSV), varicella zoster (VZV) and cytomegalo (CMV) virus infections with clinical symptoms very often accompa-

[189]

nying the renewed virus replication (Merigan, 1981); such reactivations occur with a concomitant rise in anti-viral antibody titers in the serum, a rise which offers no apparent protection against the infection but rather is a consequence of the increased antigenic load. In an exactly analogous way, immunosuppressed patients suffer a reactivation of EB virus infection with renewed viral secretion in the throat (Strauch et al., 1974) and an amplification of the anti-viral antibody response (Henle and Henle, 1981). Whilst this reactivation has generally been considered asymptomatic, recent results now suggest that the unusually high incidence of lymphoma to which these patients are subject may be a long-term and hitherto unsuspected consequence of the EB virus–host imbalance, as at least some of these lymphomas are now known to be EB virus genome-positive (Crawford et al., 1980; Hanto et al., 1981).

The above observations, stressing as they do the common ground between all 5 human herpesviruses in terms of their virus–host interactions, strongly suggest that the experimental analysis of any one such interaction will provide important lessons for the understanding of all the others. It is with this in mind that this chapter seeks to describe what has been learnt to date about the immune control of EB virus infection in man.

THE EB VIRUS MODEL

The properties which distinguish EB virus from the other human herpesviruses are its strict tropism for B-lymphocytes (Jondal and Klein, 1973) and its capacity to transform or "immortalize" these cells in vitro into permanent immunoglobulin-secreting B-lymphoblastoid cell lines (Henle et al., 1967; Pope et al., 1968; Pope, 1979). Indeed it is this unique transforming ability which has been turned to advantage in the study of cellular responses to the viral infection and which makes the EB virus model so amenable to experimental analysis. Thus, permanent target cell lines exist in which every cell carries the EB viral genome and expresses the virus-associated nuclear antigen EBNA (Reedman and Klein, 1973), a DNA-binding protein through which the virus is thought to exert its proliferative influence upon the infected cell (Klein et al., 1979). In many such cell lines, at any one time a small proportion of the cells are moving into a cycle of virus replication, accompanied by the appearance of "late" viral antigens and culminating in cell death. The proportion of lytically-infected cells can be increased in at least some lines by treatment with chemical inducing agents such as phorbol esters or sodium butyrate (zur Hausen et al., 1978; Kallin et al., 1979) and, in the absence of a fully permissive culture system, much of the biochemical analysis of virus replication has been carried out using induced cultures of this kind.

The cascade of viral protein synthesis with occurs during the lytic cycle is traditionally described in terms of those "antigens" originally defined by immunofluorescence testing, even though more recent immune precipitation studies have shown many of these "antigens" to be composed of several distinct virus-related proteins. Firstly, certain viral envelope determinants constituting the early membrane antigen (EMA) are expressed on the cell surface (Ernberg et al., 1974) before another complex family of proteins, known collectively as early antigen (EA), appears within the cell signalling the progressive inhibition of host cell macromolecular syntheses (Henle et al., 1971; Gergely et al., 1971; Kallin et al., 1979). Thereafter, viral genome replication is followed by intracellular accumulation of the viral capsid antigen (VCA) (Henle and Henle, 1966) and by expression of the complete array of viral envelope determinants which constitute the late membrane antigen (LMA) (Ernberg et al., 1974; Thorley-Lawson, 1979; North et al., 1980) and which appear on cellular membranes before virion assembly and release.

Recognition of these distinct viral antigens is more than of academic interest for each provides an independent parameter whereby the serological response of the host to EB virus infection can be characterized. Indeed, as will become apparent, the spectrum of anti-EB viral antibodies shown by any one individual can provide a valuable index of the virus–host balance which exists in that individual. After more than a decade of work dominated by these serological techniques, only recently have we begun to gain some understanding of the host's cell-mediated responses to EB virus infection and of the antigens against which they are directed. Clearly this is an area of fundamental importance for any overall view of the virus–host interaction and one that will be stressed in the following discussion of the biology of primary and persistent EB virus infections in man.

Primary EB virus infection

The available data come almost exclusively from those cases in which the primary infection is clinically manifest as IM. In this respect, it is still not clear whether the disease episode presents a true magnification of cellular events as they occur during sub-clinical infection or whether the two situations are qualitatively as well as quantitatively distinct.

Fig. 1 presents a diagrammatic view of EB virus–cell relationships as they develop during the acute phase of IM. Primary infection occurs by the oral route and the virus replicates within the oropharynx such that by the time of onset of clinical symptoms, infectious virus is regularly detectable in throat washings (Gerber et al., 1972; Miller et al., 1973). Whether the permissive cell type supporting virus replication at the site of primary infection is a B-lymphocyte or a particular type of oropharyngeal epithelium is still not known, but certainly B-cells in transit through this area must become infected and thus serve to initiate the generalized infection which is witnessed in IM. The presence of virus-infected B cells in the blood of patients with acute IM was first recognized through the high frequency of "spontaneous transformation" of their cultured lymphocytes into EB virus genome-positive lymphoblastoid cell lines (Pope, 1967). From more recent work, it would appear that most of the infected cells present in the circulation during the acute phase of the disease are in the very early stages of the infectious cycle with no detectable expression of viral antigens (Crawford et al., 1978), whilst a few are demonstrably EBNA-positive (Klein et al., 1976a) and some may even show evidence of virus-induced immunoglobulin synthesis (Robinson et al., 1981).

Humoral responses to the primary infection

During the incubation period of the disease, virus replication occurring in the oropharynx (and possibly at other sites) produces "late" viral antigens so that, by the onset of clinical symptoms, IM patients have already developed high titers of antibodies to VCA and MA, and many also become transiently anti-EA-positive; somewhat in contrast, antibodies to EBNA are usually absent at this time and only become detectable during convalescence (Henle et al., 1974). In terms of influencing the course of the infection, antibodies to certain components of the MA complex are probably the most important in that they are capable of neutralizing virus (de Schrijver et al., 1974) and thus of preventing any further dissemination of infectious virions by cell-free viraemia (Rickinson et al., 1975).

The above virus-specific humoral response is accompanied by the appearance of a battery of "irrelevant" reactivities, both auto-antibodies and a variety of heterophile antibodies, one of which, when present, is diagnostic of EB virus-induced mononucleosis and forms the basis of the Paul–Bunnell test (Henle and Henle, 1979a). It is tempting to speculate that at least some of these antibodies arise as a direct consequence of the capacity of EB virus to activate im-

CELL-VIRUS RELATIONSHIPS IN INFECTIOUS MONONUCLEOSIS

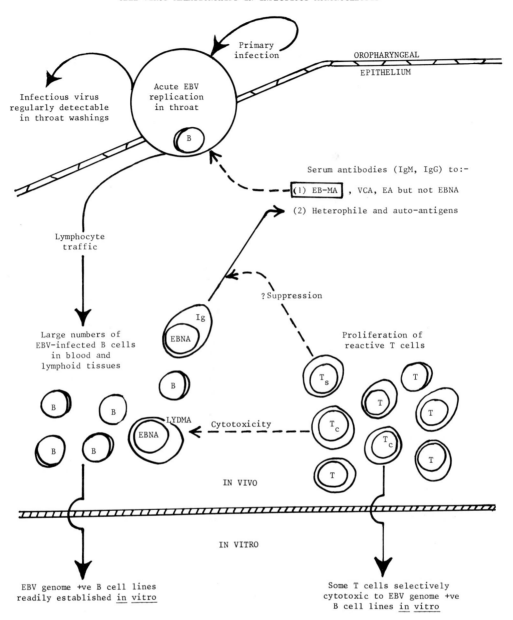

Fig. 1. A diagrammatic view of the events of primary EB virus infection leading to acute infectious mononucleosis. The various cell–virus relationships are shown in the context of the immune responses (humoral and cellular) to which they give rise. The evidence upon which this *possible* view of events is based is described in the text.

munoglobulin synthesis in infected B-cells (Rosen et al., 1977). This is still a debatable point, however, for a somewhat similar sequence of events is seen in the mononucleosis-like syndrome caused by CMV, a herpesvirus without direct B-cell-activating properties (Klemola et al., 1970).

Cellular response to the primary infection

The acute phase of IM is characterized by the appearance of large numbers of atypical lymphocytes, not only in peripheral blood, but also infiltrating many tissues (Carter, 1975). Of central importance to our view of the pathogenesis of this disease is the observation that most of these cells are not, as had been anticipated, virus-infected B-cells but in fact T-lymphoblasts reactive to the viral infection (Sheldon et al., 1973). This reactive population is heterogeneous, perhaps more so than is currently appreciated, and contains at least two (and very probably more) functional components.

(a) A cytotoxic T-cell (Tc) component. This is present in Fcγ-receptor-negative cell populations which, in in vitro chromium release assays, appear to kill EB virus genome-positive target cell lines selectively (Svedmyr and Jondal, 1975; Royston et al., 1975), although in a manner which is unusual in that target cell recognition shows no obvious HLA restriction (Lipinski et al., 1979; Seeley et al., 1981). These results were first interpreted as demonstrating the existence of a novel lymphocyte-detected membrane antigen, LYDMA, expressed on the surface of EB virus-infected cells early in the viral cycle in vivo, where it serves to elicit the primary T-cell response, as well as on all EB virus-transformed B-cell lines in vitro, rendering them sensitive to IM T-cell-mediated cytolysis (Klein et al., 1976b).

Subsequent studies have raised doubts about the EB virus-specificity of the above response and some workers have now suggested that this non-HLA-restricted cytotoxicity might represent a particular kind of "activated natural killing" induced by the acute viral infection (Klein et al., 1980; 1981). Such an in vivo response, initiated by the presence of large numbers of virus-infected B-cells and perhaps augmented by accompanying interferon release, would be similar in many respects to that which can be generated experimentally by exposing human T-cells to one of a variety of mitogenic or antigenic stimuli in vitro (Jondal and Targan, 1978; Seeley and Golub, 1978; Klein et al., 1980). Identification of the target antigen(s) for IM T-cell cytotoxicity, and of the time of its (their) appearance on B-cells post-EB virus infection, is crucial to any proper understanding of the pathogenesis of the disease.

Thus, if the relevant antigen is expressed on the B-cell surface at an early stage of the viral cycle (coincident with or soon after the appearance of EBNA), then this would imply that IM patients should exercise a very strict control over the numbers of virus-infected B cells in vivo, through the capacity of cytotoxic T-cells to destroy target B cells right at the point of onset of virus-induced B-cell proliferation. This view, broadly in line with that originally proposed on the basis of the early studies on IM T-cell cytotoxicity (Klein et al., 1976b), has been incorporated into the model of virus–cell interactions in IM which is shown in Fig. 1. If, on the other hand, expression of the relevant IM T-cell-detected target antigen is not functionally linked to the initiation of virus-induced B-cell transformation per se, but is a secondary event which may not occur until several cell divisions later, then this would leave the way open for a considerably greater expansion of the virus-infected B cell pool than that illustrated in Fig. 1. Indeed, this alternative view of the IM T-cell response, in which a relatively inefficient effector cell is dominant, might explain why the clinical course of the disease can sometimes be so unusually prolonged.

(b) A suppressor T-cell (Ts) component. The capacity of this component to inhibit B-cell activation to immunoglobulin synthesis is best revealed in vitro in the helper T-cell-dependent pokeweed mitogen (PWM)-stimulation system (Tosato et al., 1979; Haynes et al., 1979). The appearance of suppressor cells in acute IM is a most interesting example of what may be a natural homeostatic response to the stimulus of increased antibody synthesis which is induced, either directly or indirectly, by EB virus infection. Again, it remains to be seen whether this suppressor cell component of the host's T-cell response is actually effective in controlling the

viral infection. In this respect, one important point yet to be resolved by in vitro studies concerns the sensitivity of EB virus-induced polyclonal B-cell activation, an activation which is clearly helper T-cell-independent, to suppressor cells in general and to IMT cell-mediated suppression in particular (Tosato et al., 1979; Bird and Britton, 1979).

The clinical symptoms of IM can take weeks, in some cases even months, to resolve. Recovery is always accompanied by restoration of a normal blood picture free from atypical lymphocytosis, and by the establishment of a life-long EB virus-carrier state which is indistinguishable from that seen in healthy seropositive individuals whose primary infection was sub-clinical. The virus–cell interactions which permit maintenance of this carrier state are of considerable interest not only because of their relevance to the nature of "latent" infections established by other human herpesviruses, but also because they constitute the seedbed from which EB virus genome-positive malignancies may, on rare occasions, arise.

Persistent EB virus infection

The persistent nature of EB virus infection is apparent from two observations. Firstly, infectious virus can be detected in the throat washings of some 15–20 % of previously-infected individuals when a random group is surveyed at any one particular time (Gerber et al., 1972). Full prospective studies have not yet been carried out but if, as seems likely, detectable virus secretion is intermittent, then the above results would imply that most individuals support sub-clinical reactivations of persistent EB virus infection at some stage in their lives.

Secondly, cultures either of peripheral blood B-cells or of lymphoid tissues from previously-infected individuals exhibit "spontaneous transformation" to EB virus genome-positive lymphoblastoid cell lines, although at a much lower rate than is observed in cultures of B-cells from acute IM patients (Nilsson et al., 1971; Rocchi et al., 1977). Using "spontaneous transformation" as the parameter, the actual frequency of virus-infected B-cells in the blood of any one individual has proved difficult to titrate and more work is required before this potentially valuable index of the in vivo virus–host balance can be reliably monitored in the laboratory.

Humoral response to the persistent infection

Viral persistence is accompanied by the maintenance for life of stable levels of IgG antibodies to VCA, MA and EBNA, whereas antibodies to EA, at least when assayed by immunofluorescence, are not usually detectable in the serum of healthy individuals. Of these persistent reactivities, anti-MA antibodies are useful to the host in that they correlate strongly with virus-neutralizing activity (de Schryver et al., 1974) and thus offer protection against re-infection from an external source. Anti-VCA and anti-EBNA antibodies have no obviously analogous role, although to the sero-epidemiologist they provide a relatively simple means of identifying unequivocally those individuals who have already been infected with the virus.

The stability of antibody titers to the "late" viral antigens in all healthy seropositive individuals strongly implies persistent antigenic stimulation in vivo, such as might be provided by chronic or at least intermittent virus replication within the oropharynx. Consistent with this, patients under immunosuppressive treatment for renal allografts show an unusually high incidence of detectable virus replication in the throat (Strauch et al., 1974) and a concomitant rise in anti-VCA and anti-EA, but not anti-EBNA, titers (Marker et al., 1979; Cheeseman et al., 1980). The controls governing the anti-EBNA response, and indeed the nature of the cells which release EBNA in an immunogenic form in vivo, are issues which continue to arouse debate. In this context, recent results have suggested that full virus replication (at least in a non-lymphoid cell) might occur without the expression of EBNA (Volsky et al., 1981), implying that the antigen is specifically associated with the non-productive virus: B-cell interaction.

Cellular response to the persistent infection

The proven involvement of cytotoxic T-cells in the primary response to EB virus infection immediately raised the possibility of an analogous role for T-cells in the control of the life-long virus-carrier state (Klein et al., 1976b; Epstein and Achong, 1977). The first clear indication that EB virus-specific memory T-cells did indeed exist, arose from studies upon the virus-induced in vitro transformation system. Thus, whilst experimentally-infected cultures of lymphocytes from seronegative donors consistently gave rise to virus-transformed B-cell lines without interference by T-cells, in the corresponding cultures from seropositive donors outgrowth of the nascent B-cell line was frequently inhibited by a cytotoxic T-cell reaction, leading to complete regression of the cultures (Moss et al., 1978; Rickinson et al., 1981). The effector cells mediating this regression not only recognized EB virus-infected cells specifically, but did so in a classically HLA-A and -B antigen-restricted fashion (Moss et al., 1981a; Wallace et al., 1981).

In attempting to assess the importance of this memory T-cell system in the long-term control of EB virus infection, two sets of observations are particularly important.

(a) The frequency of memory T-cells (cytotoxic precursors) in peripheral blood. The phenomenon of regression has been seen in experimentally-infected cultures from virtually all healthy seropositive donors thus far tested (in excess of 100), providing that the initial number of cells seeded in these cultures is sufficiently high to ensure an adequate input of EB virus-specific memory T-cells, and providing the initial culture density permits good cell survival and efficient intercellular contact. Although the "strength" of regression (as defined by the minimum initial cell concentration required for a 50% incidence of the effect amongst replicate microtest plate cultures) can vary between individual normal donors within a 10-fold range, the level of response shown by any one particular donor is remarkably stable with repeated testing over a period of years, again suggesting a relatively constant level of antigenic stimulation. Recently, limiting dilution experiments have revealed that the frequency of EB virus-specific memory T-cells in the peripheral blood of healthy seropositive donors is remarkably high (at least one cell per 10^3 to 10^4 circulating T-cells), reinforcing the view that they constitute an extremely powerful virus-specific immunosurveillance system active in vivo (Rickinson et al., 1981).

(b) The nature of the target antigen. The surface change which reactivated memory T-cells recognize bears all the hallmarks of an EB virus-induced, lymphocyte-detected membrane antigen, LYDMA, of the kind originally invoked to explain IM T-cell cytotoxicity (Klein et al., 1976b). It is present on all EB virus-transformed lymphoblastoid cell lines thus far tested, irrespective of their degree of EMA/LMA expression, and is therefore clearly distinct from the serologically-defined virus envelope-associated cell surface antigens. Moreover, it is expressed on the membranes of virus-infected B-cells soon after the appearance of EBNA in the cell nucleus and coincident with, but not dependent upon, the initiation of cellular DNA synthesis (Moss et al., 1981b). Using the arguments outlined earlier, this suggests that memory T-cells can exercise a most efficient long-term control over the numbers of virus-infected B-cells persisting in seropositive individuals, since target cells can be destroyed at the very onset of virus-induced cell proliferation.

In the light of the above observations, it seems very probable that the LYDMA-specific memory T-cell system provides the host's first line of defence against the persistent infection. It would be naive, however, to suggest that this is the host's only form of cell-mediated response. Clearly, the species' long history of co-evolution with EB virus (as with any of the other human herpesviruses) will have selected for individuals with multiple cellular defence mechanisms against such a potentially pathogenic agent. Indeed, the existence in peripheral blood of non-antigen-specific effector cells capable of lysing EB virus-transformed target cell lines, either by antibody-dependent cellular cytotoxicity (ADCC) (Pearson and Orr, 1976) or by a non-HLA-restricted "natural killing" (NK) (Seeley et al., 1981), bears witness to this fact.

Again, it is instructive to ask what are the target structures on virus-infected cells which permit recognition and lysis by these different cellular mechanisms. The available evidence would suggest that the antibody mediating ADCC is an IgG specific for one or more components of the MA complex (Pearson et al., 1979). Interestingly, this antibody is absent during the acute phase of IM but is present in all healthy seropositive individuals (Jondal, 1976). The target role of viral envelope determinants is further substantiated by the observation that movement of virus-transformed cells into the lytic cycle is accompanied by an increasing sysceptibility to ADCC (Patarroyo et al., 1980). The target structures for NK or "activated NK" cells are still not defined, but it is important to note that in experimental systems the sensitivity of EB virus-transformed cell lines to such effectors only becomes apparent after some weeks of in vitro passage (Viallat et al., 1978; Seeley et al., 1981) and, here again, this may be increased if cells are induced to enter the later stages of the virus replicative cycle (Patarroyo et al., 1980).

Models of EB virus persistence

One of the most intriguing questions of EB virus biology concerns the nature of the virus–cell interaction whereby the virus remains "latent" in host B lymphoid tissues. There are at least 3 different ways of viewing this interaction and these alternatives are presented in Table I as a basis for discussion.

TABLE I

MODELS OF EB VIRUS PERSISTENCE IN LYMPHOID TISSUES

(i)	Long-term persistence of virus-transformed B-cells with proliferative capacity and neoplastic potential
(ii)	Long-term persistence of latently-infected B-cells without viral antigen expression
(iii)	Continual seeding of newly-infected B-cells from site of chronic virus replication in oropharynx, and continual removal by immune T-cells

One view favours the existence in lymphoid tissues of foci of proliferating EBNA/LYDMA-positive cells in which the virus–cell interaction is essentially similar to that seen in all virus-transformed cells in vitro (Klein, 1980). Most cells in the population remain under the proliferative influence of the virus, although continual movement of a small proportion of the cells into lytic cycle would serve to provide a constant source of virus structural antigens. At the same time, the overall size of this potentially neoplastic cell population is thought to be kept in check by one or more of the host's cellular defence mechanisms.

This model, though widely promulgated in the literature, is difficult to reconcile with the more recent data, outlined above, revealing the strength of the LYDMA-specific cytotoxic T-cell memory which is prevalent in all healthy seropositive individuals. If foci of virus-transformed cells do persist, as envisaged in this model, then they can only do so in immunologically-protected sites.

An alternative view of EB virus persistence envisages the establishment of a pool of "latently-infected" B-cells (Epstein and Achong, 1973) in which the virus–cell interaction is essentially similar to that whereby the neurotropic viruses HSV and VZV are harboured for life in ganglion cells. Intracellular persistence of the EB viral genome, without detectable expression of viral antigens, clearly would permit the latently-infected cell to survive in the immune host. Moreover, taking the analogy with HSV and VZV one step further, periodic reactivation of the infection in individual B cells (perhaps when sequestered in the oropharynx) would renew virus replication and serve to maintain anti-viral antibody responses.

The attraction of this model lies in its extension of the principle of latency, first developed from the study of neurotropic herpesviruses, to include the lymphotropic members of this group. In so doing, however, it necessarily invokes a new form of EB virus-B cell interaction for which there is, as yet, only circumstantial experimental evidence (Crawford et al., 1978).

A third model of the EB virus-carrier state has more recently been suggested (Moss et al., 1981b), largely as a result of the work on virus-specific T-cell surveillance which has made it clear that LYDMA-positive cells are very unlikely to be able to survive undetected in the lymphoid tissues of an immune host. In these circumstances, the viral infection may be driven back to its original site within the oropharynx where a permissive, perhaps non-lymphoid, cell clearly does exist. Chronic low-grade replication at this site, yielding levels of infectious virus in throat washings which are often below the threshold of detectability of in vitro transformation assays, would serve to maintain the virus-carrier state and, in the process, provide a constant stimulus of "late" viral antigens for humoral responses.

This model entails a novel view of EB virus persistence in lymphoid tissues which is illustrated in Fig. 2. Here, B-cells moving through the site of chronic virus replication in the throat become infected and subsequently seed out into peripheral lymphoid tissues, only to be destroyed a few days later when they reach the stage of EBNA/LYDMA expression and are recognized by cytotoxic T-cells. This balance of continual input from the throat and continual erosion by immune T-cells not only keeps the virus-infected B-cell pool at a relatively constant level in lymphoid tissues, but also provides the necessary antigenic stimuli for the maintenance of anti-EBNA antibody titers and of LYDMA-specific T-cell memory.

Although the above discussion of EB virus persistence is given particular force because this agent has the potential for host cell transformation as well as for lytic infection, many of the questions raised find their echo in any general discussion of herpesvirus latency. Are truly "latent" virus–cell interactions unique to the neurotropic herpesviruses? To what extent does subclinical reactivation of virus replication and reinfection of co-resident cells make latency a dynamic rather than a static phenomenon? Do immunologically-protected sites of chronic virus replication exist? In the absence of more data, it is not profitable to pursue these questions further in the present review but instead note what positive lessons can be learned from the above analysis of EB virus–host interactions.

198

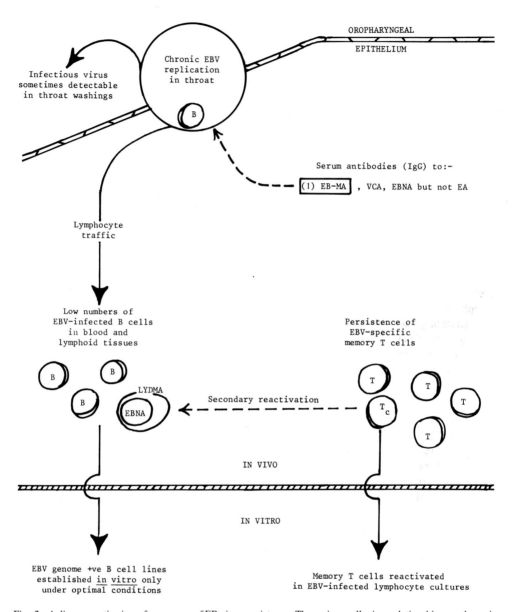

Fig. 2. A diagrammatic view of one means of EB virus persistence. The various cell–virus relationships are shown in the context of the immune responses (humoral and cellular) to which they give rise. The evidence upon which this *possible* view of events is based is described in the text.

CONCLUSIONS

Perhaps the most important lesson concerns the multiplicity of cell-mediated effector mechanisms which the host employs in controlling EB viral infection. Thus, in acute IM patients, the primary T-cell response is dominated by a non-HLA-restricted cytotoxicity (whose antigenic specificity is still obscure), whereas the most important long-term control over viral persistence appears to be mediated by HLA-restricted cytotoxic T-cells whose target antigen, LYDMA, is expressed at an early stage of the viral cycle, before virus-induced proliferation and well in advance of infectious virus release. What, if any, is the relationship between these two types of effector cell? Perhaps primary infections are usually controlled by a LYDMA specific response of the kind which is subsequently established in T-cell memory, but where this fails, a battery of less-specific and perhaps less-efficient T-cell responses are initiated, leading to the clinical manifestations of IM. To extend this argument, one might predict that the atypical lymphocytes seen in CMV-induced mononucleosis also result from an activation of less-specific second-line defences and might therefore contain reactivities functionally similar to those seen in the EB virus-induced disease.

In the wider view it would seem very likely that persistent HSV, VZV and CMV infections are under the control of a similar range of cell-mediated immune mechanisms and in this regard particular attention should be paid to the possible role of virus-specific cytotoxic T-cells. The essential unity of herpesvirus biology suggests that, just as EB virus-specific memory cells persist in the circulating T-cell pool of immune individuals, so too will analogous T-cell activities directed towards the control of all the other human herpesviruses. If these activities can be demonstrated and quantified in vitro, a proper assessment can begin to be made of their influence upon the course of herpes virus infections.

REFERENCES

Bird, A.G. and Britton, S. (1979) A new approach to the study of human B lymphocyte function using an indirect plaque assay and a direct B cell activator. *Immunol. Rev.*, 45: 41–67.
Carter, R.L. (1975) Infectious mononucleosis: model for self-limiting lymphoproliferation. *Lancet*, i: 846–849.
Cheesman, S.H., Henle, W., Rubin, R.H., Tolkoft-Rubin, N.E., Cosmi, B., Cantell, K., Winkle, S., Herrin, J.T., Black, P.H., Russel, P.S. and Hirsch, M.S. (1980) Epstein–Barr virus infection in renal transplant patients: effects of antithymocyte globulin and interferon. *Ann. Int. Med.*, 93: 39–42.
Crawford, D.H., Rickinson, A.B., Finerty, S. and Epstein, M.A. (1978) Epstein–Barr (EB) virus genome-containing, EB nuclear antigen-negative B lymphocyte populations in blood in acute infectious monucleosis. *J. gen. Virol.*, 38: 449–460.
Crawford, D.H., Thomas, J.A., Janossy, G., Sweny, P., Fernando, O.N., Moorhead, J.F. and Thompson, J.H. (1980) Epstein–Barr virus nuclear antigen-positive lymphoma after Cyclosporin A treatment in patient with renal allograft. *Lancet*, i: 1355–1356.
De Schrijver, A., Klein, G., Hewetson, J., Rocchi, G., Henle, W., Henle, G., Moss, D.J. and Pope, J.H. (1974) Comparison of EBV-neutralization tests based on abortive infection or transformation of lymphoid cells and their relation to membrane reactive antibodies (anti-MA). *Int. J. Cancer*, 13: 353–362.
Epstein, M.A. and Achong, B.G. (1973) Various forms of Epstein–Barr virus infection in man: established facts and a general concept. *Lancet*, ii: 836–839.
Epstein, M.A. and Achong, B.G. (1977) Recent progress in Epstein–Barr virus research. *Ann. Rev. Microbiol.*, 31: 421–445.
Epstein, M.A. and Achong, B.G. (1979) The relationship of the virus to Burkitt's lymphoma. In M.A. Epstein and B.G. Achong (Eds.), *The Epstein–Barr Virus*, Springer, Berlin, pp. 321–337.
Ernberg, I., Klein, G., Kourilsky, F.M. and Silvestre, D. (1974) Differentiation between early and late membrane antigen on human lymphoblastoid cell lines infected with Epstein–Barr virus. I Immunofluorescence. *J. nat. Cancer Inst.*, 53: 61–65.

Gerber, P., Nonoyama, M., Lucas, S., Perlin, E. and Goldstein, L.I. (1972) Oral excretion of Epstein–Barr virus by healthy subjects and patients with infectious mononucleosis. *Lancet*, ii: 988–989.

Gergely, L., Klein, G. and Ernberg, I. (1971) Effect of EBV-induced early antigens on host-cell macromolecular synthesis, studied by combined immunofluorescence and radioautography. *Virology*, 45: 22–29.

Hanto, D.W., Frizzera, G., Purtilo, D.T., Sakamoto, K., Sullivan, J.L., Saemundsen, A.K., Klein, G., Simmons, R.L. and Najarian, J.S. (1981) Clinical spectrum of lymphoproliferative disorders in renal transplant recipients and evidence for the role of Epstein–Barr virus. *Cancer Res.*, 41: 4253–4261.

Haynes, B.F., Schooley, R.T., Payling-Wright, C.R., Grouse, J.E., Dolin R. and Fauci, A.S. (1979) Emergence of suppressor cells of immunoglobulin synthesis during acute Epstein–Barr virus-induced mononucleosis. *J. Immunol.*, 123: 2095–2101.

Henle, G., Henle, W. and Diehl, V. (1968) Relation of Burkitt tumor associated herpes-type virus to infectious mononucleosis. *Proc. nat. Acad. Sci. U.S.A.*, 59: 94–101.

Henle, W., Diehl, V., Kohn, G., zur Hausen, H. and Henle, G. (1967) Herpes-type virus and chromosome marker in normal leukocytes after growth with irradiated Burkitt cells. *Science*, 157: 1064–1065.

Henle, G., Henle, W. and Klein, G. (1971) Demonstration of two distinct components in the early antigen complex of Epstein–Barr virus-infected cells. *Int. J. Cancer*, 8: 272–282.

Henle, G., Henle, W. and Horwitz, C.A. (1974) Antibodies to Epstein–Barr virus-associated nuclear antigen in infectious mononucleosis. *J. infect. Dis.*, 130: 231–239.

Henle, G. and Henle, W. (1979a) The virus as the etiologic agent of infectious mononucleosis. In M.A. Epstein and B.G. Achong (Eds.), *The Epstein–Barr Virus*, Springer, Berlin, pp. 297–320.

Henle, W. and Henle, G. (1979b) Seroepidemiology of the virus. In M.A. Epstein and B.G. Achong (Eds.), *The Epstein–Barr Virus*, Springer, Berlin, pp. 61–78.

Henle, W. and Henle, G. (1981) Epstein–Barr virus-specific serology in immunologically compromised individuals. *Cancer Rev.*, 41: 4222–4225.

Jondal, M. (1976) Antibody-dependent cellular cytotoxicity (ADCC) against Epstein–Barr virus-determined membrane antigens. I Reactivity in sera from normal persons and from patients with acute infectious mononucleosis. *Clin. exp. Immunol.*, 25: 1–5.

Jondal, M. and Klein, G. (1973) Surface markers on human B and T lymphocytes. II Presence of Epstein–Barr virus receptor on B lymphocytes. *J. exp. Med.*, 138: 1365–1378.

Jondal, M. and Targan, S. (1978) In vitro induction of cytotoxic effector cells with spontaneous killer activity. *J. exp. Med.*, 147: 1621–1636.

Kallin, B., Luka, J. and Klein, G. (1979) Immunochemical characterisation of Epstein–Barr virus-associated early and late antigens in *n*-butyrate-treated P$_3$HR-1 cells. *J. Virol.*, 32: 710–716.

Klein, G. (1979) The relationship of the virus to nasopharyngeal carcinoma. In M.A. Epstein and B.G. Achong (Eds.), *The Epstein-Barr Virus*, Springer, Berlin, pp. 339–350.

Klein, G. (1980) Immune and non-immune control of neoplastic development: contrasting effects of host and tumor evolution. *Cancer*, 45: 2486–2499.

Klein, G., Svedmyr, E., Jondal, M. and Persson, P.O. (1976a) EBV-determined nuclear antigen (EBNA)-positive cells in the peripheral blood of infectious mononucleosis patients. *Int. J. Cancer*, 17: 21–26.

Klein, E., Klein, G. and Levine, P.H. (1976b) Immunological control of human lymphoma: discussion. *Cancer Res.*, 36: 724–727.

Klein, G., Luka, J. and Zeuthen, J. (1979) Transformation induced by Epstein–Barr virus and the role of the nuclear antigen. *Cold Spr. Harb. Symp.*, 44: 253–261.

Klein, E., Masucci, M.G., Berthold, W. and Blazar, B.A. (1980) Lymphocyte-mediated cytotoxicity towards virus-induced tumor cells; natural and activated killer lymphocytes in man. *Cold Spr. Harb. Conf. Cell Proliferation*, 7: 1187–1197.

Klein, E., Ernberg, I., Masucci, M.G., Szigeti, R., Wu, Y.T., Masucci, G. and Svedmyr, E. (1981) T-cell response to B-cells and Epstein–Barr virus antigens in infectious mononucleosis. *Cancer Res.*, 41: 4210–4215.

Klemola, E., von Essen, R., Henle, G. and Henle, W. (1970) Infectious mononucleosis-like disease with negative heterophil agglutination test. Clinical features in relation to Epstein–Barr virus and cytomagalovirus antibodies. *J. infect. Dis.*, 121: 608–614.

Lipinski, M., Fridman, W.H., Tursz, T., Vincent, C., Pious, D. and Fellows, M. (1979) Absence of allogeneic restriction in human T cell-mediated cytotoxicity to Epstein–Barr virus-infected target cells. Demonstration of an HLA-linked control at the effector level. *J. exp. Med.*, 150: 1310–1322.

Marker, S.C., Ascher, N.L., Kalis, J.M., Simmons, R.L., Najarian, J.S. and Balfour, H.H. (1979) Epstein–Barr virus antibody responses and clinical illness in renal transplant recipients. *Surgery*, 85: 433–440.

Merigan, T.C. (1981) Immunosuppression and herpesviruses. In A.J. Nahmias, W.R. Dowdle and R.F. Schinazi (Eds.), *The Human Herpesviruses. An Interdisciplinary Perspective*, Elsevier, New York, pp. 309–316.

Miller, G., Niederman, J.C. and Andrews, L. (1973) Prolonged oropharyngeal excretion of EB virus following infectious mononucleosis. *New Engl. J. Med.,* 288: 229–232.

Moss, D.J. Rickinson, A.B. and Pope, J.H. (1978) Long-term T-cell-mediated immunity to Epstein–Barr virus in man. I Complete regression of virus-induced transformation in cultures of seropositive donor leukocytes. *Int. Int. J. Cancer,* 22: 662–668.

Moss, D.J., Wallace, L.E., Rickinson, A.B. and Epstein, M.A. (1981a) Cytotoxic T cell recognition of Epstein–Barr virus-infected B cells. I Specificity and HLA-restriction of effector cells reactivated in vitro. *Europ. J. Immunol.,* 11: 686–693.

Moss, D.J., Rickinson, A.B., Wallace, L.E. and Epstein, M.A. (1981b) Sequential appearance of Epstein–Barr virus nuclear and lymphocyte-detected membrane antigens in B cell transformation. *Nature (Lond),* 291: 664–666.

Nilsson, K., Klein, G., Henle, W. and Henle, G. (1971) The establishment of lymphoblastoid cell lines from adult and foetal human lymphoid tissue and its dependence on EBV. *Int. J. Cancer,* 8: 443–450.

North, J.R., Morgan, A.J. and Epstein, M.A. (1980) Observations on the EB virus envelope and virus-determined membrane antigen polypeptides. *Int. J. Cancer,* 26: 231–240.

Pattarroyo, M., Blazar B., Pearson, G., Klein, E. and Klein, G. (1980) Induction of the EBV cycle in B-lymphocyte-derived lines is accompanied by increased natural killer (NK) sensitivity and the expression of EBV-related antigen(s) detected by the ADCC reaction. *Int. J. Cancer,* 26: 365–375.

Pearson, G.R. and Orr, T.W. (1976) Antibody-dependent lymphocyte cytotoxicity against cells expressing Epstein–Barr virus antigens. *J. nat. Cancer Inst.,* 56: 485–488.

Pearson, G.R., Qualtiere, L.F., Klein, G., Noren, T. and Bal, I.D. (1979) Epstein–Barr virus-specific antibody-dependent cellular cytotoxicity in patients with Burkitt's lymphoma. *Int. J. Cancer,* 24: 402–406.

Pope, J.H. (1967) Establishment of cell lines from peripheral leukocytes in infectious mononucleosis. *Nature (Lond.),* 216: 810–811.

Pope, J.H. (1979) Transformation by the virus in vitro. In M.A. Epstein and B.G. Achong (Eds.), *The Epstein–Barr Virus,* Springer, Berlin, New York, pp. 205–223.

Pope, J.H., Horne, M.K. and Scott, W. (1968) Transformation of foetal human leukocytes in vitro by filtrates of a human leukaemic cell line containing herpes-like virus. *Int. J. Cancer,* 3: 857–866.

Reedman, B.M. and Klein, G. (1973) Cellular localization of an Epstein–Barr virus (EBV)-associated complement-fixing antigen in producer and non-producer lymphoblastoid cell lines. *Int. J. Cancer,* 11: 599–620.

Rickinson, A.B., Epstein, M.A. and Crawford, D.H. (1975) Absence of infectious Epstein–Barr virus in blood in acute infectious mononucleosis. *Nature (Lond.),* 258: 236–238.

Rickinson, A.B., Moss, D.J., Wallace, L.E., Rowe, M., Misko, I.S., Epstein, M.A. and Pope, J.H. (1981) Long-term T-cell-mediated immunity to Epstein–Barr virus. *Cancer Res.,* 41: 4216–4221.

Robinson, J.E., Smith, D. and Niederman, J. (1981) Plasmacytic differentiation of circulating Epstein–Barr virus-infected B lymphocytes during acute infectious mononucleosis. *J. exp. Med.,* 153: 235–244.

Rocchi, G., de Felici, A., Ragona, G. and Heinz, A. (1977) Quantitative evaluation of Epstein–Barr virus-infected peripheral blood leucocytes in infectious mononucleosis. *New Engl. J. Med.,* 296: 132–134.

Rosen, A., Gergely, P., Jondal, M., Klein, G. and Britton, S. (1977) Polyclonal Ig production after Epstein–Barr virus infection of human lymphocytes in vitro, *Nature (Lond.),* 267: 52–54.

Royston, I., Sullivan, J.L., Periman, P.O. and Perlin, E. (1975) Cell-mediated immunity to Epstein–Barr virus-transformed lymphoblastoid cells in acute infectious mononucleosis. *New Engl. J. Med.,* 293: 1159–1163.

Seeley, J.K. and Golub, S.H. (1978) Studies on cytotoxicity generated in human mixed lymphocyte cultures. I. Time course and target spectrum of several distinct concomitant cytotoxic activities. *J. Immunol.,* 120: 1415–1422.

Seeley, J., Svedmyr, E., Weiland, O., Klein, G., Moller, E., Eriksson, E., Andersson, K. and van der Waal, L. (1981) Epstein–Barr virus selective T cells in infectious mononucleosis are not restricted to HLA-A and B antigens. *J. Immunol.,* 127: 293–300.

Sheldon, P.J., Papamichail, M., Hemsted, E.H. and Holborow, E.J. (1973) Thymic origin of atypical lymphoid cells in infectious mononucleosis. *Lancet,* i: 1153–1155.

Shore, S.L. and Feorino, P.M. (1981) Immunology of primary herpesvirus infections in humans. In A.J. Nahmias, W.R. Dowdle and R.F. Schinazi (Eds.), *The Human Herpesviruses. An Interdisciplinary Approach,* Elsevier, New York, pp. 267–288.

Strauch, B., Andrews, L.-L., Siegel, N. and Miller, G. (1974) Oropharyngeal excretion of Epstein–Barr virus by renal transplant recipients and other patients with immunosuppressive drugs. *Lancet,* i: 234–237.

Svedmyr, E. and Jondal, M. (1975) Cytotoxic effector cells specific for B cell lines transformed by Epstein–Barr virus are present in patients with infectious mononucleosis. *Proc. nat. Acad. Sci. U.S.A.,* 72: 1622–1626.

Thorley-Lawson, D.A. (1979) Characterisation of cross-reacting antigens on the Epstein–Barr virus envelope and plasma membranes of producer cells. *Cell,* 16: 33–42.

Tosato, G., Magrath, I., Koski, I., Dooley, N. and Blaese, M. (1979) Activation of suppressor T cells during Epstein–Barr-virus-induced infectious mononucleosis *New Engl. J. Med.*, 301: 1133–1137.

Viallat, J., Svedmyr, E., Yefenof, E., Klein, G. and Weiland, O. (1978) Stimulation of human peripheral blood lymphocytes by autologous EBV-infected B cells. *Cell. Immunol.*, 41: 1–8.

Volsky, D.J., Klein, G., Volsky, B. and Shapiro, I.M. (1981) Production of infectious Epstein–Barr virus in mouse lymphocytes. *Nature (Lond.)*, 293: 399–401.

Wallace, L.E., Moss, D.J., Rickinson, A.B., McMichael, A.J. and Epstein, M.A. (1981) Cytotoxic T cell recognition of Epstein–Barr virus-infected B cells II. Blocking studies with monoclonal antibodies to HLA determinants. *Europ. J. Immunol.*, 11: 694–699.

Zur Hausen, H., O'Neill, F.J. and Freeze, U.K. (1978) Persisting oncogenic herpesvirus induced by the tumour promoter TPA. *Nature (Lond.)*, 272: 373–375.

Immunology of Nervous System Infections, Progress in Brain Research, Vol. 59, edited by P.O. Behan, V. ter Meulen and F. Clifford Rose

Recovery of Herpes Simplex Virus 1 ts Mutants from the Dorsal Root Ganglia of Mice

G.B. CLEMENTS and J.H. SUBAK-SHARPE

Institute of Virology, Church Street, Glasgow G11 5JR, Scotland (U.K.)

INTRODUCTION

To explain clinical observations on the behaviour of herpes simplex virus (HSV) in man and his experimental observations in rabbits, Goodpasture (1929) suggested that HSV may remain latent in neurological tissue after a primary infection. Since then and following much experimental work, HSV has been demonstrated clearly to remain latent in the sensory ganglia of experimental animals (Stevens and Cook, 1971) and man (Bastian et al., 1972; Barringer and Swoveland, 1973). Infectious virus cannot usually be demonstrated directly in latently infected individuals but can be recovered after explantation and cultivation of tissue in vitro. There is strong evidence that the virus genome is latent in neurons of ganglia (Cook et al., 1974; McLennan and Darby, 1980), but the molecular basis of latency is at present unclear.

Infectious virus recovered from a latently infected animal must have passed through at least 3 stages following the initial infection: (i) initiation of latency; (ii) maintenance of latency; and (iii) reactivation resulting in the production of virus. Investigation in experimental animals of this complex process, using ts mutants (Lofgren et al., 1977; and Watson et al., 1980) and thymidine kinase negative mutants (Field and Wildy, 1978; Tenser et al., 1979; Tenser and Dunstan, 1979) has commenced. Our present study extends these investigations to study the behaviour of the wild type and 7 ts mutants of HSV-1 in 5 different mouse strains and the distribution of latent virus in different ganglia.

MATERIALS AND METHODS

The HSV-1 strain used was the Glasgow strain 17 (Brown et al., 1972) and some of the ts mutants derived from it (Marsden et al., 1976). To propagate HSV-1, BHK C_{13} cells in burrlers were infected at a multiplicity of 1 pfu/300 cells. The virus was allowed to absorb, then 20 ml of Glasgow-modified Eagle's medium (MEM) was added, supplemented with 10% (v/v) tryptose phosphate broth and 10% (v/v) calf serum (CS). When extensive cytopathic effect became evident, cells were harvested, lysed by sonication and then centrifuged at 2000 rpm for 10 min. The resulting supernatant was assayed on BHK cells both at 31°C and 38°C in MEM containing 5% human serum to inhibit spread of the virus.

Mice were bred on site. The strains used were A, Pirbright, C57B1/6, Biozzi (high responder) and BALB/c. For s.c. inoculation the virus was diluted as appropriate with

TABLE I

INCIDENCE OF MORTALITY FOLLOWING HSV-1 INFECTION

ND, not done.

Mouse strain	$10^2–10^3$ pfu/mouse	% survival	$10^3–10^4$ pfu/mouse	% survival	$10^4–10^5$ pfu/mouse	% survival	$10^5–10^6$ pfu/mouse	% survival
Pirbright	ND	–	45/58	78	49/64	77	5/7	71
BALB/c	5/5	100	19/21	90	0/4	0	2/23	8
C57B1/6	6/6	100	13/13	100	23/24	96	18/18	100
Biozzi	12/13	94	7/8	87	33/46	72	10/10	100
A	ND	–	7/15	47	6/9	67	0/11	0

TABLE II

ISOLATION OF HSV-1 WT AND TS MUTANTS FROM SPINAL GANGLIA OF LATENTLY INFECTED MICE

ND, not done; N, no survivors.

Virus	Pfu/mouse inoculated	Mouse strain					Total	%
		Pirbright	C57Bl	Biozzi	BALB/c	A		
17 syn⁺	10^4	6/13	6/6	11/15	N	4/5	27/39	69
	10^3	3/17	6/11	3/4	2/10	6/7	20/49	41
D syn	6×10^5	6/10	0/7	3/5	3/3	0/6	12/31	39
I syn	1×10^6	10/16	15/22	10/10	3/3	6/6	44/57	77
H syn⁺	1.5×10^5	2/10	ND	ND	0/10	3/4	5/24	21
L syn	7.5×10^5	0/9	0/6	ND	3/5	ND	3/20	15
F syn	1×10^7	10/11	ND	8/12	5/10	ND	23/33	70
G syn	3.7×10^6	ND	ND	0/13	0/4	ND	0/17	0
K syn	1×10^5	3/8	ND	0/8	ND	ND	3/16	19
Total		40/94	27/52	35/54	16/41	19/28		
%		43	52	66	39	68		

phosphate-buffered saline containing 1 % calf serum (PBS). Mice were injected at weaning (3–4 weeks) with the appropriate dose of virus into the right rear footpad in 0.025 ml. The virus dilution used was titrated on C_{13} cells at 31°C at the time of inoculation. The animals were examined daily for the first two weeks after inoculation. After a minimum of 3 months the survivors were killed with chloroform and the last two thoracic ganglia, all 6 lumbar ganglia and the first and second sacral ganglia were immediately explanted from the right side. In some cases, ganglia were also explanted from the left side. The explanted ganglia were washed in about 150 μl of Eagle's medium containing 50 % foetal calf serum (EFC 50 %) and cultured in flat bottomed microtiter plates with 150 μl of EFC 50 % at 31°C in a humidified incubator under an atmosphere of 5 % CO_2 in air. The time between the death of the mouse and finishing explantation averaged 15 min.

The whole supernatant medium (150 μl) from the explants was screened twice a week for virus by addition to individual semiconfluent monolayers of BHK C_{13} cells in flat-bottomed microtiter plates at 31°C. The supernatant was replaced by 0.05 ml of fresh medium and this monitoring was continued for at least one month. The first screening was always carried out within 24–48 h after explantation. Positive cultures were recognized by the appearance of virus-induced cytopathic effect. All viruses re-isolated from mice were grown up and assayed on C_{13} cells at 31°C and 38°C to determine whether the viruses had retained the original ts phenotype.

RESULTS

Table I presents the incidence of mortality following infection of the 5 strains of mice with wild type (wt) HSV-1 virus, expressed as the percentage survival of animals at any given virus dose. The very few animals which died before the second day after inoculation or more than 14 days after the inoculation were excluded. Clinical symptoms first appeared 3 or more days after inoculation. Many animals became progressively paralyzed, a flaccid paralysis spreading from the right rear leg — severely paralyzed animals were killed. Some animals died suddenly without any visible preceding illness. Many animals became ill, irritable and transiently slightly paralyzed, but subsequently recovered fully. On inspection, no lesions could be observed at the site of inoculation in any of the animals. In respect to mortality following infection with HSV-1, the animal strains can be classified as resistant or susceptible. The resistant group comprises the Pirbright, C57B1/6 and Biozzi strains: more than 70 % of the animals survived doses of 10^5 pfu of virus. The susceptible group comprises mice of the A and BALB/c strains. The A strain mice were particularly susceptible with 53 % and 100 % of the animals dying after 10^3 and 10^5 pfu of virus respectively.

There was no mortality when HSV-1 ts mutant virus was the inoculum. No symptoms appeared in any of the animals following inoculation with doses of 10^5–10^7 pfu of HSV-1 ts mutants irrespective of mouse strain.

Latent HSV could be recovered from a number of spinal ganglia explanted from some mice 3 months or more after initial inoculation with the virus. HSV-1 wt virus was recovered from one or more ganglia of 41 % (20/49) of the mice inoculated with 10^3 pfu of virus and 69 % (27/39) of animals inoculated with 10^4 pfu (Table II). Thus, the success in recovering virus from ganglia increased with the dose of virus initially inoculated.

The anatomical distribution of the ganglia from C57B1/6 mice releasing HSV-1 ts$^+$ virus following explantation is presented in Fig. 1, which also shows a clear dose-response relationship. Increasing the virus dose resulted in both a greater proportion of animals which could be

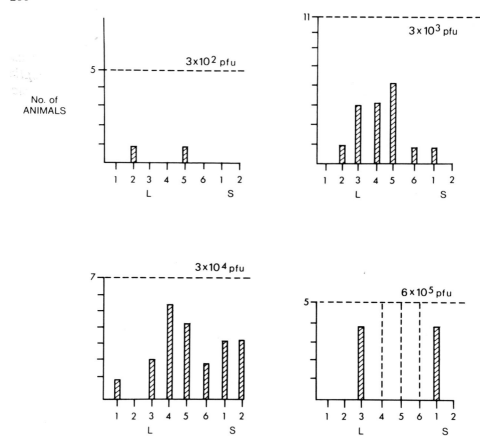

Fig. 1. The anatomical distribution of ganglia from C57B1/6 mice releasing HSV-1 ts⁺ virus following explantation. Four groups of mice were used, inoculated respectively with either 3×10^2 pfu, 3×10^3 pfu, 3×10^4 pfu or 6×10^5 pfu of virus. L1–6, lumbar ganglia; S1,2, sacral ganglia.

demonstrated to be latently infected and also in a greater proportion of ganglia from which virus could be reactivated. This applied particularly to ganglia innervating the leg (lumbar 4, 5, 6), ganglia more distant became increasingly likely to shed virus as the dose was increased. Lumbar 4, 5 and 6 ganglia of the mice inoculated with 10^5 pfu of virus were used for another purpose and not screened for release of virus. The distribution of positive ganglia in strain A mice was similar except that rather more ganglia shed virus at lower doses of virus.

Explanted ganglia first released wt virus between days 6 and 25 after being placed in culture, and no virus was recovered from any supernatant earlier than 5 days after explantation.

The recovery of ts virus from ganglia of mice initially infected with different HSV-1 ts mutants is presented in Table II. All isolates from ganglia were tested for temperature sensitivity, and with the exception of two isolates from ts I all the virus recovered from the ganglia had remained ts. Thus 6 of the tested ts mutants had retained some or all of their ability to produce latency, although, in the cases of ts K, ts L, ts H and perhaps ts D, this seems to be lowered. In the case of ts G, none of 17 mice proved positive. Of the ts mutants so far studied only I syn and F syn could be recovered at a frequency comparable to that of wt virus; the doses inoculated, however, were 100 and 1000 times greater respectively.

As far as mouse strain differences are concerned, explanted ganglia released virus from Biozzi and A strain mice in 66% and 68% of animals respectively and from 52% of C57Bl/6 mice, whereas recovery from the Pirbright and BALB/c strains occurred only in 43% and 39% of cases respectively.

DISCUSSION

These preliminary results permit the following tentative conclusions to be drawn on the basis of the mouse dorsal root ganglia model.

(1) Differences exist between mouse strains in the incidence of mortality following infection with HSV-1. These results confirm the earlier studies of Lopez (1975).

(2) The HSV-1 ts mutants D syn, I syn, H syn$^+$, L syn, F syn, G syn and K syn are avirulent.

(3) The efficiency of recovery of HSV-1 wt from ganglia is a function of the dose of virus inoculated, as is the distribution of ganglia infected latently with the virus.

(4) Differences appear to exist between strains of mice in the frequency of recovery of latent HSV from ganglia explanted.

(5) F syn, I syn, D syn, H syn$^+$, L syn, and K syn can all be reactivated from explanted ganglia. Reactivation of ts H, ts L and ts K occurs much less frequently than that of wt virus.

(6) G syn could not be recovered. It should be noted that in addition to being ts this stock has a second known lesion, being thymidine kinase negative at both permissive and restrictive temperatures.

There are some differences between these results and those reported by Lofgren et al. (1977) and Watson et al. (1980) using the same mutants. However, the animals used previously were all outbred Swiss Webster strain mice and the route of inoculation was intracerebral in the majority of cases.

REFERENCES

Barringer, J.R. and Swoveland, P. (1975) Recovery of herpes simplex virus from human sacral ganglia. New Engl. J. Med., 288: 648–650.

Bastian, F.O., Rabson, A.S., Yee, C.L. and Tralka, T.S. (1972) Herpesvirus hominis: isolation from human trigeminal ganglion. Science, 178: 306–307.

Brown, S.M., Ritchie, D.A. and Subak-Sharpe, J.H. (1973) Genetic studies with herpes simplex virus type 1. The isolation of temperature-sensitive mutants, their arrangement into complementation groups and recombination analysis leading to a linkage map. J. gen. Virol., 18: 329–346.

Cook, M.L., Bastone, V.B. and Stevens, J.G. (1974) Evidence that neurones harbor latent herpes simplex virus. Infect. Immun., 9: 946–951.

Field, H.J. and Wildy, P. (1978) The pathogenicity of thymidine kinase-deficient mutants of herpes simplex virus in mice. J. Hyg. Camb., 81: 267–277.

Goodpasture, E.W. (1929) The axis-cylinders of peripheral nerves as portals of entry to the central nervous system for the virus of herpes simplex in experimentally infected rabbits. Medicine, 7: 223–243.

Lofgren, K.W., Stevens, J.G., Marsden, H.S. and Subak-Sharpe, J.H. (1977) Temperature-sensitive mutants of herpes simplex virus differ in the capacity to establish latent infections in mice. Virology, 76: 440–443.

Lopez, C. (1975) Genetics of natural resistance to herpes virus infections in mice. Nature (Lond.), 258: 152–153.

Marsden, H.S., Crombie, I.R. and Subak-Sharpe, J.H. (1976) Control of protein synthesis in herpes virus infected cells: analysis of the polypeptides induced by wild type and sixteen temperature-sensitive mutants of HSV strain 17. J. gen. Virol., 31: 347–372.

208

McLennan, J.L. and Darby, G. (1980) Herpes simplex virus latency: the cellular location of virus in dorsal root ganglia and the fate of the infected cell following virus activation. *J. gen. Virol.*, 51: 233–243.

Stevens, J.G. and Cook, M.L. (1971) Latent herpes simplex virus in spinal ganglia of mice. *Science*, 173: 843–845.

Tenser, R.B. and Dunstan, M.E. (1979) Herpes simplex virus thymidine kinase expression in infection of the trigeminal ganglion. *Virology*, 99: 417–422.

Tenser, R.B., Miller, R.L. and Rapp, F. (1979) Trigeminal ganglion infection by thymidine-kinase negative mutants of herpes simplex virus. *Science*, 205: 915–917.

Watson, K., Stevens, J.G., Cook, M.L. and Subak-Sharpe, J.H. (1980) Latency competence of thirteen HSV-1 temperature sensitive mutants. *J. gen. Virol.*, 49: 149–159.

Immunology of Nervous System Infections, Progress in Brain Research, Vol. 59, edited by P.O. Behan, V. ter Meulen and F. Clifford Rose

Immunohistological Studies of Immunoglobulin-Containing Cells and Viral Antigens in Some Inflammatory Diseases of the Nervous System

MARGARET M. ESIRI

Department of Neuropathology, Radcliffe Infirmary, Oxford (U.K.)

INTRODUCTION

The recent development of immunoenzyme methods has enabled certain antigens to be detected within tissue sections, in many cases even after formalin fixation and paraffin-embedding (Sternberger, 1979). This has afforded the opportunity for a fresh look to be taken at some inflammatory diseases of the nervous system, and for new insight to be gained into the complexities of immunological responses within the central nervous system (CNS). It has been possible during the last few years to study a number of inflammatory diseases using the immunoperoxidase technique to detect immunoglobulin-containing (Ig) cells, and in some cases, viral antigens within CNS material. The findings are briefly reviewed below.

The material examined consisted almost entirely of sections of brains and spinal cords which had been obtained at autopsy, fixed in 10% neutral formalin and embedded in paraffin wax. In some cases, material was used after many years of storage either in formalin or in paraffin wax. Serial sections of 6μm were cut and stained by the immunoperoxidase technique (PAP) using rabbit antisera to human IgG, A and M heavy chains, and κ and λ light chains (Dakopatts). In the case of herpes simplex encephalitis (HSE) and subacute sclerosing panencephalitis (SSPE) additional sections were also stained with a rabbit antiserum to herpes simplex virus (type 1), and measles virus respectively. Details of the techniques used are to be found in earlier publications (Esiri et al., 1976; Esiri, 1980a, b; Esiri et al., 1981; Esiri, 1982). Control sections were treated with either normal rabbit serum, antilysozyme antibody, or with the above antisera preabsorbed with the appropriate antigen. With cases of SSPE, poliomyelitis and multiple sclerosis (MS) quantification of the numbers of nucleated cells with a rounded cytoplasmic outline staining strongly for each of the immunoglobulin determinants was carried out by systematically scanning equivalent areas and counting the stained cells in each of the serial sections. This was done in pathologically damaged and undamaged areas in multiple sclerosis and poliomyelitis. Results were compared by a nonparametric statistical test.

POLIOMYELITIS

Material was examined from the spinal cords and brainstems from 10 patients, 6 of whom died during the first 6 weeks of an attack of acute poliomyelitis and 4 between 4 and 8 months later (Esiri, 1980b). The highest numbers of Ig cells were found within lesions in the acute phase, but only after the first week (Table I). Counts for light chain- and heavy chain-contai-

TABLE I

MEAN (± S.D.) NUMBERS OF LIGHT CHAIN- AND HEAVY CHAIN-CONTAINING CELLS IN
LESIONS OF ACUTE AND CONVALESCENT PHASES OF POLIO

(From Esiri, 1980b, with permission).

	Heavy chains			Light chains		
G	A	M	Total	κ	λ	Total
Acute phase (n = 67)						
3.5 ± 4.1	7.2 ± 5.3	2.3 ± 4.7	13.0 ± 10.9	7.7 ± 7.6	11.1 ± 8.9	18.9 ± 14.0
(27%)	(55%)	(18%)		(41%)	(59%)	
Chronic phase (n = 79)						
1.3 ± 2.3	2.8 ± 4.6	0.36 ± 0.6	4.5 ± 6.3	3.0 ± 3.7	2.9 ± 3.8	6.0 ± 7.2
(29%)	(63%)	(8%)		(51%)	(49%)	

ning cells were significantly lower during the convalescent phase, but some cells were still present 8 months after the onset. Most of the positively stained cells were mature plasma cells and the remainder appeared to be large lymphocytes. These cells were present within perivascular inflammatory cell cuffs, and within the neighbouring damaged neuropil (Fig. 1). Cells

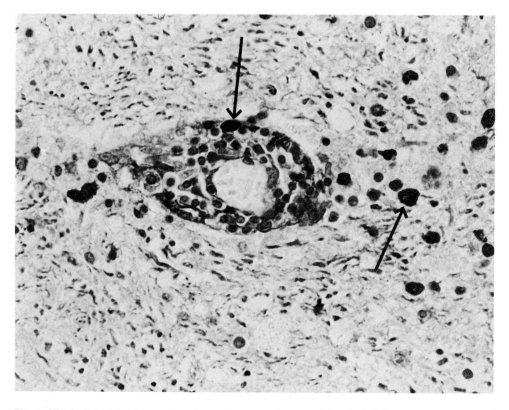

Fig. 1. Histological section from acute poliomyelitis lesion, showing staining for IgA in the cytoplasm of several plasma cells in the perivascular space and neuropil (arrows). Counterstained with haematoxylin × 600. (From Esiri, 1980b, with permission.)

containing IgA were more common than those containing IgG or IgM in both the acute phase, when they constituted 55% of the heavy chain-containing cells and the convalescent phase, when they constituted 63% of the heavy chain-containing cells demonstrated (Table I). IgM- and IgG-containing cells accounted respectively for 18% and 27% of the total seen in the acute phase and for 8% and 29% of the total in the convalescent phase. In the acute phase there were significantly more cells shown to contain light chains than heavy chains ($P < 0.01$), but this difference was not significant during the convalescent phase. There was slightly more λ than κ light chain demonstrated in the acute phase and a reversal of this ratio during the convalescent phase.

Outside the areas of damage the numbers of Ig cells were very small indeed in both acute and convalescent phases. It therefore appeared that there was a focal immune response, involving immunoglobulin-producing cells, closely localized to the areas of the CNS damaged by the polio virus. This response was maximal after the first week and during the following few weeks, and only slowly subsided, being still clearly detectable 8 months later. No attempt was made to detect polio virus antigen in this material.

HERPES SIMPLEX ENCEPHALITIS

Material has recently been examined from the brains of 29 patients with HSE who survived for periods varying from 5 days to 3 years after onset of the neurological disease (Esiri, 1982). Half the patients died within 15 days of the onset, and all but 6 within 24 days. Attention was directed particularly at those parts of the brain which are known from pathological studies to be involved in this disease (Haymaker et al., 1958; Hughes, 1969; Adams and Miller, 1973), and sections were examined for the presence of herpes simplex viral antigen as well as for the presence of Ig cells.

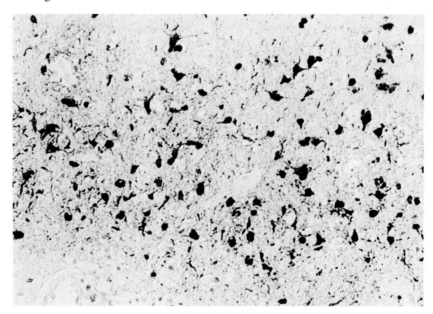

Fig. 2. Herpes simplex encephalitis. Insula cortex containing neurons and glial cells stained with an anti-herpes simplex antibody. Counterstained with haematoxylin ×200. (From Esiri, 1982, with permission.)

Viral antigen was found within the brain in all cases dying within 3 weeks of the onset of the neurological disease, but in none thereafter. Viral antigen was already most abundant in the brains of patients dying within the first week and remained plentiful during the first 16 days (Fig. 2). Inflammation and necrosis reached a peak in the third and fourth weeks when viral antigen was waning. The viral antigen was concentrated mainly in medial and inferior temporal lobes, hippocampus, amygdaloid nuclei, olfactory cortex, insulae, and cingulate gyri. It was frequently found in neurons, astrocytes and oligodendrocytes but only rarely in ependymal cells, and never found in endothelial or inflammatory cells. Viral antigen was invariably present on both sides of the brain but was more abundant on one side than the other, particularly in the first week. Viral antigen was found in the olfactory tracts (in glial cells) in 9 of 15 cases in which these were examined during the first 3 weeks of the disease. It was not seen in relation to trigeminal pathways. A particularly severe involvement of the granule cells of the dentate fascia was seen in almost all cases, and in the cases dying late in the course of the disease, this layer of cells within the hippocampus had frequently been destroyed.

The difference in amounts of viral antigen between the two cerebral hemispheres was greatest in the first week of the disease, suggesting that the viral infection may have arisen within one cerebral hemisphere and then spread to the other. With regard to the source of virus, the evidence from this study points strongly to the olfactory route although another possibility might be generation of infectious virus from a source of latent infection within the brain, perhaps within one anterior temporal lobe.

Examination of the Ig cells present in these cases showed that there were few positively stained cells present in the first week, but that by the third and fourth weeks very large numbers of Ig cells were present in perivascular spaces and neuropil. There was no significant difference at any stage of the disease between the numbers of cells containing light chains and the numbers containing heavy chains. Most of the heavy chain-containing cells stained for IgG and almost all the rest contained IgA (Table II). In 2 cases however IgM accounted for 21% and 23% of the heavy chain-containing cells. In the remaining cases IgM was present only in very small numbers of cells. The $\kappa:\lambda$ ratio varied little during the course of the disease (Table II). Occasional Ig cells were present in areas of damage within the brain in patients dying 2 and 3 years after onset of the disease.

TABLE II

PROPORTIONS (AS PERCENTAGES) OF LIGHT CHAIN- AND HEAVY CHAIN-CONTAINING CELLS IN HERPES SIMPLEX ENCEPHALITIS

Week	κ	λ	$\kappa:\lambda$	IgG	IgA	IgM	Inflammation
1 (n=2)	45	55	0.8	30	61	9	$\pm$
2 (n=8)	57	43	1.3	69	25	6	$++$
3 (n=6)	44	56	0.8	61	35	4	$+++$
4–5 (n=3)	47	53	0.9	84	15	1	$+++$
6 weeks on (n=4)	48	52	0.9	78	20	2	$+$

SUBACUTE SCLEROSING PANENCEPHALITIS

Material was examined from 5 cases of SSPE and from one case of atypical measles encephalitis in a child on immunosuppressive treatment for leukaemia. The distribution of measles virus antigen and Ig cells within the CNS have been described in detail elsewhere (Esiri et al., 1981), and will be briefly summarized here. The cases of SSPE had had a duration of illness ranging from 3 months to 7.5 years, and the child with atypical measles encephalitis died after a 2 week neurological illness. In all cases measles virus antigen was found within the brain, and in all but the longest surviving case it was very widely distributed in cerebral cortex and white matter, basal ganglia and brainstem. The virus antigen was found within neurons and oligodendrocytes but not within astrocytes, endothelial cells or inflammatory cells (Fig. 3). In

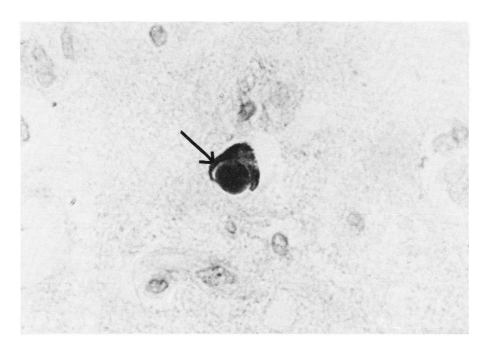

Fig. 3. Measles virus antigen in nucleus and cytoplasm of a cortical neuron from a case of SSPE (arrow). Counterstained with haematoxylin. ×800

the longest surviving case measles antigen was very scanty and confined to small foci in the cerebral cortex, subcortical white matter, hypothalamus, thalamus and brainstem. In the case of atypical measles encephalitis some multinucleate giant cells containing measles antigen were found in the hypothalamus. Ig cells were found widely distributed in all cases but varied from case to case in their frequency (Table III). They were most numerous in the cases of SSPE with short survival, and least numerous in the case of atypical measles encephalitis. Significantly more light chain-than heavy chain-containing cells were found in SSPE, but not in the case of atypical measles encephalitis. IgG was the commonest heavy chain demonstrated, although the proportion of heavy chain-containing cells containing IgG varied widely from 51 to 100%. IgA was the next most common heavy chain demonstrated. IgM contributed most significantly in the case of atypical measles encephalitis (39% of total heavy chain). In 3 cases of SSPE Ig cells were more common in grey than in white matter, and in the other two cases, which were the cases with longer survival, and the cases with the more severe white matter damage, there were more Ig cells in white than in grey matter. The $\kappa:\lambda$ ratios varied considerably, but in 4 of the 5 cases of SSPE this ratio was greater than unity (Table III).

TABLE III

SUMMARY OF IMMUNOGLOBULIN-CONTAINING CELLS IN SSPE

Data show mean cells per high power field (± S.D.). Figures in parentheses = percentages. (From Esiri et al. 1981, with permission.)

Case number	Number of areas scanned	Heavy chains				Light chains			
		G	A	M	Total	κ	λ	κ:λ	Total
1	Not applicable*	8.7 (58)	0.4 (2.6)	6.0 (39.4)	15.1	9.1 (43)	11.9 (57)	0.75	21.0
2	Grey matter (15) White matter (15) Total = 30	5.05±5.4 (69)	2.02±3.6 (28)	0.2 ±0.27 (3)	7.27±8.2	7.2 ±7.4 (57)	5.43±6.4 (43)	1.33	12.63±12.7
3	Grey matter (15) White matter (17) Total = 32	2.0 ±3.8 (92)	0.16±0.4 (8)	–	2.16±3.8	2.1 ±2.6 (53)	1.88±2.0 (47)	1.13	3.98± 4.6
4	Grey matter (9) White matter (9) Mixed (pons) (6) Total = 24	1.27±1.8 (99.7)	–	0.004±0.02 (0.3)	1.3 ±1.8	1.28±1.3 (55)	1.06±1.3 (45)	1.22	2.34± 2.3
5	Grey matter (12) White matter (12) Total = 24	0.9 ±0.9 (78)	0.09±0.09 (8)	0.17 ±0.22 (14)	1.16±1.0	1.71±1.4 (74)	0.59±0.5 (26)	2.85	2.3 ± 1.8
6	Grey matter (14) White matter Total = 29	1.78±2.5 (51)	1.72±1.7 (49)	0.01 ±0.04	3.51±3.9	2.57±3.5 (49)	2.7 ±2.8 (51)	0.96	5.27± 6.3
	Total (cases 2–6) 139								

* Cells counted in 10 selected perivascular regions. Total numbers of cells too small for statistical analysis.

TABLE IV

MEAN NUMBERS OF IMMUNOGLOBULIN-CONTAINING CELLS IN PLAQUES AND NON-PLAQUE
AREAS EXPRESSED AS NUMBER OF CELLS PER HIGH-POWER FIELD

(From Esiri 1980a, with permission).

	Heavy chain				Light chain			$\kappa{:}\lambda$ ratio
	IgG	IgA	IgM	Total	κ	λ	Total	
Non-plaque (n = 210)	0.066 (93%)	0.005 (7%)	0	0.071	0.083	0.052	0.135	1.6
Plaques								
old (n = 91)	0.239 (82%)	0.043 (15%)	0.008 (3%)	0.29	0.286	0.150	0.436	1.9
intermediate (n = 104)	0.874 (82%)	0.18 (17%)	0.019 (1%)	1.07	1.034	0.615	1.65	1.7
recent (n = 52)	1.92 (83%)	0.367 (16%)	0.019 (1%)	2.31	2.94	2.0	4.94	1.5

MULTIPLE SCLEROSIS

Autopsy material has been examined from 23 cases of MS, and the numbers of Ig cells compared in plaque and non-plaque tissue, and in plaques of varying ages, (Esiri, 1977; Esiri, 1980a). These cells were found to be much more numerous within plaques than outside them and to be more common in recent than in old plaques (Table IV). They were found in

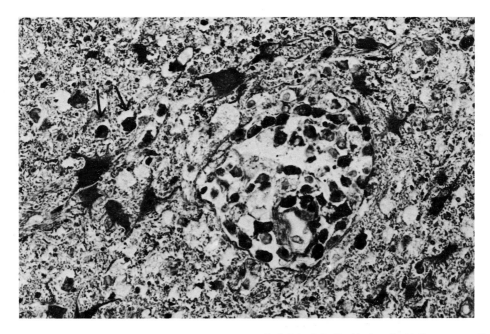

Fig. 4. Perivascular region within a recent MS plaque stained for λ light chain. Positively stained inflammatory cells are present in the perivascular space and neuropil (arrows). Astrocytes are also positively stained. Counterstained with haematoxylin. ×570. (From Esiri, 1980a, with permission.)

perivascular spaces in plaques of all ages, and within the surrounding neuropil only in recent plaques (Fig. 4). In plaques of all ages, but particularly in recent plaques, more light chain-than heavy chain-containing cells were demonstrated. There was considerable variation in $\kappa:\lambda$ ratios between different plaques even in the same case, but overall more κ than λ was demonstrated ($\kappa:\lambda$ ratio 1.7). 83% of the heavy chain found within these cells in plaques consisted of IgG and most of the remainder consisted of IgA. Sections of selected plaques were treated with an anti-measles antibody but no measles virus antigen was detected.

TABLE V

CLINICAL AND PATHOLOGICAL FEATURES FROM 5 CASES OF PERIVENOUS LEUCOENCEPHALITIS

Case number	Sex	Age (years)	Survival (days)	Clinical course	Pathology
1	M	39	3	Influenza-like illness for 10 days. Next day awoke unable to move legs. Admitted to hospital with paraplegia and sensory level at T9. Laminectomy performed but deteriorated and died	Severe perivenous inflammation with microglial and lymphocytic cells and early perivenous demyelination in brain and spinal cord. Haemorrhagic change in thoracic cord
2	F	13	4	Acute measles with rash and fever. On eighth day drowsy with stiff neck. Admitted to hospital pyrexial, with stiff neck and papilloedema. Next day had fit, required artificial ventilation and died 2 days later	As above but without haemorrhage
3	F	57	4	Rash with respiratory illness, diagnosed as "atypical pneumonia", for 13 days. Next day high fever, drowsy with headache. Admitted following day to hospital with hemiparesis. Developed coma and died 3 days later	As above, with haemorrhagic change in brain and cord
4	F	33	5		As above but without haemorrhagic changes and with some more extensive areas of demyelination
5	F	29	7	Influenza-like illness with vomiting for 8 days, followed by confusion, photophobia, neck stiffness and drowsiness. On admission to hospital had poorly reactive pupils and mild papilloedema. Developed coma, respiratory arrest and died	As above, with haemorrhagic changes in thoracic cord

PERIVENOUS ENCEPHALITIS

Material has been examined from 5 cases of perivenous leucoencephalitis. The clinical and pathological features of these cases are briefly summarized in Table V. The patients survived for 3–7 days from the onset of their neurological illness. In one case there had been an immediately preceding attack of measles (case 2). In 3 of the other 4 cases a less well defined pyrexial illness had preceded the onset of the neurological illness.

In all cases Ig cells were found within the spinal cord and/or brain, but such cells were relatively sparse in all cases, despite the presence of many mononuclear inflammatory cells within perivascular spaces and surrounding neuropil (Fig. 5). Most of the cells found to stain for heavy chains contained IgG, and most of the remainder stained for IgA. κ and λ light chain-containing cells were present in about equal numbers. A search for measles virus antigen in case 2 was negative.

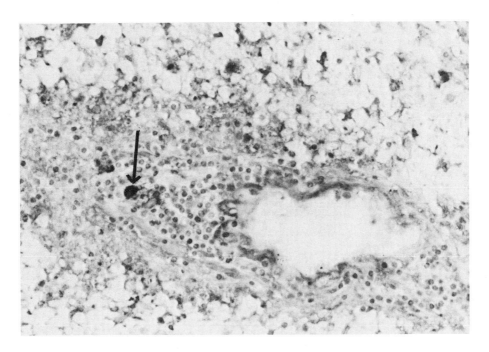

Fig. 5. Perivenous leucoencephalitis. Intense perivascular inflammation with presence of only a single cell stained for λ light chain (arrow). Counterstained with haematoxylin. ×250

CONCLUDING REMARKS

Ig cells were detected in all these 5 diseases within the CNS, and appeared to be closely confined to the areas of damage, whether these were focal (e.g. poliomyelitis, MS), or more widespread (e.g. SSPE). In HSE they were found in very large numbers in parts of the brain that had been severely damaged, but in which viral antigen was no longer detectable, whereas at an earlier stage of the disease, when viral antigen was abundant, Ig cells were only scanty. In poliomyelitis also, large numbers of Ig cells were found after the first week of the disease, i.e. following the period of viral-inflicted damage. In SSPE Ig cells and viral antigen were detectable concurrently. In all these diseases Ig cells were present in perivascular spaces and in the damaged neuropil. In MS a similar pattern was seen, with appearance of Ig cells at sites of damage, particularly recent damage, to myelin, although the Ig cell response was on a smaller scale than in the known viral diseases. By analogy with these diseases, it seems possible that a putative viral antigen may have been present prior to the appearance of these cells. In perivenous encephalitis a rather different picture was seen. A well-marked inflammatory cell response was seen, but Ig cells formed only a small part of it. Possibly many of the cells present were T-lymphocytes and microglial cells.

In all these diseases apart from poliomyelitis, IgG constituted the major heavy chain present. IgA was also present, but only exceeded IgG in poliomyelitis. IgM-containing cells were most frequently seen in acute poliomyelitis and atypical measles encephalitis, two diseases in which recent exposure to the viral antigen may be presumed. IgM was only present in comparable proportions of cells in 2 of 29 cases of HSE and 2 of 23 cases of MS. This observation perhaps favours the view that in HSE, SSPE and MS the immune response is directed towards an antigen to which the individual has been previously exposed.

In 3 diseases, acute poliomyelitis, SSPE and MS, there was an excess of light chain- over heavy chain-containing cells demonstrated. A similar but not significant trend was also present in HSE and the convalescent phase of poliomyelitis. It is possible that this discrepancy is due to an over-production of light chain by some Ig cells. This suggestion is supported by the observation of free light chains in the cerebrospinal fluid in MS and SSPE (Iwashita et al., 1974; Bollengier et al., 1975; Riberi et al., 1975; Kolar, 1977; Vandvik, 1977). No evidence was found that the apparent shortfall of heavy chain was due to the presence of IgD or IgE when selected sections were stained for these antigens.

This study provides evidence of a long-lasting immune response within the CNS in these diseases. In poliomyelitis, Ig cells were still present 8 months after onset and in HSE these cells were still present 3 years after onset. Further study of the profiles of these immune responses may be expected to provide considerable insight into the nature of immune reactions within the nervous system, not only in those diseases which are known to be caused by viruses, but also in diseases where viral antigens have not as yet been detected.

ACKNOWLEDGEMENT

This work was supported by the Medical Research Council.

REFERENCES

Adams, H. and Miller, D. (1973) Herpes simplex encephalitis: a clinical and pathological analysis of 22 cases. *Postgrad. Med. J.,* 49: 393–397.

Bollengier, F., Lowenthal, A. and Henrotin, W. (1975) Bound and free light chains in subacute sclerosing panencephalitis and multiple sclerosis serum and cerebrospinal fluid. *Zeitsch. Klin. Chem. Klin. Biochem.,* 13: 305–310.

Esiri, M.M. (1977) Immunoglobulin-containing cells in multiple sclerosis plaques. *Lancet,* 2: 478–480.

Esiri, M.M. (1980a) Multiple sclerosis: a quantitative and qualitative study of immunoglobulin-containing cells in the central nervous system. *Neuropath. appl. Neurobiol.,* 6: 9–21.

Esiri M.M. (1980b) Poliomyelitis: immunoglobulin-containing cells in the central nervous system in acute and convalescent phases of the human disease. *Clin. exp. Immunol.,* 40: 42–48.

Esiri, M.M. (1982) Herpes simplex encephalitis: an immunohistological study of the distribution of viral antigen within the brain. *J. Neurol. Sci.*, 54: 209–226.

Esiri, M.M., Taylor, C.R. and Mason, D.Y. (1976) Application of an immunoperoxidase method to a study of the central nervous system: preliminary findings in a study of formalin-fixed material. *Neuropath. appl. Neurobiol.*, 2: 233–246.

Esiri, M.M., Oppenheimer, D.R., Brownell, B. and Haire, M. (1981) Distribution of measles antigen and immunoglobulin-containing cells in the CNS in subacute sclerosing panencephalitis and atypical measles encephalitis. *J. Neurol. Sci.*, 53: 29–43.

Haymaker, W., Smith, M.G., van Bogaert, L. and Chenar, C. de (1958) Pathology of the viral disease in man characterised by nuclear inclusions. In *Viral Encephalitides*, Thomas Springfield. pp. 95–104.

Hughes, J.T. (1969) Pathology of herpes simplex encephalitis. In C.W.M. Whitty, J.T. Hughes and F.O. MacCallum (Eds.), *Virus Diseases and the Nervous System*. Blackwells, pp. 29–37.

Iwashita, H., Grunwald, F. and Bauer, H. (1974) Double ring formation in single radial immunodiffusion for kappa chains in multiple sclerosis cerebrospinal fluid. *J. Neurol.*, 297: 45–52.

Kolar, O.J. (1977) Light chains in cerebrospinal fluid in multiple sclerosis. *Lancet*, 2: 1030.

Riberi, M., Bernard, D. and Dipieds, R. (1975) Evidence for the presence of λ chain dimers in cerebrospinal fluid of patients suffering from subacute sclerosing panencephalitis. *Clin. exp. Immunol.*, 19: 45–53.

Sternberger, L.A. (1979) *Immunocytochemistry*, 2nd Edn., Wiley, New York.

Vandvik, B. (1977) Oligoclonal IgG and free light chains in the cerebrospinal fluid of patients with multiple sclerosis and infectious diseases of the CNS. *Scand. J. Immunol.*, 6: 913–922.

Immunology of Nervous System Infections, Progress in Brain Research, Vol. 59, edited by P.O. Behan, V. ter Meulen and F. Clifford Rose

Coronavirus JHM-Induced Demyelinating Encephalomyelitis in Rats: Influence of Immunity on the Course of Disease

HELMUT WEGE, RIHITO WATANABE, MAKOTO KOGA and VOLKER TER MEULEN

Institute for Virology and Immunobiology, University of Würzburg, Versbacher Str. 7, D-8700 Würzburg (F.R.G.)

INTRODUCTION

Disease processes of the central nervous system (CNS) accompanied by demyelination may be the result of a viral infection or the consequence of an immunopathological reaction directed against myelin (ter Meulen and Hall, 1978; Wisniewski, 1977; Weiner and Stohlman, 1978). In acute viral infections it has been assumed that the infection of oligodendroglial cells, leading to cell destruction, may be the main mechanism for inducing this neuropathological lesion. In the case of a persistent virus infection in oligodendroglia cells, however, it is conceivable that functional impairment of oligodendroglia cells, and/or the induction of an immune reaction to the agent which may cross-react with brain antigens, could eventually cause demyelination. Therefore, pathogenic studies on subacute or chronic demyelinating encephalomyelitides in association with viral infections may provide information on the mechanisms involved in demyelination.

In connection with this, infections by murine coronaviruses are of increasing interest (Wege et al., 1982). Strain JHM is known for its ability to cause demyelinating encephalomyelitis in different animal species (Cheever et al., 1949; Bailey et al., 1949; Weiner, 1973; Powell and Lampert, 1975; Fleury, 1980). Additionally, the virus has a tendency to cause chronic infections accompanied by demyelination (Herndon et al., 1975; Stohlman and Weiner, 1981). In rats, depending on the biological property of the virus material used, the genetic background and immune response of the host, a subacute or late demyelinating encephalomyelitis can be induced, accompanied by primary demyelination (Nagashima et al., 1978, 1979; Sorensen et al., 1980). This provides a model for analysis of the virus and host factors which interact in the pathogenesis of these diseases. In this chapter the results of our studies are summarized.

MATERIALS AND METHODS

Virus

The murine coronavirus JHM was either propagated by passage of brain homogenates from suckling mice, or grown in Sac (−) cells, and purified according to Wege et al. (1978).

Temperature sensitive mutants were selected from virus stocks, after mutagenesis with 5′-fluoruracil, by growth at 34°C and selection at 39.5°C, similar to the methods used by Haspel et al. (1978) and Robb et al. (1979).

Animals

The animals used for experiments were either outbred rats, strain Thom/Chbb (Thomae, Biberach, F.R.G.) or inbred rats, strain Lewis. Animals were inoculated into the left brain hemisphere with 0.03 ml of virus suspension using a dispenser syringe. Methods for histology, electron microscopy and virus isolation have been described in previous communications (Nagashima et al., 1978, 1979).

Immunization

For immunization, female adult rats were inoculated i.p. 4–6 times, with about 1×10^6 pfu of JHM-virus per injection. Alternatively, female rats were immunized by footpad and intradermal inoculation. The virus was purified inactivated by treatment with β-propiolactone and mixed with complete Freund's adjuvant. The animals were boosted 3 weeks later by i.m. and i.v. inoculation with purified inactivated virus. The rats were mated after the last immunization, and suckling animals born from these mothers were infected by intracerebral inoculation of JHM virus (ts6) at an age of 4–5 days.

Stimulation of lymphocytes

Lymphocytes were cultivated and stimulated with either guinea pig myelin basic protein or inactivated purified virus, according to the methods of Richert et al. (1979). Lymphoblast transformation was determined by measuring the incorporation of [^{3}H]thymidine, and adoptive transfer was performed by i.v. inoculation of $1 \times 10^7 - 1 \times 10^8$ lymphocytes according to Richert et al. (1979).

RESULTS

CNS diseases induced by JHM virus in rats

Uncloned JHM virus inoculated into the brain of suckling rats caused an acute panencephalitis (APE) which developed after a short incubation time (2–8 days) and rapidly led to death. The virus spread through all parts of the CNS, and also caused severe hepatitis. However, when JHM virus was inoculated into rats older than 21 days, two different courses, acute and subacute encephalomyelitis, were observed. After a relatively short incubation time of 6–12 days, a rapidly progressing paralytic disease occurred which was always fatal. The lesions of this acute encephalomyelitis (AE) were often necrotizing with a strong involvement of the CNS grey matter (Fig. 1A). Cell infiltrations were typical of acute inflammations and consisted mainly of polymorphnuclear lymphocytes (Fig. 1B). Viral antigens were detectable in both neurons and glia cells. Animals which showed clinical signs several weeks to months post-infection (p.i.) developed typical plaques of primary demyelination. The lesions of this subacute demyelinating encephalomyelitis (SDE) were disseminated predominantly in selected areas of the white matter including the optic nerve, midbrain and spinal cord. As illustrated in Fig. 2A, plaques were sharply demarcated. Neurons and axons were well preserved, even within the demyelinated area. Perivascular infiltrations consisted mainly of monocytes (Fig. 2B). Viral antigens were confined to glia cells. Animals which developed clinical disease after an incubation time of several months (late demyelinating encephalomyelitis, LDE) showed signs of both demyelination and remyelination on electron microscopic examination, indicating a chronic disease process. Infectious virus could be reisolated even after this long incubation time from such diseased animals.

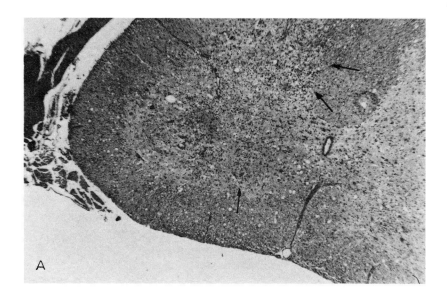

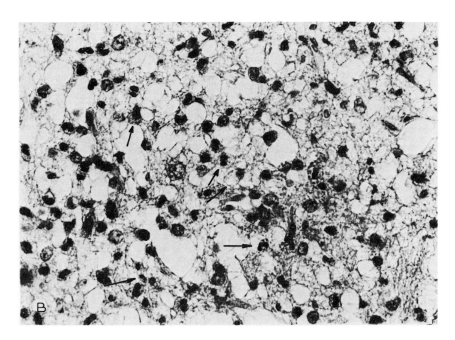

Fig. 1. Spinal cord, acute encephalomyelitis (10 days p.i.) A: widespread cell infiltrations (arrows) in necrotic area of grey matter. HE staining, × 35. B: numerous phagocytes (small arrows) including neutrophilic leucocytes (large arrows) in infiltrated area. HE staining, × 400.

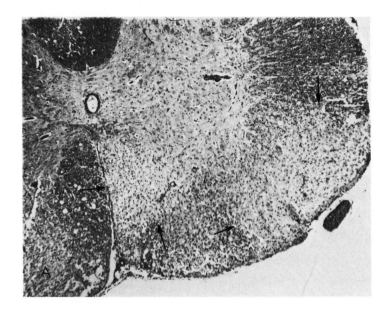

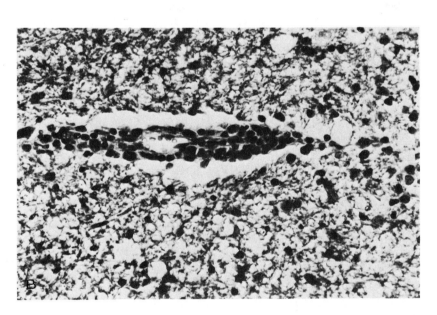

Fig. 2. Spinal cord, subacute demyelinating encephalomyelitis (25 days p.i.). A: demarcated demyelinating plaques (arrows) in white matter. Neurons are well-preserved. HE staining, ×35. B: mononuclear cell infiltration around venule. HE staining, ×400.

Influence of host age and properties of the virus on disease course

Intracerebral infection with uncloned JHM virus gave rise only to APE in suckling rats (Thomae/Chbb); in rats inoculated at an age of 21–25 days both acute, and subacute to late, encephalomyelitis developed (Table I). Cloned virus, which was adapted to grow in tissue

TABLE I

CORONAVIRUS JHM INFECTION IN RATS

Virus inoculated	Age of animals at infection	
	Suckling (< 20 days)	*Weanling (> 20 days)*
Uncloned virus	Acute panencephalitis	Acute encephalomyelitis, subacute and late demyelinating encephalomyelitis
Cloned virus	Acute panencephalitis	Acute encephalomyelitis
ts-mutants	Acute panencephalitis and subacute demyelinating encephalomyelitis depending on age of animal and mutant	Subacute and late demyelinating encephalomyelitis

culture, however, had lost the capacity to induce demyelinating diseases and led, depending on the age of the animals, to APE or AE. By contrast, temperature-sensitive mutants differed widely in their neurovirulence, and mutants were found which induced high rates of SDE in suckling rats. The results obtained with ts43, for example, are summarized in Table II: APE was only induced in rats which are inoculated within 5 days after birth. Animals inoculated with wild type virus, however, developed a typical APE which rapidly led to death, regardless of the age at infection. Animals inoculated with ts43 predominantly developed SDE especially if infected at an age of 10–15 days. With increasing age, however, the rats became resistant to the ts mutant. It is noteworthy that many animals recovered after disease periods of 1–4 weeks.

TABLE II

COMPARISON OF NEUROVIRULENCE OF JHM wt AND JHM ts43

wt, JHM wild-type virus; ts, temperature-sensitive mutant.

Age at time of infection ± 1 day	Virus 4×10^3 pfu/rat I.C.	Diseased/ total	Range of incubation time (days)	Recovery from disease	Type of disease
4	wt	7/10	3–5	none	APE
	ts43	26/26	10–17	2/13	APE< SDE
10	wt	8/10	3–6	none	APE
	ts43	22/43	14–112	11/22	SDE
15	wt	7/12	4–11	none	APE/AE
	ts43	1/12	92	–	LDE

Antiviral immunity and development of SDE

Neuropathological examination of clinically healthy rats which were dissected 30–40 days p.i., often revealed demyelinating lesions, although no infectious virus was recoverable from such animals. Further detailed studies on the kinetics of virus growth, occurrence of neutralizing antibodies and distribution and type of lesions, indicated that the development of demyelinating lesions was preceded by an AE, which did not lead to a clinically recognizable disease (Fig. 3). For this experiment, rats were infected at the age of 21–24 days with uncloned JHM virus. Groups of clinically healthy rats were randomly selected and sacrificed for investigation as shown on the time scale in Fig. 3. Within 3–12 days p.i., infectious virus could be isolated from CNS tissue of clinically healthy animals. During this early period, most of these rats revealed a neuropathologically and clinically silent AE. Later in infection, when an antiviral immune response was measurable, no infectious virus could be isolated. However, demyelinating plaques were detected in many rats which did not show a clinical disease.

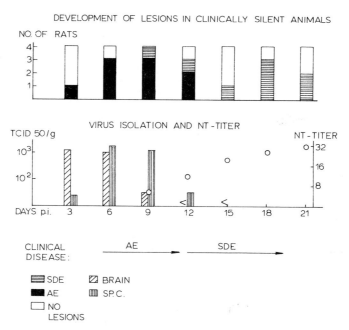

Fig. 3. Development of lesions, virus growth and antiviral immune response in clinically silents rats. Animals were infected with uncloned JHM virus at an age of 21–24 days.

These observations suggest that, in addition to the biological properties of the virus and to the host age, the antiviral immune response may modify the JHM-induced disease course. To test this hypothesis, we infected suckling rats born from mothers which were already immune against JHM virus (Fig. 4). The animals were inoculated at an age of 4–5 days with the mutant ts6. Non-immune suckling rats infected under the same conditions died within 5–15 days from a typical APE. Suckling rats born from immune mothers, however, developed high rates of SDE after prolonged incubation times. Infection of suckling rats which were born from mothers immunized by purified inactivated virus led to a similar high rate of SDE with a prolonged onset. These results indicate that the antiviral immune response can indeed modify the disease process.

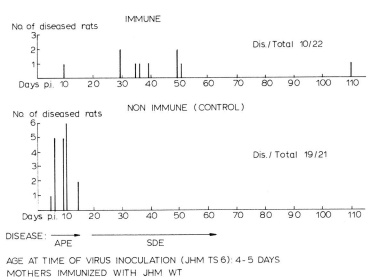

Fig. 4. Influence of maternal immunity to JHM virus on the development of CNS disease in suckling rats.

Possible involvement of reactive lymphocytes in development of SDE

In order to determine whether cell-mediated immune reactions might play a role in JHM virus-induced demyelination, experiments were performed in Lewis rats, an inbred strain which is genetically characterized and susceptible for EAE. The inoculation of JHM virus into Lewis rats led to the same disease patterns as described in the previous sections. In animals with SDE, we noticed a high number of perivascular cuffs which were not observed to such an extent during our experiments with outbred rats. Such cellular infiltrations consisted predominantly of mononuclear cells (Fig. 2B). This interesting observation prompted us to test lymphocytes from SDE animals for their ability to be stimulated with myelin basic protein (MBP) and viral antigen. As summarized in Table III, lymphocytes from Lewis rats with AE derived from peripheral blood, spleen and thymus could only be slightly stimulated by either myelin basic protein or inactivated purified virus. Animals which developed SDE after a prolonged incubation time, however, showed many perivascular cuffs in the CNS tissue and revealed an antiviral immune response indicated by neutralizing antibodies and virus-specific lymphoblast stimulation. Moreover, lymphoblasts incorporated [³H]thymidine on cultivation with myelin basic protein. Such stimulated lymphocytes were transferred to normal recipients in order to investigate the possibility of transferring the SDE disease process. Perivascular cuffs were found in several animals similar to those seen in rats with SDE (Fig. 5). Moreover, slight clinical changes consisting of weight loss, ataxic gait and hindleg paresis were observed. These preliminary results indicate that, during the disease process, lymphocytes sensitized against neuroantigens may contribute to the development of primary demyelination, in addition to the antiviral immune response.

228

TABLE III

ACUTE AND SUBACUTE CNS-DISEASE IN LEWIS RATS

Infection with JHM-virus at an age of 30 days.

	Acute encephalomyelitis	Subacute demyelinating encephalomyelitis
Onset of disease	3–9 days p.i.	12 days p.i.
Perivascular cuffing	Slight (0–4/5 sections)	Strong (> 10/5 sections)
Neutr. antibody titer	1:8	1:16–1:48
Lymphoblast Transformation in vitro		
by JHM-virus	Stimulation index ± 2	6–10 × stimulation index
by MBP	Stimulation index ⩽ 2	2–8 × stimulation index

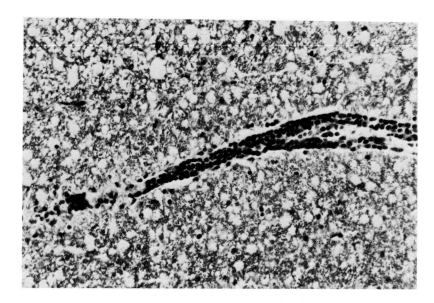

Fig. 5. Infiltration in the spinal cord consisting of mononuclear cells. Rat dissected 5 days post-adoptive transfer of lymphocytes from a rat with SDE. Stimulation by culture with MPB. HE staining, × 250.

DISCUSSION

The rate and onset of demyelinating encephalomyelitis induced in rats infected with JHM virus is influenced by biological properties of the virus, the age of the host at time of infection and the immune status of the host. This framework forms the basis for further studies on the pathogenesis of virus induced demyelination.

The uncloned virus induced both acute and subacute CNS diseases. The development of such different disease courses may be due to a genetically heterogenous virus population, consisting of clones which vary in cell tropism and growth properties. Clones which were randomly selected from tissue-culture-adapted virus were no longer capable of inducing SDE. Temperature-sensitive mutants, however, induced high rates of SDE, and the age of the animal at the time of infection was an important parameter influencing the outcome of disease. These alterations in the virulence of ts mutants are conceivably the result of impaired virus growth at the host body temperature, which enabled the animals to survive the acute stage of infection without clinical manifestation of an APE or AE. In addition, ts-mutants might be restricted in their cell tropism within the host. Knobler et al. (1981) recently demonstrated that a ts mutant of JHM virus has a predilection for replication in oligodendroglia cells, whereas wild type virus also replicates in neurons. Viral antigen was predominantly detectable only in the white matter of the CNS of animals with demyelinating encephalomyelitis or chronic infection (Weiner, 1973; Nagashima et al., 1978 and 1979; Stohlman and Weiner, 1981). Virus particles were only detectable by electron microscopy in degenerating oligodendroglia cells (Nagashima et al., 1978; Lampert et al., 1973).

Several observations indicate that the antiviral immune response may lead to conditions allowing the virus to persist in the CNS provided no clinical disease develops within the first weeks p.i. Development of SDE is probably preceded by a clinically silent AE, as our studies on the kinetics of virus growth and lesions suggest. Demyelinating plaques were only detectable at a time when no infectious virus could be isolated from clinically healthy animals and when an antiviral immune response was measurable.

Further support of the hypothesis that an immune response to the infectious process plays a pathogenic role comes from experiments with suckling rats fostered by mothers which were immune to JHM virus. Under conditions where normal rats clearly developed a fatal APE, rats reared by immune mothers developed high rates of SDE after a prolonged incubation. This type of experiment was only successful if a ts mutant was used for the challenging virus. This noteworthy shift in disease-course may not be mediated only by the continuous presence of antiviral antibodies, since lymphoid cells are also known to be transferred from the mother during the suckling period and to migrate through the gut (Seelig and Beer, 1978). It is conceivable that JHM infection, in the presence of an antiviral immunity, may confine virus replication to the more susceptible oligodendroglia cells and prevent the development of a fatal disease during the acute state of infection.

The occurrence of perivascular infiltrations in rats with SDE suggests a possible immuno-pathological mechanism in the pathogenesis of primary, virus-induced demyelination. Lymphocytes derived from these animals could be stimulated not only by virus antigen, but also by myelin basic protein. Moreover, adoptive transfer of such stimulated lymphocyte cell populations clearly led to CNS infiltration and clinical signs similar to those found in EAE. Therefore, infection of CNS tissue by JHM virus could lead to disturbances in the blood–brain barrier and breakdown or modification of myelin from infected cells, which might consequently result in sensitization of lymphoid cells against both viral and neuroantigens. These observations have to be followed by further experiments in order to characterize the functional role of different lymphocyte cell populations and their role in virus-induced demyelination.

SUMMARY

The murine coronavirus JHM is highly neurotropic for mice and rats. In rats, CNS diseases ranging from acute panencephalitis (AE) to subacute demyelinating encephalomyelitis (SDE) are observed. SDE developes after an incubation time of several weeks to months. Neuropathologically, this disease is characterized by plaques of primary demyelination in selected areas of the CNS, and perivascular infiltrations. The incidence of SDE depends on properties of the virus clone used for infection and on host factors, such as age, immune status and genetic background. First experiments indicate that during viral infection, lymphocytes are sensitized against myelin basic protein and that this may contribute to the pathogenesis of demyelinating lesions in addition to the antiviral immune response.

ACKNOWLEDGEMENTS

We thank Margaret Sturm and Hanna Wege for excellent technical assistance and Helga Kriesinger for secretarial help. This work was supported by the Deutsche Forschungsgemeinschaft and Humboldt-Stiftung.

REFERENCES

Bailey, O.T., Pappenheimer, A.M., Cheever, F.S. and Daniels, J.B. (1949) A murine virus (JHM) causing disseminated encephalomyelitis with extensive destruction of myelin II. Pathology. *J. exp. Med.*, 90: 195–212.

Cheever, F.S., Daniels, J.B., Pappenheimer, A.M. and Bailey, O.T. (1949) A murine virus (JHM) causing disseminated encephalomyelitis with extensive destruction of myelin: I. Isolation and biological properties of the virus. *J. exp. Med.*, 90: 181–194.

Fleury, H.J.A., Sheppard, R.D., Bornstein, M.B. and Raine, C.S. (1980) Further ultrastructural observations of virus morphogenesis and myelin pathology in JHM virus encephalomyelitis. *Neuropath. appl. Neurobiol.*, 6: 165–179.

Haspel, V.M., Lampert, P.W. and Oldstone, M.B.A. (1978) Temperature-sensitive mutants of mouse hepatitis virus produce a high incidence of demyelination. *Proc. nat. Acad. Sci. U.S.A.*, 75: 4033–4036.

Herndon, R.M., Griffin, D.E., McCormick, U. and Weiner, L.P. (1975) Mouse hepatitis virus-induced recurrent demyelination. *Arch. Neurol.*, 32: 32–35.

Knobler, R.L., Dubois-Dalcq, M., Haspel, M.V., Claysmith, A.P., Lampert, P.W. and Oldstone, M.B.A. (1981) Selective localization of wild type and mutant mouse hepatitis virus (JHM strain) antigens in CNS tissue by fluorescence, light and electron microscopy. *J. Neuroimmunol.*, 1: 81–92.

Lampert, P.W., Sims, J.K. and Kniazeff, A.J. (1973) Mechanism of demyelination in JHM virus encephalomyelitis. Electron microscopic studies. *Acta Neuropath.*, 24: 76–85.

Nagashima, K., Wege, H., Meyermann, R. and ter Meulen, V. (1978) Corona virus induced subacute demyelinating encephalomyelitis in rats: a morphological analysis. *Acta Neuropath.*, 44: 63–70.

Nagashima, K., Wege, H., Meyermann, R. and ter Meulen, V. (1979) Demyelinating encephalomyelitis induced by a long-term corona virus infection in rats. *Acta Neuropath.*, 45: 205–213.

Powell, H.C. and Lampert, P.W. (1975) Oligodendrocytes and their myelin-plasma membrane connections in JHM mouse hepatitis virus encephalomyelitis. *Lab. Invest.*, 33: 440–445.

Richert, J.R., Driscoll, B.F., Kies, M.W. and Alvord, E.C. (1979) Adoptive transfer of experimental allergic encephalomyelitis: incubation of rat spleen cells with specific antigen. *J. Immunol.*, 122: 494–496.

Robb, J.A., Bond, C.W. and Leibowitz, J.L. (1979) Pathogenic murine coronaviruses. III. Biological and biochemical characterization of temperature-sensitive mutants of JHMV. *Virology*, 94: 385–399.

Seelig, L.L. and Beer, A.E. (1978) Transepithelial migration of leukocytes in the mammary gland of lactating rats. *Biol. Reprod.*, 17: 730–744.

Sorensen, O., Percy, D. and Dales, S. (1980) In vivo and in vitro models of demyelinating diseases. III. JHM virus infection of rats. *Arch. Neurol.*, 37: 478–484.

Stohlman, S.A. and Weiner, L.P. (1981) Chronic central nervous system demyelination in mice after JHM virus infection. *Neurol.*, 31: 38–44.

Ter Meulen, V. and Hall, W.W. (1978) Slow virus infections of the nervous system: virological, immunological and pathogenetic considerations, *J. gen. Virol.*, 41: 1–25.

Wege, H., Müller, A. and ter Meulen, V. (1978) Genomic RNA of the murine coronavirus JHM. *J. gen. Virol.*, 41: 217–227.

Wege, H., Siddell, S. and ter Meulen, V. (1982) The biology and pathogenesis of coronaviruses. *Current Top. Microbiol. Immunol.*, 99: 165–200.

Weiner, L. (1973) Pathogenesis of demyelination induced by a mouse hepatitis virus (JHM virus). *Arch. Neurol.*, 28: 293–303.

Weiner, L. and Stohlman, S.A. (1978) Viral models of demyelination. *Neurol.*, 28: 111–114.

Wisniewski, H.M. (1977) Immunopathology of demyelination in autoimmune diseases and virus infections. *Brit. Med. Bull.*, 33: 54–59.

Immunology of Nervous System Infections, Progress in Brain Research, Vol. 59, edited by P.O. Behan, V. ter Meulen and F. Clifford Rose

Role of Macrophages in the Immunopathogenesis of Visna–Maedi of Sheep

OPENDRA NARAYAN

Department of Neurology and Comparative Medicine, Johns Hopkins University School of Medicine, Baltimore, MD 21205 (U.S.A.)

INTRODUCTION

Visna and maedi are chronic progressive diseases with prolonged incubation and clinical courses of months to years. These characteristics give rise to the name "slow diseases" (Sigurdsson and Palsson, 1958). Pathologically, the lesions are characterized by active, chronic infiltration and proliferation of mononuclear inflammatory cells in the brain and lung in addition to necrosis of parenchymal cells (Sigurdsson et al., 1962). The disease complex is caused by a persistent infection with an exogenous retro virus. These infections have been identified in sheep populations in most parts of the world and are associated with sporadic outbreaks of disease. The pneumonic form of the disease, maedi is much more prevalent than the encephalitic form, visna. In fact, visna tends to occur as a complication of maedi.

The method of replication of the virus in vivo sets the stage for slow disease, and 3 aspects can be enumerated (Narayan et al., 1977): (1) in all cases, co-cultivation of buffy coat cells with sheep fibroblasts results in syncytial cytopathic effect (CPE) of the fibroblasts and production of budding virions at the cell surfaces. In short, all infected animals are viremic; (2) explantation of diseased tissues results in similar syncytial formation and virus production by fibroblasts growing out from the explants; (3) cell-free suspensions of diseased tissues do not always cause CPE when inoculated in normal sheep fibroblasts.

These 3 phenomena are well known in this infection and are now re-examined in the light of newer findings on the replication of this virus.

Experimental infection

These retro viruses are infectious only for sheep and goats. This rules out the use of more conventional laboratory animals for pathogenetic studies. Virus inoculation of sheep via extraneural routes results in establishment of a persistent infection which can be demonstrated by CPE and virus rescue from blood leukocytes. Infection of CNS very rarely occurs despite persistent infection (Narayan, unpublished observations). Inoculation of virus into the brain results in an acute encephalitis which is followed by the typical active chronic visna lesions and persistent infection of brain and blood. The inflammatory cells in the CSF of these acutely infected animals are immunologically specific for the virus (Griffin et al., 1978). This acute encephalitis can be prevented by immunosuppression but this does not affect virus persistence in brain or blood (Nathanson et al., 1976).

Two other points need to be mentioned about the intracerebrally inoculated sheep: firstly, virus replication in brain cells is restricted (Narayan et al., 1977). This restriction may be at the

[233]

level of transcription of viral RNA (Brahic et al., 1981), thus leaving unexpressed viral genomes in some cells. Secondly, antibody responses vary according to the virus strain used. When laboratory adapted Icelandic visna viruses are used, sheep produce virus neutralizing antibodies which lead to emergence of antigenic variants of the agent (Narayan et al., 1978). When field isolates from American sheep are used, pathologic lesions and persistent infection result but no neutralizing antibody is produced (Narayan, unpublished observations).

Virus target cell

The preceding remarks highlight the essential features of the pathogenesis of visna. During the past 3 years we have directed considerable effort toward identifying the virus target cell in vivo. Studies of both naturally and experimentally infected sheep show that macrophages are invariably infected. In blood, the target cell is the monocyte and in the lung with maedi, the alveolar macrophage. Cultivation of macrophages from infected animals or virus inoculation of macrophage cultures resulted in a persistent productive infection. The main features of this macrophage infection are enumerated: (1) the cells produce limited quantities of infectious virus (10^4–10^6) for up to 3 weeks; (2) virus producing macrophages do not develop CPE; (3) virus synthesis occurs within the cytoplasm and accumulate in cytoplasmic vacuoles; (4) phagocytic functions of the infected macrophage are not impeded (Narayan et al., 1982).

The optimal method for detecting infected macrophages is by addition of fibroblasts to the culture. Syncytial CPE in the fibroblasts develops within 24 h after addition. One of the major implications of this infection is that virus is never cleared out of circulation.

Virus replication in fibroblasts occurs most efficiently when macrophages are present in the cultures. The main points of this infection are enumerated: (1) direct inoculation of fresh isolates of visna–maedi virus on fibroblasts result frequently in abortive replication; (2) addition of nonproducer fibroblasts to normal macrophages result in prompt syncytial formation and virus production by the fibroblasts; (3) in contrast to intracellular maturation of virus in macrophages, viral maturation in fibroblasts occurs at the cell membrane.

These macrophage-fibroblast reactions by field viruses help to explain some of the paradoxes of the infection in the animal and to provide suggestions for immunopathogenesis:

(1) Persistent infection in the animal can be explained by the steady state infection of macrophages.

(2) Virus induction by tissue explantation can be explained by the interaction of virus producing macrophages and fibroblasts which always abound in explant cultures.

(3) Lack of infectivity of tissue suspensions reflects the non-permissiveness of fibroblasts which are used routinely as indicator cells.

(4) Restricted virus replication in brain after i.c. inoculation may be similar to that in fibroblasts, i.e. non-macrophage cells may lack the ability to replicate virus completely. This may explain the failure of viral transcription in brain cells.

(5) The final point extends the theoretical analogy between brain cells and fibroblasts regarding the site of virus synthesis. If CNS cells replicated virus similar to fibroblasts, i.e. on membranes, then they would be targets for the known cellular immune responses in the CNS.

In summary, macrophages play crucial roles in the pathogenesis of this disease complex since they can (a) disseminate virus by the Trojan horse effect; (b) probably elude immunoelimination by intracellular production of virus; (c) control the expression of virus in non-permissively infected cells; (d) amplify the disease process by simultaneously releasing virus and lymphokines in the inflamed areas.

ACKNOWLEDGEMENTS

These studies have been supported by Grants NS 12127, NS 15721 and RR 00130 from the National Institutes of Health, and the Deutsche Forschungsgemeinschaft for a guest professorship at the Justus-Liebig-University, Giessen, F.R.G.

REFERENCES

Brahic, M., Stowring, L., Ventura, P. and Haase, A.T. (1981) Gene expression in Visna virus infection in sheep. *Nature (Lond.)*, 292: 240–242.

Griffin, D.E., Narayan, O. and Adams, R.J. (1978) Early immune responses in Visna, a slow viral disease of sheep. *J. infect. Dis.*, 138: 340–350.

Narayan, O., Griffin, D.E. and Clements, J.E. (1978) Virus mutation during "slow infection": temporal development and characterization of mutants of Visna virus recovered from sheep. *J. gen. Virol.*, 41: 343–352.

Narayan, O., Griffin, D.E. and Silverstein, A.M. (1977) Slow virus infection: replication and mechanisms of persistence of Visna virus in sheep. *J. infect. Dis.*, 135: 800–806.

Narayan, O., Wolinsky, J.S., Clements, J.E., Strandberg, J.D., Griffen, D.E. and Cork, L.C. (1982) Slow virus replication: the role of macrophages in the persistence and expression of visna viruses of sheep and goats. *J. gen. Virol.*, 59: 345–356.

Nathanson, N., Panitch, H., Palsson, P.A., Petursson, G., Georgsson, G. (1976) Pathogenesis of Visna. II. Effect of immunosuppression upon the central nervous system lesions. *Lab. Invest.*, 35: 444–451.

Sigurdsson, B. and Palsson, P.A. (1958) Visna of sheep. A slow demyelinating infection. *Brit. J. exp. Path.*, 39: 519–528.

Sigurdsson, B., Palsson, P.A. and van Bogaert, L. (1962) Pathology of Visna. *Acta Neuropath.*, I: 343–362.

Immunology of Nervous System Infections, Progress in Brain Research, Vol. 59, edited by P.O. Behan, V. ter Meulen and F. Clifford Rose

The Identification and Role of Cells Involved in CNS Demyelination in Mice After Semliki Forest Virus Infection: An Ultrastructural Study

SNEHLATA PATHAK, SHIRIN J. ILLAVIA and H.E. WEBB

Neurovirology Unit, Department of Neurology, The Rayne Institute, St. Thomas' Hospital, London SE1 7EH (U.K.)

INTRODUCTION

At a previous meeting held under the auspices of the Mansell Bequest at the Medical Society of London, Semliki Forest virus (SFV) infections in mice have been presented as a model for studying acute and chronic central nervous system (CNS) infections in man (Webb et al., 1979). Our unit has continued to work with this model, particularly as after a single intraperitoneal (i.p.) injection of an avirulent strain of SFV, mice developed patchy focal demyelination in the CNS (Suckling et al., 1978; Kelly et al., 1982) including the optic nerve (Illavia et al., 1982) and spinal cord. It is a good model because the virus which causes this effect can be given peripherally i.p., which does not break the blood–brain barrier, rather than intracerebrally (i.c.). The virus reaches high titers in blood and brain and only rarely produces a lethal, paralytic illness. Also, the effect of two and 3 i.p. injections of the virus has been studied (Chew-Lim et al., 1977, 1978; Mackenzie et al., 1978), as has the effect of using whole body irradiation (WBXRT), cyclophosphamide, anti-thymocyte serum (ATS) (Webb and Jagelman, 1979), myocrisin (sodium aurothiomalate) (Allner et al., 1974) and the type of disease produced in athymic nude mice (Jagelman et al., 1978). Extensive electron-microscopic studies have been carried out to determine the way in which the virus enters the brain (Pathak and Webb, 1974) and multiplies there, and to identify the cells involved in these processes (Pathak et al., 1976). Attempts have also been made to find out why the virulent strain of SFV L10/C1 can be seen as mature virus in adult mouse brain (over 19 days old), whereas the avirulent strain A7(74)C1 cannot be seen in a recognizable form, in spite of the fact that brain virus titers of mice infected with each strain, on the same post-inoculation day (PID), are very similar when re-titrated back into the baby mice to which both strains are lethal. Mature virus of both strains can be seen easily in the brains of mice up to the age of 14 days after i.p. or i.c. inoculation (Pathak and Webb, 1978). The only immunological manipulation so far found which produces 100% lethal disease in adult mice using the A7(74) avirulent strain is to "blockade" the mouse macrophage system with soluble gold (myocrisin–sodium aurothiomalate) inoculated i.p. When this is done the macrophages "blockaded" with myocrisin become sites of very high virus replication which reaches up to $10^{8.5}$ ICLD$_{50}$/ml (Oaten et al., 1980).

The demyelination that occurs with the avirulent strain is at its maximum between PID 14 and 21 and has largely recovered by PID 36, although evidence that the myelin has been damaged persists in that the myelin remains thin. The time at which the demyelination is starting, is the period just after virus has been cleared from the brain (PID 11) (Jagelman et al.,

238

Fig. 1 is a light micrograph and Figs. 2–10 (except Fig. 7C) are electron micrographs of the demyelinating lesion.

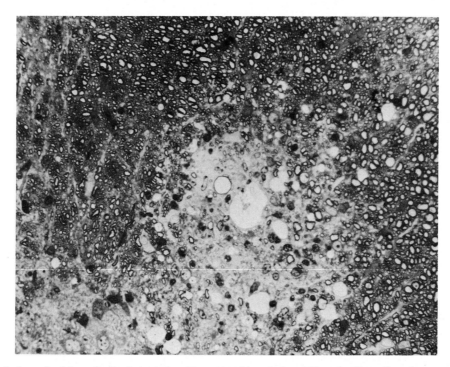

Fig. 1. Large focal demyelinating lesion in the white matter of the spinal cord. Normal well-myelinated axons can be seen around the lesion. PID 17. ×400; 1 μm Araldite section.

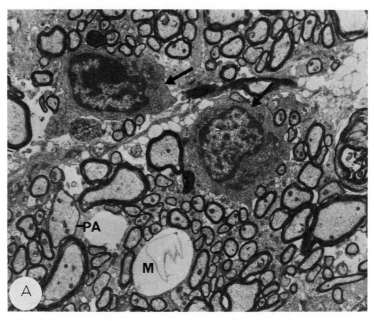

Fig. 2A.

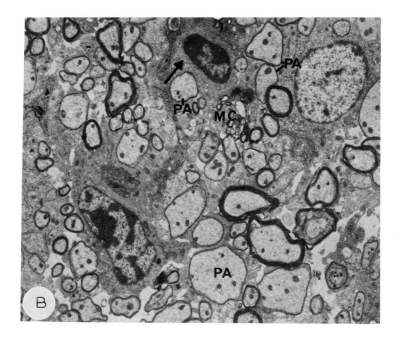

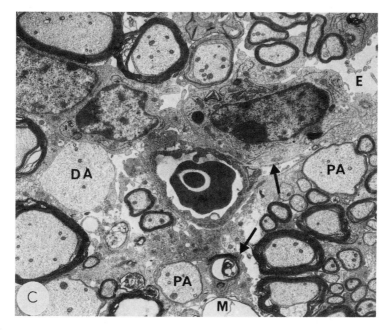

Fig. 2B, C.

Fig. 2. Different areas of the demyelinating lesion showing many infiltrating mononuclear cells and various stages of demyelination. ×3600. A: lymphoblastic cells (arrow) close to well-myelinated axons. Partially demyelinated axon (PA) and microcyst (M). B: many partially demyelinated axons (PA) close to lymphoblastic cell (arrow) and processes of macrophage (MC) with myelin debris. C: many macrophages (arrow) containing myelin debris in their cytoplasm, close to microcyst (M). Partially demyelinated (PA) and completely demyelinated axons (DA). Enlarged irregular extracellular spaces (E).

1978). It was this finding, and the fact that demyelination re-occurs after two or 3 i.p. inoculations of virus, which has made us feel that the demyelination is caused chiefly by immunological mechanisms and not by the cytolysis of oligodendrocytes, as suggested by Sheahan et al. (1981) using another avirulent strain of SFV.

In this chapter we present evidence as to the type of immunological mechanisms which may be involved in this demyelinating process, with special reference to the electromicroscopical identification and role of the cells which are present at the demyelinating sites. We also put forward an hypothesis to explain the method of formation of the spongiform (microcystic) changes which occur, and the significance of these in relation to the demyelination seen. Many infected brains and spinal cords have been examined in this laboratory by light and electron microscopy at different times after infection, and demyelinating lesions in the white matter have been seen, which were constantly present between PID 14 and 21. It has been a feature of our studies of spinal cords on PID 14 and 17 that each large focal lesion has early, middle and late stages of demyelination present together. To emphasize this point, all the pictures presented here, except one (7C), were made from one focal lesion of demyelination from the spinal cord of an infected mouse sampled on PID 17 after an i.p. inoculation. Extensive demyelinating lesions were seen in the brain of this same mouse.

MATERIALS AND METHODS

Mice

This was one of the group of 3 to 4-week-old, statistically random bred, barrier maintained, specific pathogen-free mice of either sex of a Swiss A_2G strain.

Virus

The avirulent strain of SFV, A7(74)C1, received from Dr. C.J. Bradish (Microbiological Research Establishment, Porton, Salisbury, Wiltshire, U.K.) was used. All mice were inoculated i.p. with 0.1 ml of virus containing 10^6 $ICLD_{50}$/ml. Non-inoculated mice of appropriate age were sampled as histological and EM controls.

Electron microscopy

Material was fixed and prepared as reported earlier (Pathak and Webb, 1974). Sections of 1 μm were stained with 1% Toluidine blue and examined by light microscopy. Ultrathin sections were stained with uranyl acetate and lead citrate and examined using an AEI Corinth 500 electron microscope.

RESULTS

The 1 μm sections of the infected spinal cord studied on PID 17 showed large, focal, demyelinating lesions (Fig. 1). These areas were studied by electron microscopy and showed many infiltrating mononuclear cells, microcystic changes and demyelination, along with enlarged, irregular extracellular spaces (Fig. 2A, B and C).

The lesions were limited to white matter and were not particularly concentrated around the blood vessels, although sometimes some blood vessels were seen nearby. Parenchymal tissue around some of these blood vessels showed intense swelling of the astrocytic cytoplasm attached to them, probably indicative of oedema, but no demyelination was present around such blood vessels. Mononuclear cells were numerous in the lesion areas and were identified as lymphoblastic cells and macrophages. Plasma cells were rare and polymorphs were not seen.

The lymphoblastic cells

These cells had a denser cytoplasm and nucleus than the macrophages. They showed paucity of smooth and rough endoplasmic reticulum (S.E.R. and R.E.R.) but had plenty of free, single and polyribosomes and floccular material, and generally appeared "frosted" (Figs. 3 and 4).

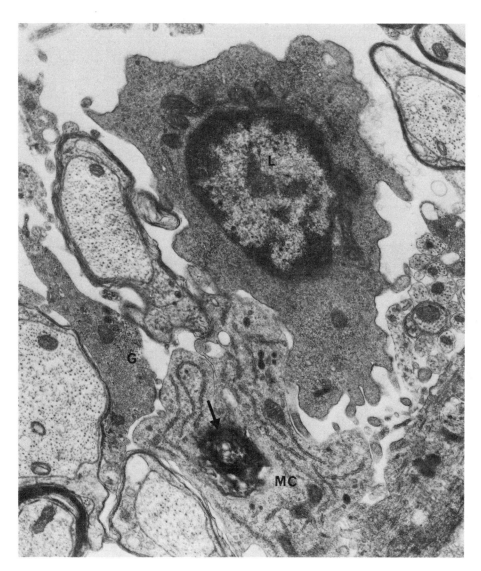

Fig. 3. Part of the lesion showing lymphoblastic cell (L) and part of a macrophage (MC) with typical R.E.R. and phagosome containing myelin debris (arrow). Process of an astrocyte (G) with many microfibrils. ×15,000.

242

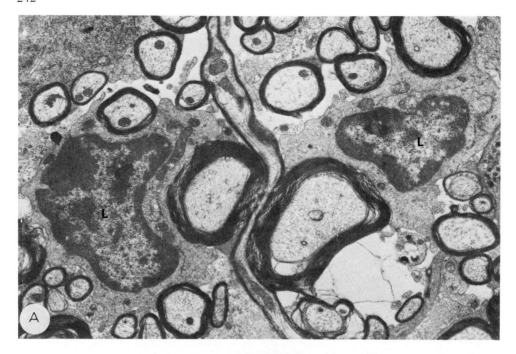

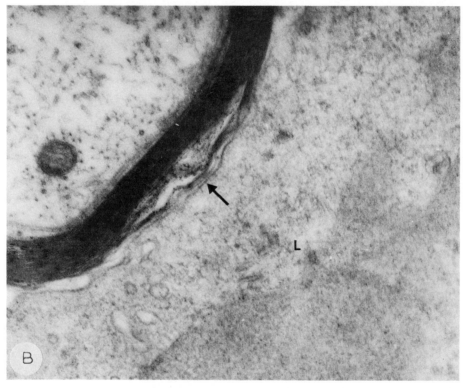

Fig. 4A, B.

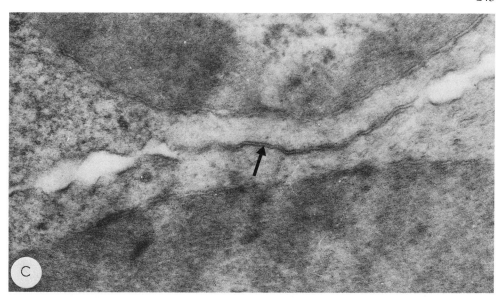

Fig. 4C.

Fig. 4.A: lymphoblastic cells (L) with prominent pseudopodial processes close to myelinated axons. ×9000. B: process of a lymphoblastic cell (L) close to a myelinated axon. A small area (arrow) showing close apposition of the plasma membranes of the lymphoblastic cell and myelin (very close contact). ×60,000. C: parts of two lymphoblastic cells showing very close contact (arrow). The cytoplasm around the contact is devoid of organelles. ×60,000.

They had large oval or lobulated nuclei, large amounts of cytoplasm, and prominent processes which were generally close to the myelin of axons (Fig. 4A). They occasionally showed very close contact with the myelin, the two plasma membranes being in close apposition (Fig. 4B). Generally, lymphoblastic cells were not seen in close contact with each other, but two such cells were seen showing a very close contact, the two plasma membranes being in close apposition. The cytoplasm around the contact was devoid of organelles (Fig. 4C). Many small processes of these cells containing floccular material, but devoid of organelles, could be seen easily in the extracellular spaces. Sometimes small ''finger-like'' processes of lymphoblastic cells were also seen projecting into the cytoplasm of astrocytes, macrophages (Fig. 5) and other cells. A few dense granules were seen in these lymphoblastic cells but phagocytic vacuoles were never seen in spite of the cells being present near damaged myelin (Fig. 6). These cells were not seen very close to naked (completely demyelinated) axons. Identical cells could be seen in the perivascular spaces and in the lumen of the blood vessels. These lymphoblastic cells appeared to differ from inactivated small lymphocytes in that they contained a large proportion of cytoplasm and larger, paler nuclei. Overall, the lymphoblastic cells were larger and paler than unactivated lymphocytes.

Macrophages

These cells showed all the characteristics of typical macrophages, e.g. ruffled membrane, filipodia and phagosomes. Here R.E.R. was in the form of long stretches which were generally full of dense material and were in parallel arrays; some S.E.R. was also present. The macrophages were very large and irregular (Figs. 3, 6 and 8). These cells could also be seen in the perivascular spaces and the lumen of the blood vessels.

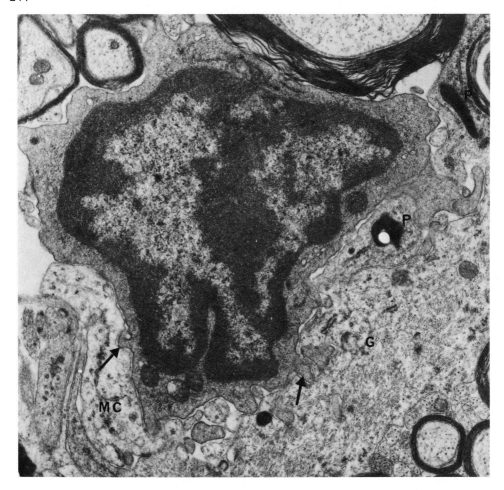

Fig. 5. Small "finger-like" processes of lymphoblastic cell (arrow) projecting into the cytoplasm of astrocyte (G) and macrophage (MC). Part of a myelinated axon is close to the lymphoblastic cell. Macrophage processes containing myelin debris (P). Small processes of lymphoblastic cell (dark) and macrophage (pale) are free in extracellular space. Well-myelinated and small unmyelinated axons in the lower right-hand corner. ×15,000.

The origin of the macrophages

The origin of these macrophages (Figs. 3, 6, 8 and 9) has been under discussion as to whether such cells are derived from microglial cells which have become phagocytic after activation, as reported in Cuprizone-induced demyelination in mice (Blakemore, 1973), or have an haematogenous origin, as reported in experimental Japanese B encephalitis (Kitamura, 1973) after using the technique of electron microscopic autoradiography on the cells of meningeal and perivascular cuffs. We see these macrophages in the parenchyma, the perivascular spaces around the blood vessels and in the lumen. We feel that certainly the majority of the macrophages have an haematogenous origin.

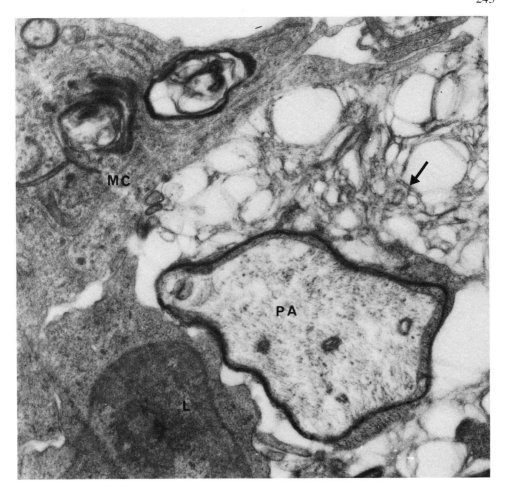

Fig. 6. Part of a lymphoblastic cell (L) close to a partially demyelinated axon (PA) and damaged vesicular form of myelin (arrow). Process of a macrophage (MC) containing myelin debris. ×24,000.

The process of demyelination

Our studies have shown that the first abnormal cells to appear in large quantities in otherwise normal white matter were lymphoblastic cells. These cells could be seen within the white matter in close contact with normal myelin or myelin which showed early signs of degeneration (Figs. 2A, 4A, B). Macrophages were rarely seen in these areas. The earliest visible demyelination process appeared to be related to the lymphoblastic contact with myelin.

One of the features of the earliest stages of myelin degeneration was the separation of the myelin lamellae, leading to the formation of intramyelinic vacuoles (microcysts), the axons appearing quite intact. At this stage, macrophages could be seen in intimate contact with some

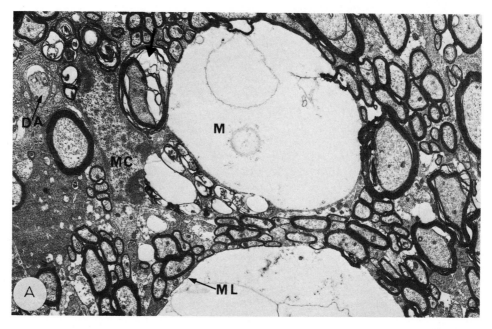

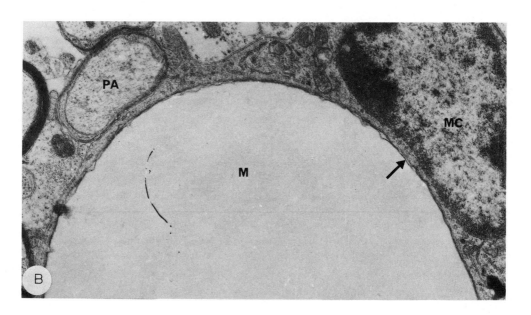

Fig. 7A, B.

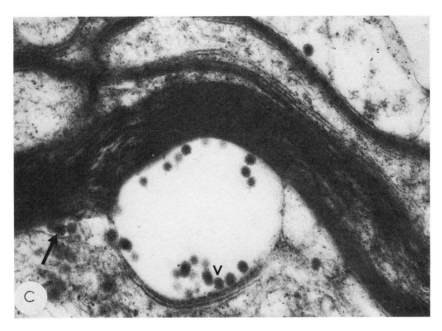

Fig. 7C.

Fig. 7.A: part of the lesion showing microcyst (M) close to a myelinated axon with intramyelinic vacuoles (arrow). Macrophage (MC) containing myelin debris is close to microcyst. Part of another microcyst showing traces of myelin lamella (ML) lining the cyst. Completely demyelinated axon (DA) surrounded by the processes of macrophage. ×3600. B: Large process from macrophage (MC) closely applied to microcyst (M). Thin myelin lining (arrow) is seen clearly. Partially demyelinated axon (PA) near microcyst. ×15,000. C: part of a myelinated axon showing mature virus particles (V) in a cyst, possibly in the oligodendrocyte tongue. Mature virus (arrow) can also be seen in the periaxonal space. Adult mouse brain, PID 2, virulent strain. ×60,000.

of these cysts and sometimes their long pseudopodia could be seen encircling them (Figs. 7A, B and 8). Lymphoblastic cells were also present nearby. Abnormal myelin can be seen as coiled masses, lamellar arrays and in a vesicular form in the more advanced areas of the lesion sometimes near thinly myelinated and naked axons. All these forms of degenerated myelin could also be seen phagocytosed in macrophages (Fig. 9). Processes of macrophages within the lamellae of myelin sheaths, suggesting stripping of myelin, were not seen, but some thinly myelinated and large naked (completely demyelinated) axons were seen surrounded by macrophage processes (Figs. 2C and 7A).

In an advanced lesion area, lymphoblastic cells and macrophages were frequently seen in close association with each other, and occasionally small "finger-like" processes of lymphoblastic cells were seen projecting into the cytoplasm of these macrophages without any obvious damage being caused. Sometimes a lymphoblastic cell was seen nearly surrounded by a macrophage (Fig. 9). The significance of this type of association between these two cells in the demyelinating process is not clear as yet, but suggests that macrophages may have an important role in addition to phagocytosis.

248

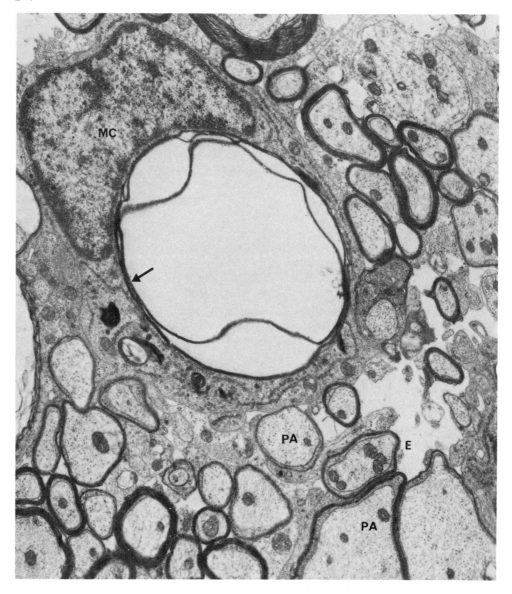

Fig. 8. Macrophage (MC) enclosing a large cyst containing myelin (arrow). Partially demyelinated axons (PA). Enlarged extracellular spaces (E). ×12,000.

Formation of the intramyelinic microcysts

The early close and effective contact of a lymphoblastic cell with the myelin, though temporary, may somehow damage it (Fig. 4A and B). This may lead to the separation of myelin lamellae at intraperiod and/or dense lines. Extracellular fluid may then enter into the spaces so formed, resulting in large intramyelinic vacuoles or microcysts (Fig. 7A and B) and also, possibly, the vesicular form of myelin (Figs. 6 and 9). Some of these microcysts may

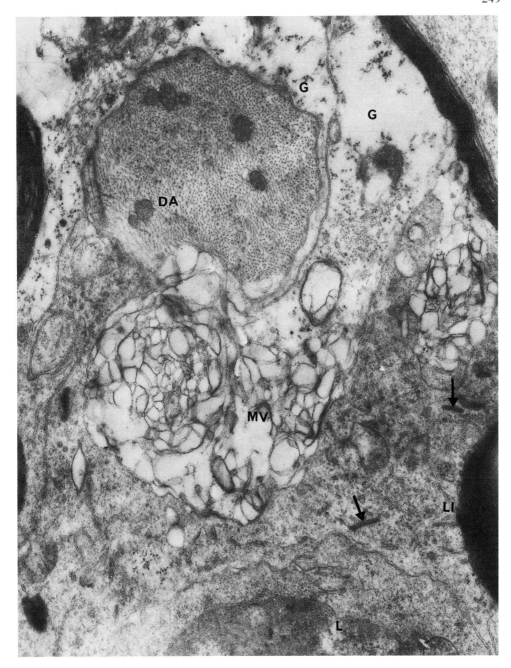

Fig. 9. Vesicular form of myelin (MV) surrounded by the processes of a macrophage containing myelin debris (arrow) and lipid (LI) in the cytoplasm. Completely demyelinated axon (DA) surrounded by the processes of an astrocyte (G) containing microfibrils and glycogen. Part of a lymphoblastic cell (L) which is surrounded by macrophage. ×24,000.

eventually burst, due to internal fluid pressure, leaving the damaged myelin in the extracellular spaces. Myelin is highly elastic and after the rupture of the microcyst, with retraction of the surrounding myelin, this myelin may assume coiled forms.

Formation of periaxonal microcysts

Other microcysts appear due to the enlargement of the periaxonal space. In some areas, a few myelinated axons showed the myelin sheath and axon intact but the periaxonal space enlarged. A hypothesis for the method by which this may happen is made from seeing the sites of replication of a virulent strain of SFV (L10/C1) in adult mice. It must be remembered that although avirulent SFV A7(74) multiplies to similar titers in adult mouse brains, it cannot be visualized in a mature form at electron microscopical level. There is every reason from our studies in mice 14 days old and younger, however, (Pathak and Webb, 1978) to believe that the sites of virus multiplication are the same with each strain. Using the virulent strain L10/C1 in adult mice, intense virus replication can be seen in neurons (Pathak et al., 1976), in oligo-dendrocytes (Pathak, unpublished observation) and, sometimes, virus particles were seen in the cyst in the inner tongue of the oligodendrocytes and in the periaxonal spaces (Fig. 7C). The large amount of viral antigen at these sites may produce an osmotic fluid intake, with cyst formation and those cysts may rupture, causing demyelination. In the lesion described here it was the first type of microcyst (intramyelinic), which was more common.

Some of the spongiform areas consist of large, irregular, extracellular spaces near demyeli-nated and thinly myelinated axons (Figs. 2C and 8). They may have arisen from the rupture of microcysts. Some enlargement of the extracellular spaces, as seen in the neuropil in the lesion areas, could be due to inflammatory oedema.

Astrocytes

These cells show prominent processes containing microfibrils and glycogen and can be easily seen in the lesion areas, particularly surrounding demyelinated axons (Fig. 9). It could be that they have some function related to protection of axons and to their remyelination. Some of these cells at the lesion showed swelling and vacuolization. Sometimes the astrocytes had small "finger-like" projections of the lymphoblastic cells within them (Fig. 5) and these may have been causing some damage. Some of the swelling and vacuolization could be secondary to inflammatory oedema. Kelly et al. (1982) have suggested that lymphoblastic projections into the astrocytes are damaging these cells and may, indirectly, be causing myelin damage. Although some astrocytes had a small amount of myelin debris within the cytoplasm we do not think they are the cells chiefly involved in the phagocytosis of myelin.

Oligodendrocytes

These cells generally appeared normal, and although a few were vacuolated, they were not particularly associated with the lesion area. Large axons with thin myelin sheaths were seen close to the processes of normal oligodendrocytes (Fig. 10).

Neurons

These cells generally appeared normal. No virus particles were seen at any time in the tissue. As stated previously, it has been cleared from the brain by PID 11.

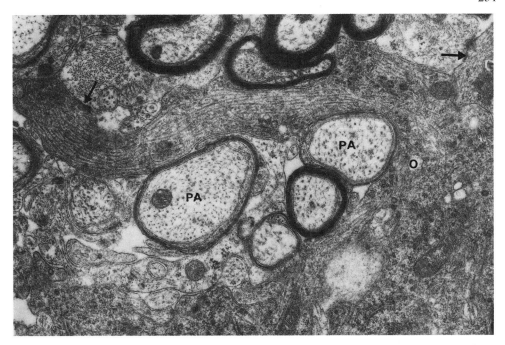

Fig. 10. Process from a normal oligodendrocyte (O) close to well-myelinated and thinly myelinated axons (PA). Normal astrocytic processes showing dense connections (arrow). ×24,000.

DISCUSSION

In the literature contributory evidence from other experimental models can be found to suggest that the lymphoblastic cells (activated lymphocytes) may play an initial and important role in the pathological process and demyelination.

In vitro models

Zinkernagel and Doherty (1974) have indicated by analysis in vitro in lymphocytic choriomeningitis (LCM) virus infection of mice that cytotoxic T-cells act alone and can cause cell death in "one hit" phenomena which require close, if transient, association between lymphocyte and target cells.

Sanderson and Glauert (1977, 1979) have described sensitized cytotoxic T-cells (pale T-cells) and suggested that their projections, which might develop as a result of contact with specific antigen, are related to the mechanism of killing of mastocytoma cells in culture. Their sensitized cytotoxic T-cells are quite similar in appearance to the lymphoblastic cells described by us.

Sanderson and Glauert (1977) have also described small point contacts and close continuous contacts which are seen commonly between cytotoxic T-cells and tumour cells in culture. They reported that the two plasma membranes were in close apposition but were intact and were 7 nm apart, and no specialized junctions were observed. They have also reported "finger-like" projections (but these were not seen very often) and suggested that close contacts may induce the formation of projections. Sanderson (1976) has also reported that T-cells move very rapidly and argued that continual T-cell contact is not necessary for the final lysis of the cells and that once any close contact has been made the final lysis is difficult to stop.

Ferluga and Allison (1974) have reported that in culture, sensitized T-cells kill mastocytoma cells rapidly. First, they have an effective contact with the tumour cells. The plasma membrane of the target cell becomes leaky to ions but not to cytoplasmic proteins. This allows an increased passive ion influx into the target cell once the lymphocyte has moved away. The final lytic event is due to osmotic effects and does not require the presence of the effector cell. Similarly, in our material a close and effective contact of lymphoblastic cells with myelin, though temporary, may lead to the formation of intramyelinic vacuoles (microcysts).

In vivo models

Dal Canto and Lipton (1975) have shown with Theiler's virus given i.c. to mice, that extensive lesions were seen in the white matter of the spinal cord in the absence of visible virus particles. The inflammatory cells at these sites consisted of lymphocytes, plasma cells and monocytes. Myelin stripping by mononuclear cells was seen. Oligodendrocytes were normal. They report that it is a primary demyelination and suggest that it is immune-mediated. Lipton and Dal Canto (1976) further report that immunosuppression of mice with cyclophosphamide and rabbit antiserum to mouse thymocytes eliminated mononuclear cell infiltrates in the spinal cord and prevented the occurrence of demyelination. Their experiments with antisera support the view that demyelination is T-cell-dependent.

Tanaka et al. (1975) described lymphoid cells, which are somewhat similar in appearance to the lymphoblastic cells described here. They have suggested that these cells are mainly responsible for the degeneration of white matter in the experimental parainfluenza-type 1 virus-induced encephalopathy in mice and that it is a virus-induced cell-mediated immune response.

Hapel (1975) has shown that the inflammatory response and the elimination of virus from the mouse brain after i.c. infection with Bebaru virus, a group A arbovirus, is T-cell-dependent. He also states that immune serum does not play a major part in the inflammatory process.

Berger (1980), using an avirulent strain of SFV in CBA and nude mice and giving cyclophosphamide as an immunosuppressant, concluded that either antibody or immune T-cells can trigger pathology, but that there is also some participation from non-immune, bone-marrow-derived, mononuclear cells, probably of the monocyte-macrophage lineage.

Some workers have reported that demyelination in the CNS seems to be due to the direct cytolytic effect of virus on oligodendrocytes. Lampert et al. (1973) and Fleury et al. (1980) have shown that after i.p. and i.c. infection of mice with the JHM strain of mouse hepatitis virus, demyelination in brainstem and spinal cord seems to be due to the direct cytolytic effect of virus on oligodendrocytes which contained virus particles and showed degeneration. The immune system does not appear to be involved here. Macrophages had stripped myelin nonspecifically from axons which remained intact.

Recently, Sheahan et al. (1981) have reported demyelination in the brain and spinal cord of mice following i.p. infection with a mutant strain (M136) of SFV. Here oligodendrocytes degenerate and they have suggested that demyelination is primarily due to destruction of oligodendrocytes by this mutant virus. This is in contrast to what happens with the avirulent strain we have used where the demyelinating areas are shown associated with infiltrating cells and the oligodendrocytes appear generally intact.

Therefore, we feel that in our model, although virus multiplication may occur in oligodendrocytes, it does not appear to lead to cytolysis of these cells and thus does not play a direct part in the demyelination process. We also feel that immune serum factors are not important. Our evidence strongly suggests that the cell-mediated immune system plays the most important role in the pathological process, including the demyelination. In our SFV infections of athymic nude mice, minimum demyelination occurs within the first 28 days after infection, suggesting that the demyelination is T-cell-dependent (Jagelman et al., 1978). Demyelination is reproduced if these mice are reconstituted with normal spleen cells before virus infection (Suckling et al., 1982). Reconstitution studies at present being carried out in the laboratory strongly suggest that, if the spleen cells used for reconstitution are depleted of T-cells, the demyelination is significantly reduced. The lymphoblastic cells described by us appear to be very similar to the activated T-lymphocytes (lymphoblasts) described by Roitt (1977). It is possible that these highly mobile cells produce damage when they make close contact with the myelin possibly by the secretion of some cytotoxic substances. These may damage the myelin, making it more permeable to ions and thereby causing osmotic imbalance and cystic development within it, with eventual rupture. As projections from these lymphoblastic cells were not seen penetrating the myelin, it would seem that direct cell insertion is unlikely to be the cause of myelin breakdown.

We conclude that the demyelination appears to be initiated by the lymphoblastic cells which we have described here and which are likely to be of the T-lymphocyte group.

ACKNOWLEDGEMENTS

The authors thank the St. Thomas' Hospital Charitable Funds and Philip Fleming Charitable Trust for their financial assistance and Mrs. Sandra Hayhoe for her excellent technical assistance.

REFERENCES

Allner, K., Bradish, C.J., Fitzgeorge, R. and Nathanson, N. (1974) Modifications by sodium aurothiomalate of the expression of virulence in mice by defined strains of Semliki Forest virus. J. gen. Virol. 24: 221–228.

Berger, M.L. (1980) Humoral and cell mediated immune mechanisms in the production of pathology in avirulent Semliki Forest virus encephalitis. Infect. Immun. 30: 244–253.

Blakemore, W.F. (1973) Demyelination of the superior cerebellar peduncle in the mouse induced by cuprizone. J. neurol. Sci. 20: 63–72.

Chew-Lim, M., Suckling, A.J. and Webb, H.E. (1977) Demyelination in mice after two or three infections with avirulent Semliki Forest virus. Vet. Path. 14: 67–72.

Chew-Lim, M., Scott, T. and Webb, H.E. (1978) An ultrastructural study of cerebellar lesions induced in mice by three inoculations of avirulent Semliki Forest virus. Acta neuropath. 41: 55–59.

Dal Canto, M.C. and Lipton, H.L. (1975) Primary demyelination in Theiler's virus infection. An ultrastructural study. Lab. Invest. 33: 626–637.

Ferluga, J. and Allison, A.C. (1974) Observations on the mechanism by which T-lymphocytes exert cytotoxic effects. Nature (Lond.), 250: 673–675.

Fleury, H.J.A., Sheppard, R.D., Bornstein, M.B. and Raine, C.S. (1980) Further ultrastructural observations of virus morphogenesis and myelin pathology in JHM virus encephalomyelitis. Neuropath. appl. Neurobiol., 6: 165–179.

Hapel, A.J. (1975) The protective role of thymus derived lymphocytes in arbovirus-induced meningoencephalitis. Scand. J. Immunol., 4: 267–278.

Illavia, S.J., Webb, H.E. and Pathak, S. (1982) Demyelination induced in mice by avirulent SFV. I. Virology and effects on optic nerve. Neuropath. appl. Neurobiol., 8: 35–42.

Jagelman, S., Suckling, A.J., Webb, H.E. and Bowern, E.T. (1978) The pathogenesis of avirulent Semliki Forest virus infections in athymic nude mice. *J. gen. Virol.*, 41: 599–607.

Kelly, W.R., Blakemore, W.F., Jagelman, S. and Webb, H.E. (1982) Demyelination induced in mice by avirulent SFV. II. An ultrastructural study of the focal demyelination in the brain. *Neuropath. appl. Neurobiol.*, 8: 43–53.

Kitamura, T. (1973) The origin of brain macrophages — some considerations on the microglia theory of Del Rio-Hortega. *Acta Path. Jap.*, 23: 11–26.

Lampert, P.W., Sims, J.K. and Kniazeff, A.J. (1973) Mechanism of demyelination in JHM virus encephalomyelitis — Electron microscopic studies. *Acta neuropath.*, 24: 76–85.

Lipton, H.L. and Dal Canto, M.C. (1976) Theiler's virus induced demyelination-prevention by immunosuppression. *Science*, 192: 62–63.

Mackenzie, A., Suckling, A.J., Jagelman, S. and Wilson, A.M. (1978) Histopathological and enzyme histochemical changes in experimental Semliki Forest virus infection in mice and their relevance to Scrapie. *J. comp. Path.*, 88: 335–344.

Oaten, S.W., Jagelman, S. and Webb, H.E. (1980) Further studies of macrophages in relationship to avirulent Semliki Forest virus infections. *Brit. J. exp. Pathol.*, 61: 150–155.

Pathak, S. and Webb, H.E. (1974) Possible mechanisms for the transport of Semliki Forest virus into and within mouse brain. An electronmicroscopic study. *J. neurol. Sci.*, 23: 175–184.

Pathak, S. and Webb, H.E. (1978) An electron-microscopic study of avirulent and virulent Semliki Forest virus in the brains of different ages of mice. *J. neurol. Sci.*, 39: 199–211.

Pathak, S., Webb, H.E., Oaten, S.W. and Bateman, S. (1976) An electron-microscopic study of the development of virulent and avirulent strains of Semliki forest virus in mouse brain. *J. neurol. Sci.*, 28: 289–300.

Roitt, I.M. (1977) *Essential Immunology*, 3rd Edn., Blackwell, Oxford, pp. 47–59.

Sanderson, C.J. (1976) The mechanism of T-cell mediated cytotoxicity. II. Morphological studies of cell death by time-lapse microcinematography. *Proc. roy. Soc. B.*, 192: 241–255.

Sanderson, C.J. and Glauert, A.M. (1977) The mechanism of T-cell mediated cytotoxicity. V. Morphological studies by electron microscopy. *Proc. roy. Soc. B.*, 198: 315–323.

Sanderson, C.J. and Glauert, A.M. (1979) The mechanism of T-cell mediated cytotoxicity. VI. T-cell projections and their role in target cell killing. *Immunology*, 36: 119–129.

Sheahan, B.J., Barrett, P.N. and Atkins, G.J. (1981) Demyelination in mice resulting from infection with a mutant of Semliki Forest virus. *Acta neuropath.*, 53: 129–136.

Suckling, A.J., Jagelman, S. and Webb, H.E. (1978) Virus associated demyelination: a model using avirulent Semliki Forest virus infection of mice. *J. neurol. Sci.*, 39: 147–154.

Suckling, A.J., Jagelman, S. and Webb, H.E. (1982) Immunoglobulin synthesis in nude (nu/nu), nu/+ and reconstituted nu/nu mice infected with a demyelinating strain of Semliki Forest virus. *Clin. exp. Immunol.*, 47 in press.

Tanaka, R., Iwasaki, Y. and Koprowski, H. (1975) Experimental parainfluenza-type-1-virus-induced encephalopathy in the adult mouse: An ultrastructural study of early lesions. *Amer. J. Path.*, 79: 335–346.

Webb, H.E., Chew-Lim, M., Jagelman, S., Oaten, S.W., Pathak, S., Suckling, A.J. and MacKenzie, A. (1979) Semliki Forest virus infections in mice as a model for studying acute and chronic central nervous system virus infections in man. In F.C. Rose (Ed.), *Clinical Neuroimmunology*, Blackwell, Oxford, pp. 369–390.

Webb, H.E. and Jagelman, S. (1979) Viral infections of the CNS in the immune compromised host with special reference to certain paraneoplastic syndromes. In J.M.A. Whitehouse and H.E.M. Kay (Eds.), *CNS Complications of Malignant Disease*, MacMillan, London, pp. 258–280.

Zinkernagel, R.M. and Doherty, P.C. (1974) Characteristics of the interaction in vitro between cytotoxic thymus derived lymphocytes and target monolayers infected with lymphocytic choriomeningitis virus. *Scand. J. Immunol.*, 3: 287–294.

Immunology of Nervous System Infections, Progress in Brain Research, Vol. 59, edited by P.O. Behan, V. ter Meulen
and F. Clifford Rose

Some Interactions of Virus and Maternal/Foetal Immune Mechanisms in Border Disease of Sheep

R. M. BARLOW

Moredun Research Institute, Edinburgh EH17 7JH, Scotland (U.K.)

INTRODUCTION

Border disease (BD) is a congenital disorder of lambs which, in its typical form, is characterized by poor viability, low birth weight, tremor, and in smooth-coated breeds by an unusually coarse, hairy, birth-coat (Barlow and Dickinson, 1965). The outstanding pathological feature is a deficiency of myelin in the central nervous system (CNS). BD is caused by a placenta-crossing pestivirus, closely related to the viruses of mucosal disease or bovine virus diarrhoea (BVD) and swine fever or hog cholera (HC) (Acland et al., 1972; Hadjisavvas et al., 1975; Vantsis et al., 1976, Plant et al., 1976).

In recent years new clinico-pathological features of BD virus infection have been recognized. These blend with features of the other pestivirus diseases to form a spectrum such that the distinction between BD, BVD and HC is more a matter of emphasis than of fundamental difference. The mechanisms responsible for this spectrum of changes are poorly understood, though host response is beginning to emerge as a crucial factor.

In the foetal sheep, immunological responsiveness with respect to BD viral antigens may be considered to develop about midgestation, i.e. 70–90 days gestation (Zakarian et al., 1975; Gardiner et al., 1980). Thus, in considering the host response it is first necessary to indicate the events which take place in the pregnant ewe and then to examine in more detail the consequences for the foetus of infections initiated after 90 or before 70 days gestation.

The nature of the inocula used in these experimental studies is summarized in Table I.

TABLE I

INOCULA MENTIONED IN TEXT

Inocula	Description
IIB	a pool of brain tissue from newborn severe hairy-shaker lambs — second experimental passage in sheep yielding cytopathic virus in tissue culture (Barlow, 1972).
BP-77	a pool of brain tissue of newborn severe hairy-shaker lambs — first sheep/sheep passage of IIB (Barlow et al., 1979)
H-77	homogenized brain of a hairy-shaker lamb from a field outbreak of BD yielding a non cytopathic virus in tissue culture (Barlow et al., 1979)
NADL Strain BVD	U.S. strain of BVD virus, cytopathic and passaged many times in tissue culture (supplied by Dr. Malmquist, Ames, IA).

INFECTION OF THE EWE

Infection of the pregnant ewe

Following parenteral injection of infective material the ewe exhibits no clinical malaise, but a transient neutropenia and a mild febrile response may occur within 6–11 days (Shaw et al., 1967; Vantsis et al., 1979). Within about 10 days a focal or diffuse placentitis with caruncular necrosis develops (Barlow, 1972, 1982), and may contribute to the foetal death and abortion which follow in some cases. If the pregnancy is sustained the placentitis heals in about 25 days. Neutralizing antibody appears in maternal serum from about 11–14 days after infection (Vantsis et al., 1980).

Infections of the foetus after 90 days gestation

Following maternal infection, virus crosses the placenta and invades the foetus. Within about 15–21 days a disseminated nodular periarteritis (Fig. 1) develops in many foetal tissues, but is particularly marked in the CNS where it affects mainly small distributing arteries and arterioles in meninges and brain substance (Zakarian et al., 1975, 1976). The lesions have a tendency to bilateral symmetry. Specific immunofluorescence staining (Fig. 2) indicates that viral antigen in brain is located in the vessel walls and perivascular tissues (Gardiner et al., 1980). Although viral antigen tends to disappear in a few months, the lesion can persist without obvious morphological change for about one year into postnatal life.

The periarteritic form of BD infection is subclinical and affected lambs have precolostral serum neutralizing antibody. Their capacity to excrete infective virus has not been investigated.

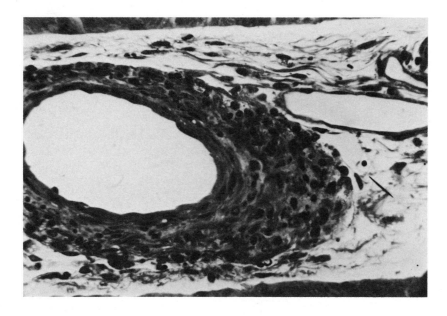

Fig. 1. Periarteritis in a meningeal arteriole. The media and adventitia are infiltrated by mononuclear cells and a lymphocyte is adherent to the endothelium. An adjacent venule is not involved. (Perfusion fixation H & E × 400.)

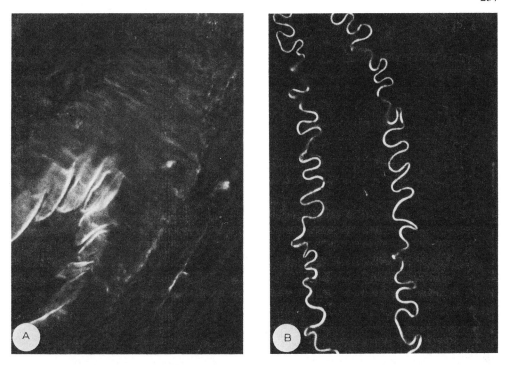

Fig. 2. Indirect fluorescent antibody staining of cerebral vessels (Cryostat sections, × 650; courtesy of A. C. Gardiner). A: BD viral antigen in media and adventitia. B: autofluorescence in elastic laminae of control animal.

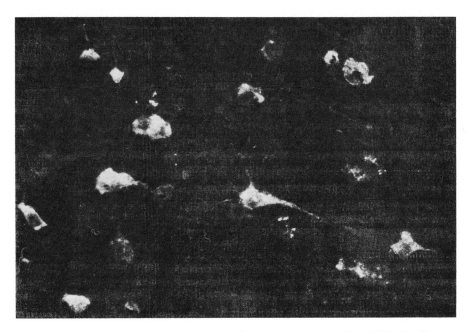

Fig. 3. Indirect fluorescent antibody staining of nerve cells and processes in newborn BD lambs. (Cryostat section, × 960; courtesy A. C. Gardiner.)

Infection of the foetus before 70 days gestation — usual effects

Most of our work has been carried out with experimental infections of pregnant ewes at 50–54 days gestation. Following foetal invasion, viral antigen is widely distributed in foetal tissues (Terpstra, 1978). In the CNS, immunofluorescence has shown it to be located principally in nerve cells and processes (Gardiner, 1980) where it may persist until at least 5 months after birth (Fig. 3). The virus does not appear to be cytotoxic and typically no inflammatory reaction occurs. The main pathological change is interference with the active process of myelination of the CNS resulting in congenital hypomyelinogenesis (Fig. 4) (Barlow and Storey, 1977). This is associated clinically with varying degress of tremor, and in some breeds also with hairiness of the fleece (Derbyshire and Barlow, 1976). Precolostral sera from ''hairy-shaker'' lambs do not contain BD virus-neutralizing antibody (Plant et al., 1977; Vantsis et al., 1979), but antimyelin antibodies have been described (Patterson et al., 1977).

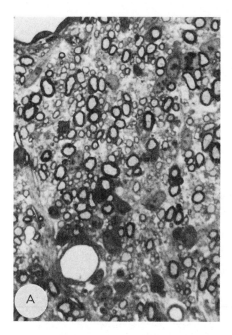 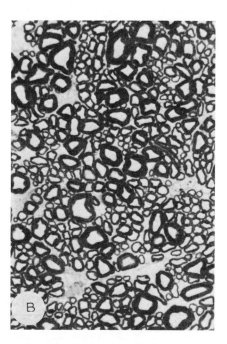

Fig. 4. TS dorsal funiculus spinal cord 135-day foetuses. (Araldite — Toluidine blue — thionine, × 960). A: BD. B: control.

Over a period of 16–20 weeks post-partum, the tremor and hypomyelinogenesis gradually resolve (Barlow and Dickinson, 1965, Sweasey and Patterson, 1979). Passively acquired colostral antibody wanes and recovered hairy shaker lambs again become seronegative for BD virus neutralizing antibody. They continue, however, to excrete virus for life. Thus in a practical sense they are tolerant to the infecting strain of virus. As adults they may have low fertility but both sexes can pass the infection to their progeny and flockmates (Gardiner and Barlow, 1981).

Infections of the foetus before 70 days gestation — alternative effects

In a number of BD infections, initiated at 50–54 days gestation, pathological changes have resulted which were markedly different from those described above. Within 21 days of infection a necrotizing encephalitis developed which was centered upon the subependymal mantle layer and the external granular layer of the cerebellum (Figs. 5 and 6). These lesions

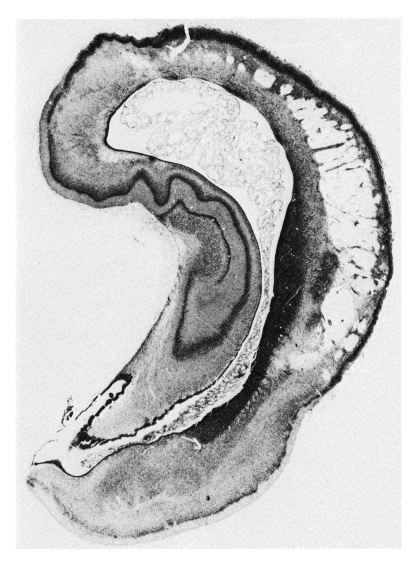

Fig. 5. TS posterior cerebrum 75-day foetus with necrosis and inflammation of the subependyma and primordial white matter. (H & E, × 12).

were heavily infiltrated with macrophages and lymphocyte-like cells (Figs. 7 and 8) and resulted in a range of gross intracranial malformations in those foetuses which were carried to term (Clarke and Osburn, 1978; Barlow, 1980). Malformations included hydranencephaly,

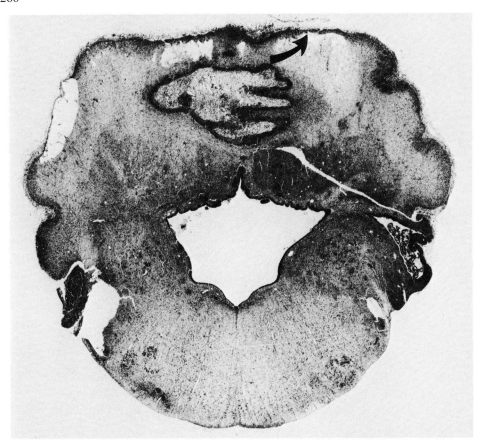

Fig. 6. TS. Brainstem 75-day foetus with liquefactive necrosis of cerebellum (H & E, × 12).

porencephaly and cerebellar hypo- or dysplasia (Fig. 9). Lambs in which these manifestations were most severe did not show hypomyelinogenesis, hairiness or tremor, though some also had severe skeletal abnormalities. BD virus or viral antigen could not be demonstrated in their tissues and at first it was considered that the inoculum might have become contaminated with another virus. Considerable effort has been expended in the search for this hypothetical second virus, but without success, and since the majority of such lambs were shown to have specific BD virus neutralizing antibody in their precolostral sera (A.C. Gardiner and P. Nettleton, personal communication) it is tentatively concluded that infection with BD virus had occurred, but had been controlled by intense foetal inflammatory and immune responses, apparently taking place precociously at a gestational age at which the foetus is normally immunologically unresponsive to this virus.

The reasons for this "alternative" BD pathology (AP) are incompletely understood, but AP does not appear to be a random event. It has not been observed following the infection of fully susceptible pregnant ewes with the IIB pool virus (Table I). Most predictably, it has occurred when this inoculum has been either incubated in vitro with immune serum to another pestivirus

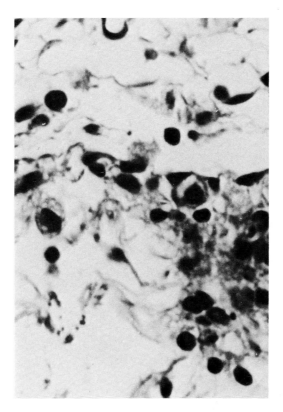

Fig. 7. Detail of necrotic external granular layer at point arrowed in Fig. 6. There is some necrotic debris and a macrophage present. (H & E, × 1060).

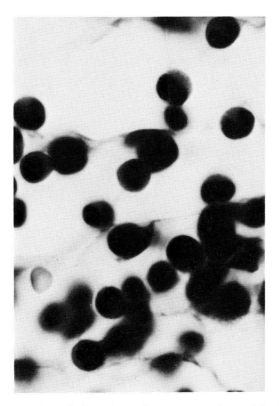

Fig. 8. Infiltrate of mononuclear cells in meninges adjacent to arrowed area of Fig. 6. (H & E, × 1500).

strain, or injected into pregnant sheep with previous experience of another strain (Tables II and III). The data in Table IV indicate that whereas experience of a particular strain of BD virus conferred solid immunity to rechallenge with the homologous strain in the next pregnancy, resistance to a heterologous challenge virus was incomplete and AP was likely to occur. It would thus appear that "incomplete neutralization" by "poor-fit" antibody may be involved in the production of AP, the virus being processed in some way, either in vitro, or in the maternal host, prior to invasion of the foetus.

TABLE II

RESULTS OF INOCULATION OF CHEVIOT EWES AT 54 DG WITH BD IIB BRAIN POOL FOLLOWING IN VITRO INCUBATION WITH NORMAL CALF SERUM (NCS) OR CALF BVD (NADL STRAIN) ANTISERUM (BVD)

BD, Border disease — non-inflammatory hypomyelinogenesis; AP, alternative pathology, inflammatory and necrotizing; DG, days of gestation.

Inoculation	Ewe number	Pathology of progeny				
		Cerebral cavitation	Cerebellar dysplasia	Spinal inflammation	Spinal hypomyel	Diagnosis BD/AP
BII+NCS	B120	?	?	–	+++	BD
	B120	?	?	–	+++	BD
	B134	–	–	–	+++	BD
	B155	–	–	–	++	BD
	B166	Aborted – no histology				
BII+BVDS	B168	++++	+++	+	?	AP
	B168	++++	++++	++	–	AP
	B104	–	–	–	++	BD
	B107	+++	++	–	–	AP
	B143	++++	+++	–	–	AP
	B143	++++	+++	–	–	AP

TABLE III

INFECTION OF PREGNANT CHEVIOT EWES WITH NADL, BVD VIRUS AT 54 DG AND CHALLENGE IN NEXT PREGNANCY WITH BD IIB BRAIN POOL

Adapted from Barlow et al. (1980). See Table II for key to abbreviations.

Ewe number	Progeny	
	First pregnancy	Second pregnancy
1	BD	BD
2	AP	Normal
3	Normal	AP
4	AP	Normal
5	Aborted	Aborted
6	AP	Normal

Further reference to Table III indicates that the BP77 virus (Table I) was perhaps a more virulent strain as it almost completely overrode the immunity conferred by the H77 strain (Table I) whilst the latter appeared to have the capacity to produce AP in the foetus of a seronegative ewe. Table V provides further examples of this last phenomenon: it can be seen that whilst BP77 caused typical BD in all 4 breeds of sheep tested, H77 only did likewise in sheep with Blackface blood, infection in the other breeds resulting in apparently normal progeny or progeny with AP. These results suggest that the previous immunological experience of the ewe and/or her genetic constitution in conjunction with a particular strain of virus may cause similar alterations to the pathological outcome of infection, though not necessarily through the same mechanisms.

TABLE IV

CHALLENGE OF SERONEGATIVE AND SEROPOSITIVE EWES WITH 2 STRAINS OF BD AT 54 DG

Adapted from Vantsis et al. (1980). See Table II for key to abbreviations.

Status	Challenge	Number	Ewes aborting	Ewes with live progeny		
				Normal	Affected	BD/AP
Sero-negative	H77	11	4	1	6	5 BD 1AP
	BP77	13	4	0	9	All BD
Sero-positive	H77 (Homologous)	12	0	12	0	All normal
	BP77 (Homologous)	9	2	7	0	All normal
	H77 (Heterologous)	11	1	5	5	2 BD, 3 AP
	BP77 (Heterologous)	12	0	1	11	All BD

TABLE V

RESULTS OF CHALLENGE OF PREGNANT EWES OR 4 BREEDS AT 54 DG
WITH BP77 OR H77 STRAINS OF BD

Adapted from Barlow et al. (1979). See Table II for key to abbreviations.

Challenge		Breeds			
		Dorset horn	Bl. Leicester × Blackface	Blackface	Cheviot
BP77	Number of ewes	13	4	5	4
	Number with progeny (status)	11(BD)	4(BD)	4(BD)	1(BD)
H77	Number of ewes	8	3	4	4
	Number with progeny (status)	3(AP) 1(normal)	3(BD)	2(BD)	1(AP) 1(?normal)

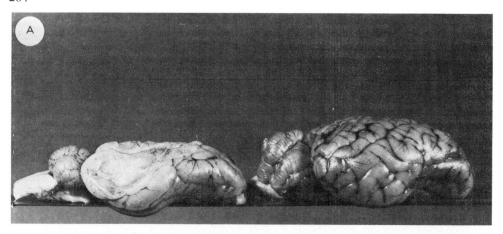

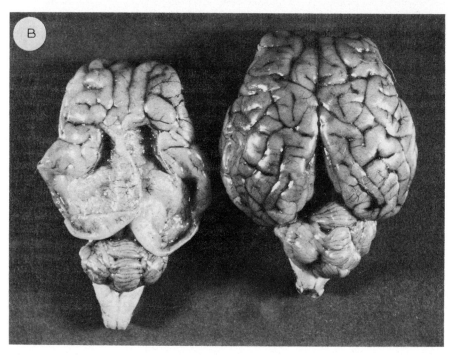

Fig. 9. Brain with hydranencephaly and cerebellar hypoplasia. A normal control is on the right. A: lateral view. B: dorsal view.

Responsiveness in the tolerant sheep

Recovered hairy shaker lambs are ill-thriven and difficult to rear (Sweasey and Patterson, 1979). Tissue cultures of clotted blood from these lambs frequently yield non-cytopathic virus (Terpstra, 1978; Westbury et al., 1979) even when the IIB pool which is cytopathic in tissue culture (Vantsis et al., 1976) has been used to establish the infection. Such lambs often develop fatal enteric or respiratory disorders and many deaths are associated with the stress of weaning.

Recent studies in our laboratory have failed to implicate any of the common causes of ovine gastroenteritis and pneumonia in our experimental cases, but cytopathic and non-cytopathic BD viruses have been isolated from the tissues, the cytopathic variant predominating in most instances.

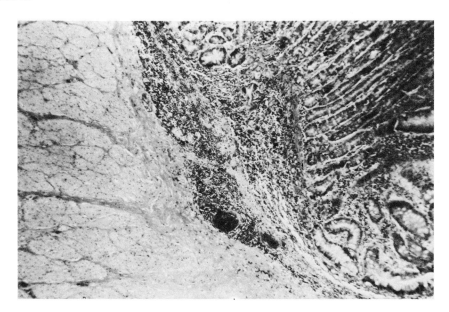

Fig. 10. Hyperplastic typhlocolitis. All coats are thickened and the lamina propria is heavily infiltrated by macrophages. (H &E, × 100).

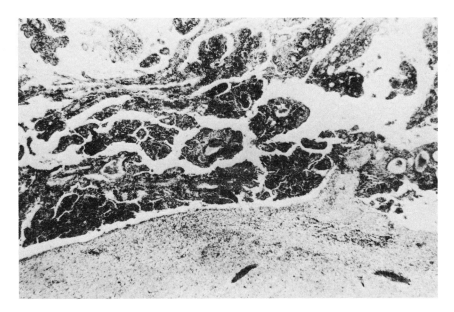

Fig. 11. Periventricular encephalitis with heavy mononuclear cell infiltration of adjacent choroid plexus. (H & E, × 100).

266

In these lambs the associated pathological change is one of generalized lymphoproliferation. This is manifested by hyperplastic typhlocolitis (Fig. 10) and terminal ileitis, pneumonitis, mycarditis, interstitial nephritis, thyroiditis and pancreatitis. There is splenomegaly and enlargement of lymph nodes. In the CNS there is periventricular encephalitis, meningitis and choroiditis (Figs. 11 and 12). In some lesions plasma cells can be identified among the lymphoid infiltrates, but only exceptionally have affected lambs developed neutralizing antibodies.

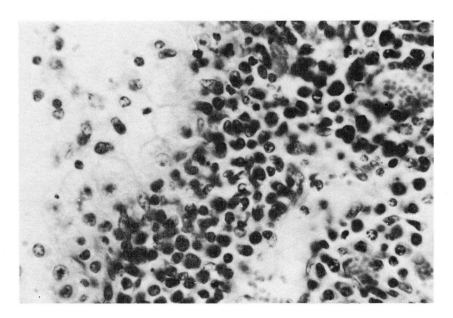

Fig. 12. Inflammatory infiltration of choroid plexus. At left center is vacuolated choroidal ependyma. (H & E, × 600).

We have reproduced this lymphoproliferative disorder experimentally and in high incidence by the injection of a further dose of the BD virus strain which produced the original disease. Following "superinfection", depression, diarrhoea and respiratory distress developed in 2–3 weeks and the animals became moribund in a further week without the production of detectable neutralizing antibody.

However, when recovered hairy-shaker sheep were superinfected with heterologous virus they remained well, antibodies to the second strain of virus were present 3 weeks after infection and histological examination at this time revealed only mild lymphoid infiltrations in some organs.

These results suggest that the tolerant state in recovered hairy shaker lambs includes a delicate balance between virus and host which must involve attenuation of viral (cyto) pathogenicity by means other than conventional immunological mechanisms or the restriction of tissue substrates suitable for viral replication. Stress or deliberate administration of homologous virus upsets the balance, the virus regaining (cyto) pathogenicity and the host mounting a florid but apparently impotent, immunoinflammatory response. The tolerance must be highly specific since only superinfection with a heterologous strain stimulates the production of antibody; thus, presumably the antibody is directed selectively against unshared antigenic determinants.

COMMENT

The phenomena of alternative foetal pathologies and lymphoproliferative disease which have been described here are aspects of pestivirus–host relationships which relate to the question of tolerance.

It is suggested that the typical form of BD virus infection which results in the hairy-shaker lamb may be regarded as a tolerant condition as the individual is persistently infected but does not produce either a humoral or a cellular immune response.

In the alternative form of pathology (AP), which results in gross intracranial malformations, this tolerant state either does not develop or is broken at an early stage, the foetus responding with a necrotizing and mononuclear cell inflammatory reaction in the granuloprival layers of the developing CNS. Antiviral antibody is produced and infection appears to be eliminated before birth. Prominent among the factors which give rise to this altered response is the involvement of heterologous "poor-fit" antibody in the experimental system and it is clear that the virus is processed in some way, in vitro, or in the maternal host. Though the ovine placenta is impermeable to circulating maternal antibody, even when damaged in the typical form of BD, it is not unreasonable to speculate that virus, complexed with "poor-fit" antibody, might cross to the foetus, changing the usual pattern of infection and stimulating a response in the foetal host.

At the other end of the age range, where lymphoproliferative disease has been provoked by stress or superinfection by homologous virus, the tolerant state appears also to have been threatened. Changes in the cytopathogenicity of the virus are accompanied by massive infiltrations of the tissues with mononuclear cells suggesting an immunological basis, though virus neutralizing antibody is not developed prior to the death of the host. In this form of disease it would appear that tolerance may have been broken or at least shaken. The mechanisms involved are at present obscure but are readily amenable to exploration by experiment.

ACKNOWLEDGEMENTS

I am grateful to my colleagues A. C. Gardiner and P. Nettleton for their collaboration in this work and for allowing me to draw upon as yet unpublished data.

REFERENCES

Acland, H.M., Gard, G.P. and Plant, J.W. (1972) Infection of sheep with a mucosal disease virus. *Aust. Vet. J.*, 48: 70–71.

Barlow, R.M. (1972) Experiments in Border disease. IV. Pathological changes in ewes. *J. comp. Path.*, 82: 151–157.

Barlow, R.M. (1980) Morphogenesis of hydranencephaly and other intracranial malformations in progeny of pregnant ewes infected with pestiviruses. *J. comp. Path.*, 90: 87–98.

Barlow, R.M. (1982) Maternal pathology. In: R.M. Barlow and D.S.P. Patterson (Eds.), Border disease of sheep: a pestivirus-induced teratogenic disorder. A collaborative review. *Suppl. Zbl. Vet. Med., Advances in Veterinary Medicine, Vol. 36,* Paul Parey, Berlin, pp. 53–55.

Barlow, R.M. and Dickinson, A.G. (1965) On the pathology and histochemistry of the central nervous system in Border disease of sheep. *Res. vet. Sci.*, 6: 230–237.

Barlow, R.M. and Storey, I.J. (1977) Myelination of the ovine central nervous system with special reference to Border disease. I. Qualitative aspects. II. Quantitative aspects. *Neuropath. appl. Neurobiol.*, 3: 237–253 and 255–265.

Barlow, R.M., Vantsis, J.T., Gardiner, A.C. and Linklater, K.A. (1979) The definition of Border disease; problems for the diagnostician. *Vet. Rec.*, 104: 334–336.

268

Barlow, R.M., Rennie, J.C., Gardiner, A.C. and Vantsis, J.T. (1980) Infection of pregnant sheep with the NADL strain of bovine virus diarrhoea virus and their subsequent challenge with Border disease IIB pool., *J. comp. Path.*, 90: 67–72.

Clarke, G.L. and Osburn, B.I. (1978) Transmissible, congenital demyelinating encephalopathy of lambs. *Vet. Path.*, 15: 68–82.

Derbyshire, M.B. and Barlow, R.M. (1976) Experiments in Border disease. IX. The pathogenesis of the skin lesion. *J. comp. Path.*, 86: 557–570.

Gardiner, A.C. (1980) The distribution and significance of Border disease viral antigen in infected lambs and foetuses. *J. comp. Path.*, 90: 513–518.

Gardiner, A.C. and Barlow, R.M. (1981) Vertical transmission of Border disease infection. *J. comp. Path.*, 91: 467–470.

Gardiner, A.C., Zakarian, B. and Barlow, R.M. (1980) Periarteritis in experimental Border disease. III. Immunopathological observations. *J. comp. Path.*, 90: 469-474.

Hadjisavvas, T.H., Harkness, J.W., Huck, R.A. and Stuart, P. (1975) The demonstration by interference tests of an infectious agent in fetuses from ewes inoculated with Border disease tissue. *Res. vet. Sci.*, 18: 237–243.

Patterson, D.S.P., Sweasey, D. and Harkness, J.W. (1977) Anti-myelin antibodies in the serum of lambs with experimental Border disease. *J. Neurochem.*, 29: 763–765.

Plant, J.W., Acland, H.M. and Gard, G.P. (1976) A mucosol disease virus as a cause of abortion, hairy birth coat and unthriftiness in sheep. *Aust. vet. J.*, 52: 57–62.

Plant, J.W., Gard, G.P. and Acland, H.M. (1977) Transmission of a mucosal disease virus infection between sheep. *Aust. vet. J.*, 53: 574-577.

Shaw, I.G., Winkler, C.E. and Terlecki, S. (1967). Experimental reproduction of hypomyelinogenesis congenita of lambs. *Vet. Rec.*, 81: 115–116.

Sweasey, D. and Patterson, D.S.P. (1979) Congenital hypomyelinogenesis (Border disease) of lambs. Postnatal neuochemical recovery in the central nervous system. *J. Neurochem.*, 33: 705–711.

Terpstra, C. (1978) Detection of Border disease antigen in tissues of affected sheep and in cell cultures by immunofluorescence. *Res. vet. Sci.*, 25: 350–355.

Vantsis, J.T., Barlow, R.M., Fraser, J., Rennie, J.C. and Mould, D.L. (1976) Experiments in Border disease. VIII. Propagation and properties of a cytopathic agent. *J. comp. Path.*, 86: 111–120.

Vantsis, J.T., Linklater, K.A., Rennie, J.C. and Barlow, R.M. (1979) Experimental challenge infection of ewes following a field outbreak of Border disease. *J. comp. Path.*, 89: 331–339.

Vantsis, J.T., Barlow, R.M., Gardiner, A.C. and Linklater, K.A. (1980) The effects of challenge with homologous and heterologous strains of Border disease virus on ewes with previous experience of the disease. *J. comp. Path.*, 90: 39–45.

Westbury, H.A., Napthine, D.V. and Straube, E. (1979) Border disease; persistent infection with the virus. *Vet. Rec.*, 104: 406–409.

Zakarian, B., Barlow, R.M. and Rennie, J.C. (1975). Periarteritis in experimental Border disease. I. The occurrence and distribution of the lesions. *J. comp. Path.*, 85: 443–460.

Zakarian, B., Barlow, R.M., Rennie, J.C. and Head, K.W. (1976) Periarteritis in experimental Border disease. II. Morphology and histochemistry of the lesion. *J. comp. Path.*, 86: 477–487.

Immunology of Nervous System Infections, Progress in Brain Research, Vol. 59, edited by P.O. Behan, V. ter Meulen and F. Clifford Rose
© *1983 Elsevier Science Publishers B.V.*

Some Pathogenetic Aspects of Borna Disease

RUDOLF ROTT and KNUT FRESE

Institut für Virologie und Veterinär-Pathologie, Justus-Liebig-Universität Giessen, D-6300 Giessen (F.R.G.)

INTRODUCTION

Borna disease (BD) is a chronic encephalomyelitis occurring naturally in horses and sheep and is endemic in certain areas of Germany and Switzerland. The disease occurs only sporadically and large groups of animals are never affected. BD has attracted considerable interest because it has characteristics which are typical of persistent virus infections of the central nervous system (CNS). It is characterized by a long incubation period and a progressive development with gradual loss of coordination and certain sensory afflictions.

Histopathological lesions are only seen in the nervous system. In the CNS they are characterized by non-purulent meningoencephalitis and myelitis. Perivascular infiltrations in the grey matter are the main changes observed. A necrotizing encephalitis is rarely seen (for review see Heinig, 1969).

Animals with clinical disease always have infectious virus in the CNS as well as high amounts of antibodies in both serum and cerebrospinal fluid (CSF). These antibodies react in serological binding tests but do not neutralize infectivity (Ludwig et al., 1977; unpublished results).

THE CAUSATIVE AGENT

The causative agent of BD has not been characterized so far. It is intimately associated with cell membranes and is extremely hydrophobic. It can be inactivated by ultraviolet light and certain detergents.

The virus replicates in cultures of embryonic rabbit and rat brain cells or after cocultivation of infected brain cells with several permanent cell lines. It is especially interesting that virus which is produced in permanent cell lines after cocultivation with infected brain cells is immediately adapted to these cells. All cell types infected with BD virus have the characteristics of a persistent infection without showing a cytopathic effect. The virus seems to be strictly cell associated. Maximal virus yields are obtained 10–12 days after infection. With fluorescent antibodies virus antigen can be seen in the cell nucleus (Ludwig et al., 1973; Herzog and Rott, 1980). This fluorescent antibody assay is used both for detecting and quantitating of virus as well as measuring antibodies.

[269]

TABLE I

BORNA DISEASE IN EXPERIMENTAL INFECTED ANIMALS

From Heinig (1969) and Sprankel et al. (1978)

Host species	Incubation period (weeks)	Percent of diseased animals	Pathology	Antibody response in diseased animals
Horse	4–20	60	Encephalomyelitis	+
Sheep	> 6	50	Encephalomyelitis	+
Rabbit	4– 6	95	Encephalomyelitis	+
Rat	4–32	30	Encephalomyelitis	+
Guinea pig	4–56	50	Encephalomyelitis	+
Chicken	4–60	80	Encephalomyelitis	+
Rhesus monkey	> 6	80	Encephalomyelitis	+
Tree shrew	4– 7	Rare	Encephalomyelitis	+

TABLE II

DISTRIBUTION OF BD VIRUS-SPECIFIC ANTIGENS IN RABBITS AFTER INTRACEREBRAL INFECTION

Location	Days after infection															
	8	8	10	10	12	12	14	14	27	28	39	39	40	42	47	50
Cortex	−	+	−	−	−	+++	+	++	+++	++	+	++	+++	+	+++	+++
C. quadrigemina	−	−	−	−	−	−	−	++	++	++	++	+	+++	−	+++	+++
Hippocampus	−	−	−	−	−	−	+++	++	++	+++	+	+++	++	−	+	++
B. olfactorius	−	−	−	−	+++	−	+	−	+++	++	+	−	+	−	++	+++
Cerebellum	−	−	−	−	−	+++	+	−	−	−	+	++	++	+++	+++	+++
M. oblongata	−	−	−	−	−	−	−	+	−	−	+	−	−	+	+	+
M. spinalis	−	−	−	−	−	−	+	+	+	+	+	+	++	+	+	+
P. chorioidei	−	−	−	−	−	−	−	−	−	−	−	−	+	−	−	+
G. trigeminale	−	−	−	−	−	−	+	+	+++	+++	+	+	+++	++	+	+
N. ischiadicus	−	−	−	−	−	−	−	−	−	−	−	−	−	−	−	−
Intestine	−	−	−	−	−	−	−	−	−	+	−	−	+	−	−	+
Stomach	−	−	−	−	−	−	−	−	−	−	+	−	+	−	−	−
Pancreas	−	−	−	−	−	−	−	−	−	−	−	+	+	−	−	−
Adrenals	−	−	−	−	−	−	−	−	−	−	++	+++	+++	+++	−	−
Lacrimal g.	−	−	−	−	−	−	−	−	−	−	−	−	−	+	−	−
Nasal mucosa	−	−	−	−	−	−	−	−	−	−	−	−	−	−	−	−
Lung	−	−	−	−	−	−	−	−	−	−	−	−	−	−	−	−
Heart	−	−	−	−	−	−	−	−	−	−	−	−	−	−	−	−
Liver	−	−	−	−	−	−	−	−	−	−	−	−	−	−	−	−
Spleen	−	−	−	−	−	−	−	−	−	−	−	−	−	−	−	−
Kidney	−	−	−	−	−	−	−	−	−	−	−	−	−	−	−	−
Testes	−	−	−	−	−	−	−	−	−	−	−	−	−	−	−	−
Parotis	−	−	−	−	−	−	−	−	−	−	−	−	−	−	−	−
Ln. parotid	−	−	−	−	−	−	−	−	−	−	−	−	−	−	−	−

HOST RANGE

BD virus has a broad host range in experimental animals (Table I). Infection occurs regularly only after intracerebral inoculation. The experimental animal of choice is the rabbit. In this species the incubation period lasts for 4–6 weeks and the clinical signs and pathological changes are similar to those seen in the natural disease in horses and sheep. The rabbits usually die within one week after the onset of detectable disease. In other species the incubation periods vary greatly and clinical symptoms are often less distinct than in the rabbits (Heinig, 1969). In tree shrew *(Tupaia glis)*, an animal which has been placed on the phylogenetic root of primates, the infection tends to be subclinical. It is of special interest that in this animal species behavioral alterations can be noted, although typical locomotor disorders are absent. These alterations are especially expressed as an exaggeration of all the components of the normal social behaviour (Sprankel et al., 1978).

PATHOGENESIS OF BORNA DISEASE IN RABBITS

Some indications on pathogenesis of BD have been obtained in experimentally infected rabbits (unpublished results). Virus specific antigen becomes detectable about 12 days after i.c. inoculation. This can be seen in the cortex and olfactory bulbs. It spreads to other areas of the brain including the hippocampus, midbrain and cerebellum. Neurons in the retina, trigeminal ganglia, and the autonomic ganglia also have antigen in the late infection. In addition, cells of the adrenal medulla are also infected (Table II).

The neurotropism of the virus suggests dissemination via nerve pathways. Since retinal neurons are invariably infected in this disease there was an opportunity to demonstrate that the optic nerve was the viral conduit: coagulation of the optic nerve prevented the retinopathy (Krey et al., 1979b).

Inflammatory changes consisting of mononuclear cell infiltrations are first seen in the meninges and the cortex during the first weeks after infection. A pleocytosis occurs at this time and persists throughout the infection. Inflammatory lesions in the parenchyma are diffusely disseminated in the neuropil, and are concentrated in perivascular spaces. Inflammatory lesions are also seen among neuronal tissues of the peripheral nervous system where viral antigen could be detected. This includes the retina, spinal and autonomic ganglia, and the medulla of the adrenal gland. Inflammatory cells consist of lymphocytes of varying sizes including immunoglobulin secreting cells, and a few macrophages.

It could be speculated that the close proximity of inflammatory cells to neurons might be important in the pathogenesis of the disease. Some support for this comes from examination of the retina of affected rabbits. Although viral antigen was present in nearly all neurons, neuronal death was only recognized in areas near blood vessels where cellular infiltrates were dense (Krey et al., 1979a,b). Furthermore, it is of interest that all animals with clinical disease have virus specific antibodies in serum and CSF. Antibody titers in the CSF frequently exceed those in serum, suggesting local production in the CNS (Ludwig et al., 1977). Whether these antibodies have any significance for the disease is not clear.

SUMMARY

In summary, BD is a slowly progressive disease resulting from a persistent infection of the entire nervous system. Viral dissemination seems to occur only via nerve conduits, perhaps by axonal transport. Neurons throughout the nervous system are targets for infection. The lesions of the disease are mainly inflammatory and their localization in the grey matter suggests reactivity to infected neurons. The specific immunologic parameters of the disease, however, have yet to be elucidated.

ACKNOWLEDGEMENT

Supported by the Deutsche Forschungsgemeinschaft (Sonderforschungsbereich 47).

REFERENCES

Heinig, A. (1969) Die Bornasche Krankheit der Pferde und Schafe. In H. Röhrer (Ed.), *Handbuch der Virusinfektionen bei Tieren, Vol. 4*, Fischer, Jena, pp. 83–148.

Herzog, S. and Rott, R. (1980) Replication of Borna disease virus in cell cultures. *Med. Microbiol. Immunol.*, 168: 153–158.

Krey, J., Ludwig, H. and Boschek, C.B. (1979a) Multifocal retinopathy in Borna disease virus infected rabbits. *Amer. J. Ophthalmol.*, 87: 157–164.

Krey, H., Ludwig, H. and Rott, R. (1979b) Spread of infectious virus along the optic nerve into the retina in Borna disease virus-infected rabbits. *Arch. Virol.*, 62: 161–166.

Ludwig, H., Becht, H. and Groh, L. (1973) Borna disease (BD), a slow virus infection: biological properties of the virus. *Med. Microbiol. Immunol.*, 158: 275–289.

Ludwig, H., Koester, U., Pauli, G. and Rott, R. (1977) The cerebrospinal fluid of rabbits infected with Borna disease virus. *Arch. Virol.*, 55: 209–223.

Sprankel, H., Richardz, K., Ludwig, H. and Rott, R. (1978) Behavior alterations in tree shrew (*Tupaia glis*, Diard 1820) induced by Borna disease virus. *Med. Microbiol. Immunol.*, 165: 1–8.

Immunology of Nervous System Infections, Progress in Brain Research, Vol. 59, edited by P.O. Behan, V. ter Meulen and F. Clifford Rose
© *1983 Elsevier Science Publishers B.V.*

Immunological Studies in Demyelinating Encephalitis Associated with Vaccinia Virus and Canine Distemper Virus Infection

A.J. STECK and M. VANDEVELDE

Department of Neurology, Centre Hospitalier Universitaire Vaudois, 1011 Lausanne, and Institute of Comparative Neurology, University of Berne, Berne (Switzerland)

INTRODUCTION

A number of viral models of demyelination are now being studied. Infection with a virus can cause the direct death of the oligodendrocytes leading to demyelination. Virus models of demyelination more pertinent to multiple sclerosis (MS) involve damage to the myelin-oligo-dendrocyte compartment resulting from the involvement of the immune system. Examples include vaccinia virus, which belongs to a group of viruses associated with postinfectious encephalomyelitis (Johnson, 1980) and canine distemper virus, an agent related to measles virus (Hall et al., 1980) causing a neurologic disease in dogs associated with demyelination in the central nervous system (CNS).

It has been suggested that an infectious agent in conjunction with a suspected sensitization to brain components may be involved in the etiology of MS (Nathanson and Miller, 1975; Boese, 1980). Accordingly, the interaction between viruses, host tissues and the immune system must be considered in the investigation of demyelinating diseases. We will review here data on the humoral response to the myelin-oligodendrocyte compartment in mice infected with vaccinia virus (Steck et al., 1981) and present recent results of the immune response to myelin basic proteins in dogs with canine distemper virus infection (Vandevelde et al., 1982).

VACCINIA VIRUS INFECTION

We have investigated the appearance of autoantibodies to brain antigens following intracranial infection of mice with two different strains of vaccinia virus: a neurotropic strain (WR) which is characterized by a high mortality after intracranial infection with concomitant rapid multiplication of virus in brain and a non-lethal dermotropic strain (Elstree) which does not replicate in nervous tissue (Turner, 1967).

Mice injected with the neurotropic strain of vaccinia virus developed a high titer of antimyelin antibody. Binding values averaged 7500 cpm at a 1:10 dilution, which represents a 15-fold increase over the values for sera obtained 4 days after inoculation with the neurotropic strain or for sera obtained from mice inoculated with the dermotropic strain. To dissect this immune response further, we looked for antibodies against markers of the myelin-oligodend-rocyte compartment. The neurotropic strain induced the production of antibodies against myelin basic protein (mbp), a specific marker of the myelin membrane (Fig. 1), and against

276

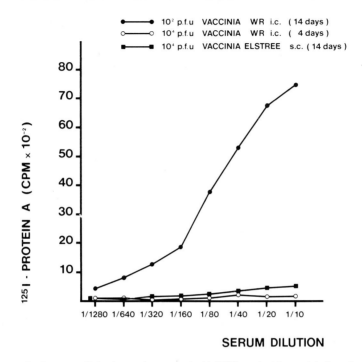

Fig. 1. Serum antibodies to myelin basic protein measured with [^{125}I]protein A in vaccinia-inoculated mice. Methods are described in Steck et al., 1981.

galactocerebroside (Fig. 2), a cell surface marker for oligodendrocytes (Raff et al., 1978). When oligodendrocytes isolated from calf brain were used as target cells, a significant titer of binding antibodies was again found only in sera obtained on the fourteenth post-inoculation day with the neurotropic strain. Binding values with this serum averaged 17,000 cpm at 1:20 dilution, which represents an 8-fold increase over the other sera. In contrast, when neurons isolated from rat brain were used, no difference in binding was observed between the sera of animals infected with the neurotropic or the dermotropic strains (data not shown).

We have presented evidence for the ability of the neurotropic strain to elicit an immunological reaction that appears directed essentially towards the myelin-oligodendrocyte compartment. Viruses can show tropism restricted to one group of cells. That oligodendrocytes can be directly attacked by the neurotropic strain of vaccinia virus is suggested by recent experiments in which dissociated neworn mouse brain cells were infected with different strains of vaccinia virus. It was found, using an indirect immunofluorescence technique, that the neurotropic strain of vaccinia virus infected oligodendrocytes, whereas the dermotropic strain did not (Beranek et al., 1982). Astrocytes were not infected by vaccinia strains. Sensitization could thus result from replication of virus within oligodendrocytes with subsequent release of hidden immunogens such as the mpb.

GALACTOCEREBROSIDE BINDING ANTIBODIES

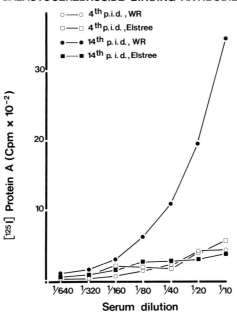

Fig. 2. Serum antibodies to galactocerebroside measured with [^{125}I]protein A in vaccinia-inoculated mice. Galactocerebroside was coated on microtiter plates in chloroform: methanol 2:1 and the organic phase was evaporated before saturating the wells with a solution of 2% bovine serum albumin.

CANINE DISTEMPER VIRUS INFECTION

Although it appears that oligodendrocytes can be directly attacked by vaccinia virus, viral induced demyelination may be enhanced as a result of a local immune reaction. Such may be the case in the demyelinating encephalitis associated with canine distemper virus.

Dogs with canine distemper encephalitis were examined using immunological techniques, including demonstration of antibodies against canine distemper virus in the serum and against myelin basic protein in serum and in cerebrospinal fluid (CSF). The brains were examined pathologically and immunoglobulin was demonstrated in lesions by means of immunohistological techniques (Table I). Dogs with acute canine distemper encephalitis had none or low antibody levels against canine distemper virus or mbp and there was no immunoglobulin in demyelinating lesions. Both dogs with chronic canine distemper encephalitis had very high antibody titers against mbp in the CSF and demyelinating lesions contained immunoglobulin.

This marked increase of antibody titer to mbp in the CSF of dogs with chronic canine distemper encephalitis supports the association between chronic demyelination and a local immune reaction. This demonstrates that the CNS, from an immunological point of view, partly reacts as a separate entity, which means that lymphocytes present within the brain react on their own and yield an immune response independent from that outside the CNS. Since white matter destruction is far more extensive in inflammatory that in noninflammatory lesions, demyelination in chronic canine distemper encephalitis may be enhanced by a local immune reaction.

278

TABLE I

IMMUNOLOGICAL AND PATHOLOGICAL FINDINGS IN DEMYELINATING ENCEPHALITIS ASSOCIATED WITH CANINE DISTEMPER VIRUS INFECTION

Antibodies against canine distemper virus (CDV) expressed in serum dilution. Antibodies against mbp in serum or CSF are expressed in cpm.

Dog	Lesion type	CDV inclusion bodies	Immunopathologic findings	Serum anti-CDV antibody (titer)	Serum anti-MBP antibody (CPM)	CSF anti-MBP antibody (CPM)
1	Acute	Present	Negative	Negative	1170	156
2	Acute	Present	Negative	1/36	1025	458
3	Acute	Present	Occasional Ig + cell	1/48	3238	610
4	Chronic	Present	Large number of Ig + cells. Ig bound to myelin	1/324	7026	8939
5	Chronic	Absent	Several Ig + cells. Ig bound to myelin	1/48	2683	2589
6	Old Sclerotic	Absent	Few Ig + cells in lesion	?1/62	3773	710

CONCLUSION

The presence and the role of vaccinia and canine distemper virus induced autoimmunity to the myelin-oligodendrocyte compartment is still unknown. The demonstration of myelin-bound immunoglobulins in demyelinating lesions of canine distemper virus-infected dogs together with an elevation of anti mbp antibodies in the CSF suggest that these antibodies could be contributing factors in the pathogenesis of demyelination and serve to amplify the basic lesion, particularly in chronic disorders.

ACKNOWLEDGEMENTS

The authors thank Mrs. G. Perruisseau and Mrs. N. Page for expert technical assistance and Mrs. A.-M. Vodoz for secretarial help. This work was supported by Grants 3.957-0.80 (to A.J.S.), and 3.805-79 (to M.V.) from the Swiss National Fund, and by a fund from the Swiss Multiple Sclerosis Society.

REFERENCES

Beranek, C.F., Schaefer, R., Bologa, L. and Herschkowitz, N. (1982) Viral tropisms in mouse brain cell cultures. *Med. Microbiol. Immunol.*, 170: 201–207.

Boese, A. (Ed.) (1980) *Search for the Cause of Multiple Sclerosis and other Chronic diseases of the Central Nervous System*, Verlag Chemie, Denfield Beach, FL.

Hall, W.W., Lamb, R.A. and Choppin, P.W. (1980) The polypeptides of canine distemper virus: synthesis in infected cells and relatedness to the polypeptides of other morbilliviruses. *Virology*, 100: 433–449.

Johnson, R.T. (1980) Neurologic diseases associated with viral infections. *Postgrad. Med.*, 50: 159–163.

Leibowitz, S. and Kennedy, M.C. (1978) Galactocerebroside is a specific cell-surface antigenic marker for oligodendrocytes in culture. *Nature (Lond.)*, 274: 813–816.

Nathanson, N. and Miller, A. (1975) Epidemiology of multiple sclerosis: critique of the evidence for a viral etiology. *Amer. J. Epidemiol.*, 107: 451–461.

Raff, M.C., Mirsky, R., Fields, K.L., Lisak, R.P., Dorfman, S.H., Silberberg, D.H., Gregson, N.A.,

Steck, A.J., Tschannen, R. and Schaefer, R. (1981) Induction of antimyelin and antioligodendrocyte antibodies by vaccinia virus — an experimental study in the mouse. *J. Neuroimmunol.*, 1: 117–124.

Turner, G.S. (1967) Respiratory infection of mice with vaccinia virus. *J. gen. Virol.*, 1: 399–402.

Vandevelde, M., Kristensen, F., Kristensen, B., Steck, A.J. and Kihm, U. (1982) Immunological and pathological findings in demyelinating encephalitis associated with canine distemper virus infection, *Acta Neuropathol.*, 56: 1–8.

Immunology of Nervous System Infections, Progress in Brain Research, Vol. 59, edited by P.O. Behan, V. ter Meulen and F. Clifford Rose

Experimental Control of Cerebral Amyloid in Scrapie in Mice

H. FRASER and MOIRA E. BRUCE

ARC and MRC Neuropathogenesis Unit, West Mains Road, Edinburgh EH9 3JQ, Scotland (U.K.)

INTRODUCTION

Scrapie is an infectious neurological disease of adult sheep and goats, sometimes transmissible to laboratory animals which develop the clinical disease after incubation periods of many months. Numerous strains of the causal agent have been distinguished, on the basis of incubation period and neuropathological characteristics, in inbred mice (Dickinson, 1976; Dickinson and Fraser, 1977; Fraser and Dickinson, 1973). The neuropathology of scrapie is largely degenerative with no inflammatory association (Fraser, 1979a, b), complementing the apparent failure of the immune system to respond to the infection and the absence of any demonstrable antigenicity in strains of agent studied so far (Gardiner, 1966; Porter et al., 1973; Fraser and Hancock, 1977; Fraser and Dickinson, 1978). Scrapie is by far the most extensively studied and best understood member of a group of diseases, the "infectious degenerative encephalopathies", which also include Creutzfeldt–Jakob disease and kuru in man, and transmissible mink encephalopathy (Marsh, 1976), caused by similar agents with unconventional properties, now designated "virinos" (Dickinson and Outram, 1979), to distinguish them from conventional viruses and from viroids.

In one major respect experimental murine scrapie has a much wider relevance in that it provides a set of particularly appropriate research models for the study of cerebral amyloidosis, for which no other model is known. Amyloid-containing argyrophilic plaques, occurring in the experimental disease with only certain scrapie agents, are a valid equivalent to those occurring in Alzheimer's disease and in cerebral amyloidosis in other dementias of known infectious origin (Fraser and Bruce, 1973; Bruce and Fraser, 1975; Wisniewski et al., 1975). Experimental scrapie infections of mice provide a number of predictable models to study amyloidosis in the central nervous system (Bruce et al., 1976; Fraser, 1976) and it is this that justifies the inclusion in a symposium on CNS immunity of a paper on a disease lacking immunological response in the infected hosts or antigenicity in its causal agents. The wider negative reason which warrants the inclusion of scrapie is as a reminder that chronic CNS infection can occur without conventional immune response: this raises a point which will not be dealt with here, namely, whether there might be a positive disarming of the immune responses in this class of disease.

The two major unanswered questions concerning cerebral amyloid in general and in scrapie in particular, are its molecular identity and its origin (Fraser, 1979b): whether it is related to any of the known defined amyloid types, whether it is generated locally or systemically, and if locally, whether it is derived from cells of neuroectodermal or mesenchymal origin? If systemically, what possible mechanisms of local processing might cause its deposition? The most plausible interpretation points to its originating within the brain itself (Bruce and Fraser, 1981). Its chemical identity can only be speculated about: is it analogous to the known AA of secondary amyloid (Benditt, 1976), to the light chain type, associated with the plasma cell dysgenesias (Glenner and Terry, 1973), to the hormone-derived amyloid varieties (Pearce et al., 1972) and does it contain the P-component common to amyloid extracts generally (Dyck et al., 1980)?

Passage studies with particular scrapie-agents, which produce large numbers of amyloid plaques in all mouse strains studied, have highlighted two important aspects of scrapie which bear on our understanding of strain variation. One is the occurrence of a sudden mutational change in agent properties, in which the incubation periods become greatly shortened compared with passages prior to breakdown, coincident with a change in lesion distribution and a reduction in the frequency of amyloid plaques (Bruce and Dickinson, 1979). The second is the occurrence of asymmetrically distributed focal lesions in the mid- and forebrains, in regions where, before the mutation, lesions are otherwise absent, but in which after the mutation, lesions occur symmetrically and with some intensity (Fraser, 1979c). Studies of cerebral amyloidosis in scrapie and of the biology of the strains of agent responsible for it, are contributing to understanding the pathogenesis of a variety of similar diseases in other mammals.

EXPERIMENTAL PROTOCOLS FOR THE STUDY OF CEREBRAL AMYLOID IN MURINE SCRAPIE

The approach to work on the biology of scrapie and cerebral amyloidosis has been developed to obtain a broad overview of the diversity of agent properties. A variety of inbred mouse strains and crosses are used. By far the most important factor controlling variation in the biology of scrapie in mice is the Sinc gene and inbred strains have been selected with different allelic configurations, in which the pathogenesis of scrapie shows different consequential patterns. The extent to which amyloid deposition in the brain is influenced by these genetic differences varies, depending upon the scrapie-strain/host-strain combination studied.

VM mice, and strains derived from them, carry the p7 alleles of Sinc which control the incubation period of scrapie. Others, such as C57BL, carry the s7 allele, and in some studies F_1 crosses between VM and C57BL are used, and these have the Sinc s7p7 genotype; for full details of this system, see Dickinson and Meikle (1971). The details of the agents and isolates studied are described elsewhere (Bruce et al., 1976). In addition, standardized systems have been developed to establish consistent and unbiased incubation period measurements and histopathological indices, upon which strain-typing characteristics are based (Dickinson et al., 1968; Fraser and Dickinson, 1973; Fraser, 1976). The incubation period characteristics of some of the important strains, which show wide variety in terms of the cerebral amyloidosis they induce, are listed in Table I.

MORPHOLOGICAL OBSERVATIONS OF CEREBRAL AMYLOID IN MURINE SCRAPIE

The most typical type of lesion associated with scrapie is a vacuolar degeneration affecting the grey matter, and sometimes the white matter, the nature and variation of which has been

TABLE I

INCIDENCES OF PLAQUES AND INCUBATION PERIODS FOR BEST-STUDIED
COMBINATIONS OF SCRAPIE STRAIN AND MOUSE GENOTYPE

Mice were injected i.c. with 10^{-2} dilution of scrapie mouse brain. Scrapie strain: (C), passaged in C57BL; (V), passaged in VM. Mouse strain: C, C57BL; V, VM; X, C57BL $\times$ VM F_1-cross.

Scrapie strain	Passages studied	Mouse strain	n	Mean incubation period (days + S.E.)	% with plaques in H & E sections
ME7	4–12	C	78	161 ± 1	1.3
(C)		X	15	250 ± 3	13.3
		V	47	333 ± 2	51.1
ME7	4–12	C	45	166 ± 1	4.4
(V)		X	18	250 ± 3	11.1
		V	80	312 ± 4	55.0
87A	2–5	C	37	351 ± 4	78.4
(C)		X	5	552 ± 23	100
		V	23	600 ± 5	100
87V	3–6	C	23	430 ± 17	78.3
(V)		X	5	564 ± 18	60.0
		V	53	294 ± 2	96.2
22C	4–9	C	55	178 ± 1	0
(C)		X	7	270 ± 8	0
		V	23	449 ± 3	0
22A	4–7	C	82	459 ± 4	39.0
(V)		X	35	564 ± 8	80.0
		V	98	195 ± 1	0
79A	2–5	C	28	152 ± 1	0
(C)		X	24	234 ± 4	0
		V	22	293 ± 6	0
79V	2–7	C	35	239 ± 2	0
(V)		X	17	323 ± 4	0
		V	36	267 ± 4	0

extensively described and reviewed elsewhere (Fraser, 1976, 1979b, c). In contrast to the regular occurrence of vacuolation, cerebral amyloidosis and amyloid plaques are only found with certain scrapie strains (Bruce et al., 1976), and when present they are readily detected with haematoxylin and eosin (Fig. 1) although methods of staining based on the Masson's trichrome technique have proved to be most useful for studying their morphological variation. Based on these two simple methods, various forms of cerebral amyloid have been distinguished (Bruce and Fraser, 1975), either as diffuse deposits often associated with needle scars, or as discrete forms designated "amorphous", "stellate", "shadowy" and "giant" plaques, although various intermediate forms also exist. These plaques can occur in both grey and white matter, and are frequent in the cerebral cortex, hippocampus, corpus callosum, thalamus and adjacent to the lateral ventricles (Fig. 2). In a recent study of attempted primary isolations into mice from 5 cases of Icelandic scrapie a variety of bizarre forms of amyloid deposition was found, and plaques occurred in hitherto unusual locations such as the suprachiasmatic nucleus, the raphé of the mesencephalic tegmentum in the vicinity of the oculomotor complex, and close to the locus coeruleus in the medulla/pons (Fraser, in press).

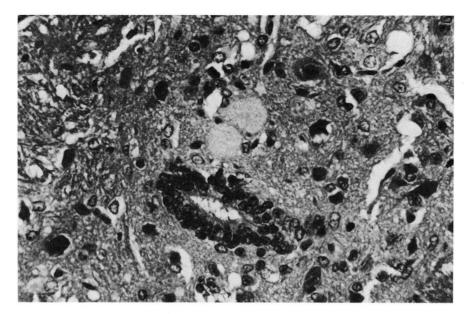

Fig. 1. Cerebral amyloid plaque in spinal cord of VM mouse injected with the 87V scrapie strain. Haematoxylin and eosin, magnification: × 420.

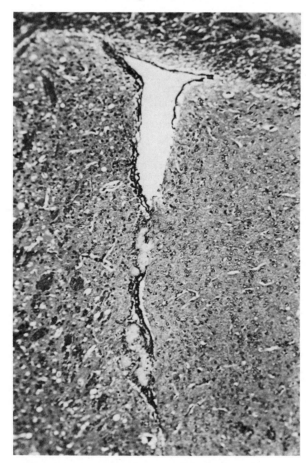

Fig. 2. Cerebral amyloid plaques associated with lateral ventricles in VM mouse injected intracerebrally with 87A. P.T.A.H., magnification: × 105.

The distribution of amyloid plaques in the well-studied model systems differs in relation to several important biological and experimental variables (see below). There is no apparent association with vacuolar degeneration in either grey or white matter, except in the important instance when asymmetrical foci of vacuolation, seen with some "wild-type" agents, is associated with amyloid. Otherwise, plaques occur in areas of severe vacuolation as well as in areas free from this type of pathology (Bruce, 1980).

An association with small blood vessels is frequent (Fig. 3) and sometimes resembles the "plaque-like" angiopathy described by Scholz (1938) which has also been identified in so-called atypical Alzheimer's disease (Corsellis and Brierley, 1954) and in the Gerstmann–Sträussler syndrome (Masters et al., 1981). However, in general, the most typical, discrete forms of murine amyloid plaques show all the features associated with human senile plaques, and their similarity can most clearly be seen in silver sections of murine scrapie brain (Fig. 4). The 3 main components of senile plaques, extracellular amyloid, with surrounding microglia and degenerating neuritic processes (Kidd, 1964; Terry and Wisniewski, 1970) are also readily detected ultrastructurally in amyloid plaques in scrapie (Bruce and Fraser, 1975; Wisniewski et al., 1975).

THE IDENTIFICATION AND ANALYSIS OF SOME FACTORS INFLUENCING THE OCCURRENCE AND VARIATION OF AMYLOID PLAQUES IN MURINE SCRAPIE

Different experimental conditions impose striking effects on the occurrence, frequency and distribution of amyloid plaques within the brain, and variation due to agent strain, host genotype and age, inoculation route and dose have all been studied (Bruce, 1980).

Scrapie strain differences are outstandingly the most important biological variable influencing the occurrence of amyloid plaques: with some strains amyloidosis has not been observed, whereas with others the intensity of amyloidosis and the frequency of plaques are extremely high (Bruce et al., 1976). A number of well-defined scrapie strains, and some isolates not yet well characterized, have been studied mainly in 3 mouse genotypes, C57BL (Sinc^{s7}), VM (Sinc^{p7}) and their F$_1$ cross, all injected intracerebrally, and the percentage incidence of plaques is shown in Table I. It is evident that two strains, 87V and 87A, produce high plaque incidences, whereas 22C, 79A and 79V produce none, an absence which is confirmed when the more sensitive staining methods based on Masson's trichrome are used.

It emerges from Table I that host-genotype can significantly influence the occurrence of plaques for some scrapie strains, such as 22A and ME7, and the incidences correspond to the ranking of incubation periods in different genotypes. This relationship with incubation period, however, was not found to be a consistent finding, as those agents which do not induce amyloid plaques have incubation periods within the range of those that do, and experimental procedures which prolong incubation, such as dilution or boiling of agent, or the use of peripheral injection routes, produce fewer plaques. Whether there exists for cerebral amyloidosis anything analagous to the single gene difference found in A/J mice to determine resistance to systemic amyloidosis, remains to be seen (Wohlgethan and Cathcart, 1979), although recent work with a Sinc^{p7} strain derived from VM mice is highly suggestive that there are genes independent of Sinc which also control cerebral amyloidosis.

Studies with 4 strains, 87A and 87V, both with a high amyloid plaque frequency in all mouse genotypes, ME7 with a lower frequency, and 79A with which plaques are not associated, as well as with uninfected extremely aged mice, have shown that the occurrence of plaques is not influenced by age (Bruce and Fraser, 1982). Peripheral routes of infection prolong incubation

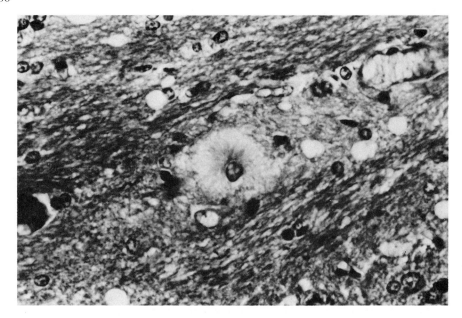

Fig. 3. Cerebral amyloid plaque associated with a capillary in the corpus callosum. Masson's trichrome, magnification: × 660.

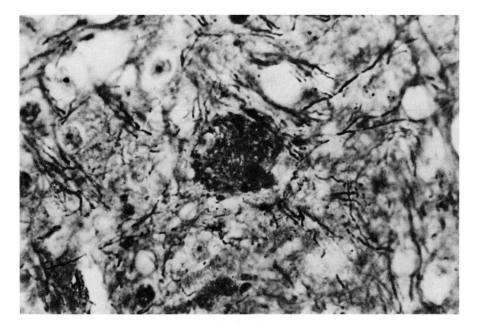

Fig. 4. Cerebral amyloid plaque. Bodian's silver method, × 420.

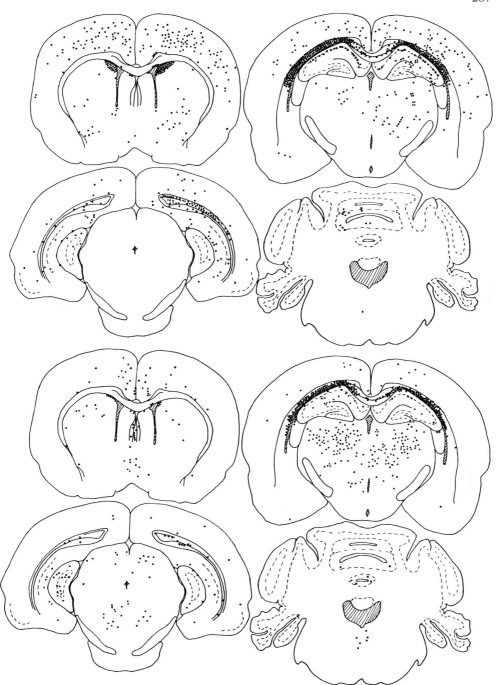

Fig. 5. Distribution maps of amyloid plaques in sections of VM mice injected intracerebrally with 87V (above, compiled from 53 mice) and 87A (below, compiled from 23 mice) scrapie strains. Each dot represents one plaque. Haematoxylin and eosin. The ME7 and 22A agents have been studied with identical methods, and show similar distribution patterns to that of 87A. The 87V agent shows a distinct pattern of plaque distribution in both C57BL and VM mice (Bruce, 1980).

periods, compared with the intracerebral route, but induce smaller numbers of plaques and the distribution of plaques is also quite different — following intracerebral injection, plaques are associated with areas closely associated with the lateral ventricles such as the corpus callosum and hippocampus, whereas they are absent from these regions with peripheral routes (Bruce and Fraser, 1981). Also, following intracerebral injection, plaques are a relatively early lesion, beginning by one-third of the incubation period, well before degenerative vacuolation appears (Bruce, 1981).

Strains of scrapie agents differ in their heat stability, and some can withstand prolonged boiling or even exposure to much higher temperatures with only moderate losses of infectivity (Dickinson and Taylor, 1978), although it has been shown that boiling does influence pathogenesis, and that boiled agent injected intracerebrally may undergo a peripheral cycle of replication before intracerebral events can proceed, unlike unheated agent in which intracerebral events proceed independently of peripheral pathogenesis (Dickinson and Fraser, 1969). With plaque-inducing agents, boiling consistently resulted in an altered distribution of plaques in the brain, more resembling that which followed peripheral injection routes with unboiled inocula (Bruce, 1980).

Dilution of inoculum increases the mean duration and spread of incubation periods, thus offering the opportunity to study the influence that such incubation period differences might have on the occurrence of plaques. Numerous titration experiments (22A and 87V intracerebrally) have been analyzed for the effect on plaque occurrence of different dilutions of inoculum and of differences in incubation period within single dilutions, and a very consistent effect has emerged: the number of amyloid plaques decreases with dilution of agent, but *within* each dilution group those individuals with the longer incubation periods have more plaques than those with shorter ones. Plaques have never been seen in the uninfected mice at or beyond the terminal dilutions, whereas they always occur in infected mice, even at the terminal dilutions (Bruce, 1980). This and the observation that plaques are seen after injection of boiled inocula, demonstrate that the occurrence of cerebral amyloid, when it does occur, is a specific concomitant of scrapie neuropathogenesis, and is not due to the presence of an undetected conventional virus in the scrapie passage lines.

There are also important differences in the distribution of plaques within the brain, depending upon strain and mouse genotype. For instance, Fig. 5 shows the composite analysis of their distribution in coronal brain sections in VM mice. The most dense accumulation is found in the cerebral cortex and forebrain with the 87V strain, compared with 87A with which plaques are more prevalent in the thalamus. Analogous differences in plaque distribution also characterize other strains such as ME7 and 22A (Bruce, 1980). There is no obvious association of amyloid plaque distribution with the distribution of vacuolar degeneration, and the two lesions appear to occur independently of one another.

CONCLUSIONS

There are two major neuropathological changes in scrapie: a degenerative vacuolation and cerebral amyloidosis. Although a great deal has been learnt about factors controlling these changes, there is still a paucity of knowledge of the primary disorders involved in their etiology at the molecular level. A major question which any eventual synthesis must answer is the basis of the independence or dissociation between these two lesions, both topographically within the brain, and between different agent systems. Why do some agent-strains fail to induce amyloid plaques, and why is there so much variation in the frequency and distribution between the strains which do produce plaques?

There is some evidence pointing to a local rather than a systemic origin of the amyloid in the brain, but it is not possible to exclude formally either a mechanism of local processing of systemically-produced precursors, or systemic co-factors. The questions can legitimately be raised, in a volume on immunity in the CNS, whether immunity in a broad sense has a role in the pathogenesis of cerebral amyloid in scrapie, and whether any analogy can be drawn with the systemic amyloidoses where immunological disorders — either neoplastic or failures of immunoregulation — are usually involved. Does an "immune origin" necessarily imply generation from immune cells, usually conceived as lymphoid in origin, or can the molecular events leading to immune recognition and response be vested, in a vestigial form, in other somatic cells such as neuroectoderm? A major physiological contrast between neuroectodermal and lymphoidal cells is that they occupy extreme poles in the spectrum of proliferative capacity, the former having almost none, whereas the function of the latter is integrally dependent upon a capacity to undergo a clonal expansion in response to antigen recognition. However, in secondary amyloidosis this clonal proliferation is exhausted, which points to a plausible parallel with fully differentiated neuroectoderm whose proliferative capacity is likewise "eclipsed". Such a mechanism need not exclude a local processing of a systemic precursor, or the involvement of systemic co-factors.

Whatever eventual explanation of the amyloid plaque in experimental scrapie in mice turns out to be, it can be seen now to have both intrinsic importance in basic neurobiology, as well as far-reaching implications for understanding the parallel phenomenon in Alzheimer's disease and other dementias.

REFERENCES

Benditt, E.P. (1976) The structure of amyloid protein AA. In O. Wegelius and A. Pasternack (Eds.), *Amyloidosis*, Academic Press, New York, pp. 323–358.

Bruce, M.E. (1980) *The Neuropathology of Scrapie in Mice, With Special Reference to Cerebral Amyloidosis and Agent Stability*. Ph. D. Thesis, Open University.

Bruce, M.E. (1981) Serial studies on the development of cerebral amyloidosis and vacuolar degeneration in murine scrapie. *J. comp. Pathol.*, 91: 589–597.

Bruce, M.E. and Dickinson, A.G. (1979) Biological stability of different classes of scrapie agent. In W.J. Hadlow and S.B. Prusiner (Eds.), *Slow Transmissible Diseases of the Nervous System, Vol. 2*, Academic Press, New York, pp. 71–86.

Bruce, M.E. and Fraser, H. (1975) Amyloid plaques in the brains of mice infected with scrapie: morphological variation and staining properties. *Neuropath. appl. Neurobiol.*, 1: 189–202.

Bruce, M.E. and Fraser, H. (1981) Effect of route of infection on the frequency and distribution of cerebral amyloid plaques in scrapie mice. *Neuropath. appl. Neurobiol.*, 7: 289–298.

Bruce, M.E. and Fraser, H. (1982) Effect of age on cerebral amyloid plaques in murine scrapie. *Neuropath. appl. Neurobiol.*, 8: 71–74.

Bruce, M.E., Dickinson, A.G. and Fraser, H. (1976) Cerebral amyloidosis in scrapie in the mouse: effect of agent strain and mouse genotype. *Neuropath. appl. Neurobiol.*, 2: 471–478.

Corsellis, J.A.N. and Brierley, J.B. (1954) An unsual type of pre-senile dementia (atypical Alzheimer's disease with amyloid vascular change). *Brain*, 77: 571–587.

Dickinson, A.G. (1976) Scrapie in sheep and goats. In R.H. Kimberlin (Ed.), *Slow Virus Diseases of Animals and Man*, North-Holland, Amsterdam, pp. 209–239.

Dickinson, A.G. and Fraser, H. (1969) Modification of the pathogenesis of scrapie in mice by treatment of the agent. *Nature (Lond.)*, 222: 892–893.

Dickinson, A.G. and Fraser, H. (1977) Scrapie: pathogenesis in inbred mice: an assessment of host-control and responses involving many strains of agent. In: V. ter Meulen and M. Katz (Eds.), *Slow Virus Infections of the Central Nervous System*, Springer, New York, pp. 3–14.

Dickinson, A.G. and Meikle, V.M.H. (1971) Host-genotype and agent effects in scrapie incubation: change in allelic interaction with different strains of agent. *Molec. gen. Genet.*, 112: 73–79.

Dickinson, A.G. and Outram, G.W. (1979) The scrapie replication-site hypothesis and its implications for pathogenesis. In W.J. Hadlow and S.B. Prusiner (Eds.), *Slow Transmissible Diseases of the Nervous System, Vol. 2*, Academic Press, New York, pp. 13–31.

Dickinson, A.G. and Taylor, D.M. (1978) Resistance of scrapie agent to decontamination. *New Engl. J. Med.*, 299: 1413–1414.

Dickinson, A.G., Meikle, V.M.H. and Fraser, H. (1968) Identification of a gene which controls the incubation period of some strains of scrapie in mice. *J. comp. Pathol.*, 78: 293–299.

Dyck, R.F., Lockwood, C.M., Kershaw, M., McHugh, N., Duance, V.C., Baltz, M.L. and Pepys, M.B. (1980) Amyloid P-component is a constituent of normal human glomerular basement membrane. *J. exp. Med.*, 152: 1162–1174.

Fraser, H. (1976) The pathology of natural and experimental scrapie. In R.H. Kimberlin (Ed.), *Slow Virus Diseases of Animals and Man*, North-Holland, Amsterdam, pp. 267–305.

Fraser, H. (1979a) Scrapie: a transmissible degenerative neurological disease. In P.O. Behan and F. Clifford Rose (Eds.), *Progress in Neurological Research with Particular Reference to Motor Neurone Disease*, Pitman, London, pp. 194–210.

Fraser, H. (1979b) The pathogenesis and pathology of scrapie. In D.A.J. Tyrell (Ed.), *Aspects of Slow and Persistent Virus Infections*, Martinus Nijhoff, The Hague, pp. 30–58.

Fraser, H. (1979c) Neuropathology of scrapie: the precision of the lesions and their diversity. In W.J. Hadlow and S.B. Prusiner (Eds.), *Slow Transmissible Diseases of the Nervous System, Vol. 1*, Academic Press, New York, pp. 387–406.

Fraser, H. and Bruce, M.E. (1973) Argyrophilic plaques in mice inoculated with scrapie from particular sources. *Lancet*, i: 617.

Fraser, H. and Dickinson, A.G. (1973) Scrapie in mice; agent-strain differences in the distribution and intensity of grey matter vacuolation. *J. comp. Pathol.*, 83: 29–40.

Fraser, H. and Dickinson, A.G. (1978) Studies of the lymphoreticular system in the pathogenesis of scrapie: the role of spleen and thymus. *J. comp. Pathol.*, 88: 563-473.

Fraser, H. and Hancock, P.M. (1977) An investigation of the macrophage electrophoretic mobility test in the diagnosis of scrapie in sheep. *J. comp. Pathol.*, 87: 267–274.

Gardiner, A.C. (1966) Cell-diffusion reactions of tissues and sera from scrapie-affected animals. *Res. vet. Sci.*, 7: 190–195.

Glenner, G.G. and Terry, W.D. (1973) The immunological origin of amyloid fibril proteins. In H. Peeters (Ed.), *Protides of the Biological Fluids, 20th Colloquium*, Pergamon, Oxford, pp. 55–62.

Kidd, M. (1964) Alzheimer's disease — an electron-microscopic study. *Brain*, 87: 307–320.

Marsh, R.F. (1976) In R.H. Kimberlin (Ed.), *Slow Virus Diseases of Animals and Man*, North-Holland, Amsterdam, pp. 359–380.

Masters, C.L., Gajdusek, D.C. and Gibbs, C.J. (1981) Creutzfeldt–Jakob disease virus isolations from the Gerstmann–Sträussler syndrome. *Brain*, 104: 559–588.

Pearse, A.G.E., Ewen, S.W.B. and Polak, J.M. (1972). The genesis of apudamyloid in endocrine polypeptide tumours: histochemical distinction from immunoamyloid. *Virchows Arch. B*, 10: 93–107.

Porter, D.D., Porter, H.G. and Cox, N.A. (1973) Failure to demonstrate a humoral immune response to scrapie infection in mice. *J. Immunol.*, 111: 1407–1410.

Scholz, W. (1938) Studies of the pathology of brain vessels. II. The productive degeneration of the small arterioles and capillaries. *ZeitsGesampte. Neurol. Psychiat.*, 162: 694–715.

Terry, R.D. and Wisniewski, H. (1970) The ultrastructure of the neurofibrillary tangle and the senile plaque. In G.E.W. Wolstenholme and M. O'Connor (Eds.), *Alzheimer's Disease and Related Conditions*, Churchill, London, pp. 145–165.

Wisniewski, H.M., Bruce, M.E. and Fraser, H. (1975) Infectious etiology of neuritic (senile) plaques in mice. *Science*, 190: 1108–1110.

Wohlgethan, J.R. and Cathcart, E.S. (1979) Amyloid resistance in A/J mice is determined by a single gene. *Nature (Lond.)*, 278: 453–454.

Immunology of Nervous System Infections, Progress in Brain Research, Vol. 59, edited by P.O. Behan, V. ter Meulen and F. Clifford Rose

Age-Dependent Paralytic Viral Infection in C58 Mice: Possible Implications in Human Neurologic Disease

WILLIAM H. MURPHY, JOHN F. NAWROCKI and LARRY R. PEASE

The Department of Microbiology and Immunology, The University of Michigan School of Medicine, Ann Arbor, MI 48109 (U.S.A.)

INTRODUCTION

Using an age-dependent motor neuron disease in C58 mice as an experimental model, we have been analyzing the specific ways that aging, viral infection, genetic factors and immune deficiency act together to predispose mice to paralytic disease. Since the background work recently was reviewed (Murphy et al., 1980) this report will be confined largely to a discussion of the findings that appear to provide some fresh insights into the basic mechanisms that may be important in the pathogenesis of the age-dependent neurologic diseases of man of suspected viral etiology.

LACTIC DEHYDROGENASE VIRUS

Lactic dehydrogenase virus (LDV) is widespread in both domestic and wild mice and causes life-long infection (Rowson and Mahy, 1975). Immune complexes typically are found (Oldstone and Dixon, 1971) in the plasma of infected mice. LDV does not cause significant pathologic changes in the tissues of infected mice under ordinary circumstances (Rowson and Mahy, 1975). The main properties of LDV (Brinton-Darnell and Plagemann, 1975) are summarized in Table I. Nawrocki et al. (1980) and Martinez et al. (1980) reported that LDV, derived from line Ib transplantable leukemia, causes a fatal inflammatory motor neuron disease when inoculated into C58 mice which were 9 or more months of age, and in younger C58 mice, providing that they are immunosuppressed first by X-irradiation or drugs. LDV strains differ markedly in their neuropathogenicity (Nawrocki et al., 1980) ranging from those that are highly paralytic to those that cause inapparent infection (Table II).

GENETIC EVIDENCE FOR THE DUAL VIRUS INFECTION HYPOTHESIS

Nineteen inbred strains of mice have been tested (Duffey et al., 1976; Pease and Murphy, 1980) for their susceptibility to paralytic LDV infection. Of these, only the C58, AKR, C3H/Fg and PL/J strains were susceptible. All of the naturally susceptible strains are characterized by a high natural incidence of leukemia. None of the non-leukemic strains were susceptible to paralytic LDV infection. These results suggested that, the genes of the major histocompatibility complex which regulate the susceptibility to viral-induced leukemia

(Steeves and Lilly, 1977), might also regulate the susceptibility of mice to paralytic LDV infection. To test this hypothesis a series of genetic experiments were carried out (Pease et al., 1982) to determine how the H-2 haplotype and Fv-1 genotype of mice affected susceptibility. In studies of F_1 hybrid mice, C58 females were crossed with either resistant or susceptible males. Table III shows that susceptibility was independent of the $H-2^k$, $H-2^b$ or $H-2^d$ haplotypes. Only Fv-$1^{n/n}$ mice were susceptible. In Fv-$1^{n/n}$ mice susceptibility was age-dependent.

TABLE I

MAIN PROPERTIES OF LACTIC DEHYDROGENASE VIRUS

Common viral infection of mice
Common in virus stocks and transplantable tumors
Without pathologic effect
Grows only in mice
Enveloped: 55 nm
RNA infectious: 5×10^6 daltons (48S)
VP1 — core protein — 15,000 daltons
VP2 — envelope protein — 18,000 daltons
VP3 — envelope protein — 24,000–44,000 daltons
Buoyant density = 1.12–1.13 g/cm³

TABLE II

RELATIVE NEUROPATHOGENICITY OF LDV STRAINS

Indicator C58 mice 7- to 9-months-old received 600R of whole-body X-irradiation. The next day mice received an i.p. injection of approximately 10^8 ID_{50} of each test virus. Mice were observed for paralysis for 60 days.

LDV strain	Incidence of paralysis	Mean days to paralysis
Ib-LDV	13/13	15
R-LDV	6/14	26
W-LDV	0/14	

TABLE III

SUSCEPTIBILITY OF F_1 HYBRID MICE TO PARALYTIC LDV INFECTION

All mice received 550R of whole-body X-irradiation 24 h before the i.p. injection of 10^8 ID_{50} of Ib-LDV. The female is listed first in each cross. Mice were scored for paralysis over a 30-day period. Paralysis was confirmed histologically. Data are from 2–6 replicate experiments. S, susceptible; R, resistant.

F_1 hybrid	Susceptibility of parents:		H-2 type of hybrid	FV-1 type of hybrid	Incidence of paralysis at:		
					6 months	9 months	12 months
C58 × AKR/Boy	S	S	k/k	n/n	24/29		13/15
C58 × AKR-H-2^b/ Boy	S	S	k/b	n/n	13/34		12/14
C58 × DBA/2J	S	R	k/d	n/n	2/8	5/8	
C58 × C3H/HeJ	S	R	k/k	n/n	2/8	7/12	
C58 × C57BL/10Sn	S	R	k/b	n/b	0/26		0/10
C58 × B10.BR	S	R	k/k	n/b	0/20		0/14

TABLE IV

SUSCEPTIBILITY OF BACKCROSS PROGENY TO PARALYTIC LDV INFECTION

Mice were infected and scored for paralysis as described in Table III. The female in each cross is listed first. Data are from 3–6 replicate experiments. C58 and B10.BR mice are H-2$^{k/k}$. B10 is congenic to B10.BR but is H-2$^{b/b}$. S, susceptible; R, resistant.

Group	Backcross progeny	Phenotype of parents	H-2 type	Fv-1 type	Incidence of paralysis in mice at age of:		
					6 months	9 months	12 months
1	C58 × (C58 × B10)	S × R	k/k or k/b	n/n or n/b	18/53		6/12
2	(C58 × B10) × C58	R × S	k/k or k/b	n/n or n/b	1/93		1/20
3	C58 × (C58 × BALB)	S × R	k/k or k/d	n/n or n/b		13/32	
4	(C58 × BALB) × C58	R × S	k/k or k/d	n/n or n/b		0/15	
5	C58 × (C58 × B10.BR)	S × R	k/k	n/n or n/b	20/46		7/15
6	(C58 × B10.BR) × C58	R × S	k/k	n/n or n/b	28/77		8/16

To obtain direct genetic evidence that the Fv-1 genotype of mice regulated susceptibility to paralytic LDV infection, backcross progeny of the appropriate genotypes were tested for susceptibility. As shown in Table IV, reciprocal crosses were made between susceptible C58 mice (male or female) and resistant F_1 hybrids (male or female). When group 2 in Table IV is compared to group 1, a much lower incidence of disease is found in the testcross progeny that nursed on the resistant C58 × B10 mothers. Analogous results are seen when group 3 is compared to group 4. Since the frequency of disease in mice is not influenced by sex (Duffey et al., 1976), such results represent a non-Mendelian resistance effect mediated by the C58 × B10 mothers in group 2, and the C58 × BALB mothers in group 4. When B10.BR mice were used in place of B10 (compare groups 1 and 2 with 5 and 6), no maternal resistance was found. Since B10.BR mice are H-2^k and B10 mice are H-2^b, the results indicate that the H-2^b haplotype had a significant effect on maternal resistance in the (C58 × B10) × C58 backcross. In the experiments summarized in Table IV, Mendelian theory predicts that 50% of the mice would be Fv-$1^{n/n}$. In mice old enough to be fully susceptible, and where maternal effects were excluded, 50% of the mice were susceptible to paralytic LDV infection.

The alleles for glucose-6-dehydrogenase (Gdp-1) isoenzymes a and b are tightly linked to Fv-1 (Rowe and Sato, 1973). These markers, therefore, were used to test directly whether susceptible and resistant mice were of the Fv-1 genotypes (Fv-$1^{n/n}$ or Fv-$1^{n/b}$) predicted on the basis of Mendelian inheritance. When kidney extracts of the appropriate testcross progeny (group 3, Table IV) were typed individually for the inheritance of Gdp-1^a (C58 derived) or Gpd-1^b (BALB-derived) alleles, the results showed (Pease et al., 1982) that 12/13 susceptible mice were homozygous for the C58 derived Gpd-1^a (Fv-1^n) allele. All 5 resistant mice were Gpd$^{a/b}$ (Fv-$1^{n/b}$). These results confirmed that mice which inherited an Fv-1^b allele were resistant. Linkage group analysis of the testcross progeny in groups 5 and 6 in Table IV further confirmed (Pease et al., 1982) that a single gene (Fv-1) outside the major histocompatibility complex regulated susceptibility to paralytic LDV infection. Considered together, the results summarized above provide reasonable evidence that coinfection by LDV and endogenous C-type retrovirus(es) was required to elicit paralytic disease.

AGE EFFECTS ON RECONSTITUTION OF IMMUNOLOGIC COMPETENCE

As C58 mice age, they spontaneously lose (Murphy et al., 1980; Duffey et al., 1978; Duffey et al., 1976) a protective, 350R resistant, cortisone-sensitive, adherent, Thy 1.2$^+$, T-cell subpopulation. This loss appears to correlate (Murphy et al., 1980) with a decrease in the ability of old C58 mice to clear LDV from their tissues. We proposed that the loss in clearance resulted from a deficiency in the antibody response to virus. The mechanisms responsible for such a defect in immunologic function, may have been an increase in suppressor T-cells, or a loss in T-helper or T-amplifier functions. We therefore began an analysis of the afferent response to determine how T-cell subpopulations changed with age and how such changes affected the protective antibody response to LDV infection. Because LDV is extraordinarily infectious it was necessary first to quantify the dose–response of X-irradiated indicator C58 mice of different ages to LDV infection. Fig. 1 shows that the PD$_{50}$ (dose of virus that paralyzed 50% of indicator mice) of LDV was $< 10^1$ for 12-month-old mice, about $10^{1.5}$ for 7- and 9-month-old mice, and approximately $10^{3.5}$ for 4-month-old mice. Three-month-old X-irradiated mice were highly resistant to paralytic infection. These results indicate that there were major differences in the immunologic competence among mice of the different age groups even after 600R of whole body X-irradiation. Thus, X-irradiated mice cannot be considered "immunologically inert" (Pilarski and Cunningham, 1975). The differential susceptibility of X-irradiated indicator mice of different ages, therefore, has to be controlled carefully in the design of experiments.

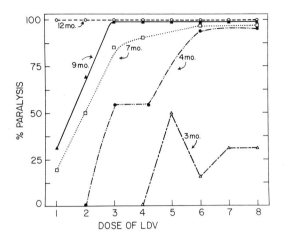

Fig. 1. Dose-effects of LDV on X-irradiated mice of different ages. Indicator mice received 600R of whole body X-irradiation 24 h before the i.p. injection of graded $\log_{10}$-doses of LDV. Mice were scored for paralysis for 60 days. Data are from 2 replicate experiments (10–20 mice per data point).

To analyze the afferent response it also was necessary to develop a model that permitted quantification of T-cell subpopulations in mice of different ages. In brief, 7-month-old X-irradiated indicator mice were reconstituted with normal spleen cells (NSC) obtained from donors of different ages. Recipient mice then were challenged with 10^3 ID_{50} of LDV. The PD_{50} values (Fig. 2) for NSC obtained from 2- and 7-month-old mice were $10^{6.5}$ and $10^{7.1}$, respectively. With 12-month-old donors a dose of 3×10^7 NSC afforded only 40 % protection.

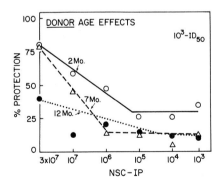

Fig. 2. Effects of spleen cell donor age on protection of indicator mice from LDV infection. Spleen cells obtained from donors of different ages were injected i.p. into 7-month-old indicator mice that had received 600R of whole body X-irradiation 24 h previously. Indicator mice challenged 24 h later by the i.p. injection of 10^3 ID_{50} of LDV were scored for paralysis for 60 days. Data are from 3 replicate experiments (20–30 mice per data point).

Table V shows how age affected the loss of the 350R resistant T-cell subpopulation. At 2 months of age X-irradiation of donors increased the protective effect of NSC. At 7 and 12 months of age 350R pretreatment eliminated protection. The results for 2-month-old X-irradiated mice suggested that 350R of whole body X-irradiation either enhanced immunity (had an immunostimulatory effect) or reduced suppression. Enhancement of immunity could have resulted from the activation of NK cells (Heberman and Ortaldo, 1981).

TABLE V

AGE AND X-IRRADIATION EFFECTS ON PD_{50} VALUES OF NORMAL SPLEEN CELLS

Experiments were carried out as described for Fig. 2 except that spleen cell donors received 350R of whole body X-irradiation 24 h before normal spleen cells were harvested from donors. PD_{50} = dose of normal spleen cells that protected 50% of indicator mice from paralysis.

Age of spleen cell donor	PD_{50} values		Effects of 350R
	Normal	*X-irradiated*	
2 months	$10^{6.5}$	$10^{5.1}$	Increased protection
7 months	$10^{7.1}$	$\gg 3 \times 10^7$	Eliminated protection
12 months	$> 3 \times 10^7$	No protection	Not applicable

A parallel study was carried out to determine how the age of indicator recipients affected the ability of NSC from 2-month-old mice to reconstitute such animals. The experiment described in Fig. 2 was repeated except that recipient indicator mice were either 5, 7 or 12 months old.

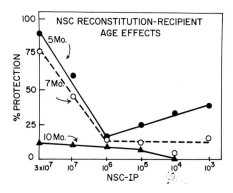

Fig. 3. Effect of recipients' age on reconstitution by spleen cells from normal 2-month-old mice. Experiments were carried out as described for Fig. 2 except that the age of the X-irradiated (600R) recipients was varied. Results are from 3 replicate experiments (10–30 mice per data point).

The results summarized by Fig. 3 show that the PD_{50} values of NSC in 5- and 7-month-old recipients ($10^{6.9}$ and $10^{7.0}$, respectively) did not differ significantly. Moreover, the slopes of the protection curves were essentially the same. In contrast, 2-month-old NSC had virtually no protective effect in 10-month-old indicator mice. One way to explain these results is to propose that 10-month-old mice suppressed the immunologic activity of the injected 2-month-old normal spleen cells. An alternative hypothesis is that there may not have been enough residual immunologic competence in 10-month-old indicator mice to permit reconstitution by 2-month-old NSC (see Fig. 1 and Pilarski and Cunningham, 1975). To summarize, having defined virus dose-effects, and donor and recipient age-effects, it now is possible to quantify the Lyt phenotypes of normal spleen cells as a function of age and then attempt to link such changes with the neutralizing antibody response to LDV infection.

THE NEUTRALIZING ANTIBODY RESPONSE TO LDV INFECTION

LDV, like lymphocytic choriomeningitis virus (Oldstone and Dixon, 1969), characteristically causes life-long infection. Infectious immune complexes persist in the plasma of infected mice throughout life (Notkins et al., 1966). Although sera from mice chronically infected with LDV have neutralizing activity (Notkins et al., 1966), and the neutralizing activity is associated with the immunoglobulin fraction (Nawrocki et al., 1980), the capacity of the various immunoglobulin subfractions to neutralize LDV had not been determined. We therefore compared the relative capacity of whole immune serum and the IgG and IgM immunoglobulin fractions to neutralize LDV in vivo. The most effective way of demonstrating neutralizing activity was to inject test sera i.v. into mice 24 h before i.p. challenge with virus (Nawrocki et al., 1980). In young immunocompetent mice neutralizing antibody was detectable (Table VI) within 10 days after immunization and reached peak levels at 15 days.

TABLE VI

KINETICS OF THE NEUTRALIZING ANTIBODY RESPONSE TO LDV

Mice (not X-irradiated) were "immunized" by the i.p. injection of 10^8 ID_{50} of LDV. Sera were collected by retrorbital bleeding on the days indicated. Five-month-old indicator mice received 600R of whole body X-irradiation 24 h before the i.v. injection of a 1:10 dilution of heat inactivated (56°C for 1 h) immune serum pooled from each age group. The next day mice were challenged by the i.p. injection of 10^5 ID_{50} of LDV. Mice were scored for paralysis for 60 days. In control mice not receiving antiserum, the incidence of paralysis was 36/40 (90%). Results are from 2–4 replicate experiments.

Age of immune serum donors	Time in days after immunization	Fraction of mice protected
2 months	7	14/26 (30%)
	10	17/20 (85%)
	15	13/13 (100%)
	30	15/15 (100%)
12 months	7	9/17 (53%)
	15	3/12 (25%)
	30	5/12 42%)

Although neutralizing antibody was detectable in 12-month-old disease-susceptible mice at 7 days, usually less than 50% of mice were protected. Table VII shows that both the IgM and IgG serum fractions were protective. When survival data were plotted as a function of time, the

298

results showed (Fig. 4) that IgM either protected mice or did not, i.e. there was no delay in deaths as seen with the IgG serum fraction. Considered together, these results show that young mice rapidly produce neutralizing antibody to LDV involving both the IgM and IgG subclasses. Old, disease-susceptible mice are deficient in this regard. We are analyzing whether the described immunologic deficiency in old mice can be linked directly to T-cell subpopulation changes with age. One cannot, however, exclude the possibility of other immunologic deficiencies, such as in macrophage functions. This is particularly important for LDV since it preferentially replicates in macrophages (Rowson and Mahy, 1975).

TABLE VII

RELATIVE NEUTRALIZING ACTIVITY OF WHOLE SERUM, IgG AND IgM SERUM FRACTIONS

Serum was obtained from 2-month-old mice that had received an immunizing i.p. injection of 10^7 ID_{50} of LDV 35 days previously. After inactivation at $56°C$ for 1 h antiserum was fractionated on a protein A Sepharose column. The fractionated serum was precipitated with 45 % saturation of ammonium sulfate and dialyzed against 0.85 % NaCl solution ($4°C$) for 24 h (change every 6 h). Whole and fractionated sera were made up to a concentration of 1 mg protein/ml. Neutralization tests were carried out as described in Table VI except that 7-month-old indicator mice were used. Indicator mice received a 1 ml i.v. injection of each test serum. In control mice not receiving antiserum, 10 % (1/10) failed to develop disease.

Serum fraction	Fraction of mice protected
Whole serum	7/7 (100 %)
IgG	4/7 (57 %)
IgM	4/7 (57 %)

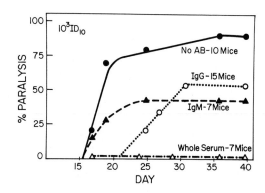

Fig. 4. Effects of whole serum, IgG and IgM immunoglobulin fractions on the survival of indicator mice challenged with 10^5 ID_{50} of LDV.

THE PERSISTENT INFECTION MODEL

These experiments were carried out to determine how the age of mice at the time of LDV infection affected the natural occurrence of paralytic disease. Thus, un-irradiated mice of different ages were infected with 10^8 ID_{50} of LDV and scored for paralysis over the next 18 months. Since a very high percentage of C58 mice develop spontaneous leukemia by 12 months of age, large numbers of animals are lost from experiments. Although results are still incomplete, the data in Table VIII nevertheless show that paralytic disease occurred in mice persistently infected for 9 or more months. The incidence of spontaneous paralytic disease in mice infected at 1 month of age was about 5 %. The data also suggest that the older the mice at the time of infection, the greater the frequency of disease.

TABLE VIII

NATURAL OCCURRENCE OF PARALYSIS AFTER LDV INFECTION

Mice of the listed ages were injected i.p. with 10^8 ID_{50} of LDV. Total number of paralyzed mice/total number surviving at the indicated times.

Age when infected	Months after infection					
	0	6	9	12	15	18
Newborn	0/95	0/95	(In progress)			
1 month	0/75	0/75	0/73	1/55	4/20	4/0
3 months	0/84	0/78	0/61	(In progress)		
6 months	0/82	0/51	1/32	(In progress)		
12 months	0/21	11/19	12/15	12/0		

In a parallel study we analyzed the selective effects of disease susceptible (C58) and resistant (BALB) mice on LDV virus populations. The avirulent strain of W-LDV (see Table II) was passed in C58 mice to determine whether they selected for neurovirulence. The neuroparalytic Ib-LDV strain was passed in BALB mice to test whether they selected for avirulence. The data in Table IX show that C58 mice selected for neurovirulence. Selection was most rapid in the 12-month-old mice that had been X-irradiated before passage. The results were less clear-cut (data not shown) when 7-month-old indicator mice were used. Nevertheless, one must be cautious in drawing conclusions unless the effects of the age of the passage and the indicator animals are carefully controlled. This point is illustrated more clearly by the data in Table X. When 7-month-old indicator animals were used BALB mice clearly selected for avirulence. Selection was less evident when assays for paralysis were done in 10-month-old indicators. Interestingly, as virus was passed serially in BALB mice, the median time for paralysis shifted from approximately 15–20 days to 25–40 days. Considered together the data in Tables IX and X show that selection for, or against, neurovirulence can be documented, providing that the age of the passage and indicator mice are carefully controlled.

DISCUSSION AND COMMENTS

An advantageous feature of the described experimental model is that the balance between paralytic and inapparent infection is a very delicate one. By carefully manipulating experimental conditions it therefore is possible to critically analyze how age-dependent changes in immunologic competence, viral infection, and genetic factors interact to determine the outcome of infection, i.e. one can focus on how each element in a complex, multifactorial disease determines susceptibility or resistance. The genetic studies, for example, provide an

TABLE IX

PASSAGE OF AVIRULENT W-LDV IN C58 MICE SELECTS FOR NEUROVIRULENCE

Mice used for passage: 10^8 ID_{50} of W-LDV (see Table II) was injected i.p. into either normal 12-month-old mice that had received 600R of whole body X-irradiation 24 h earlier or not. Plasma collected from such mice 5 days later was diluted 10^{-2} and 1 ml (approximately 10^7 ID_{50}) injected i.p. into the next passage of mice. Paralysis was scored over 40 days. Mice paralyzed: 10-month-old indicator mice received 600R of whole-body X-irradiation 24 h before the i.p. injection of a 10^{-2} dilution of a plasma specimen pooled from 6–7 mice per passage.

Passage number	Age of mice used for passage	Fraction of mice paralyzed
1	12 months	0/10
	12 months-XR	0/6
3	12 months	1/10
	12 months-XR	2/8
7	12 months	2/10
	12 months-XR	8/9
10	12 months	4/10
	12 months-XR	7/7

TABLE X

PASSAGE OF NEUROVIRULENT Ib-LDV IN BALB MICE SELECTS FOR AVIRULENCE

Experiments were carried out as described in Table IX except that passages were made in 9-month-old BALB mice. Control virus (Ib-LDV) before passage caused paralysis in 9/10 7-month-old and in 3/3 10-month-old indicator mice.

Passage number	Fraction of mice paralyzed in indicator that were:	
	7 months old	10 months old
1	6/10 (60%)	8/8 (100%)
5	2/8 (25%)	5/7 (71%)
7	0/8 (0%)	7/10 (70%)
10	1/10 (10%)	5/10 (50%)

insight into a hitherto unsuspected role that endogenous retroviruses may play in the so-called slow virus infections (ter Meulen, 1977). The evidence is reasonably sound that dual infection by LDV and the C-type endogenous viruses was required to elicit paralytic LDV infection in C58 and other leukemia-prone mice. Thus, only leukemia-prone $Fv-1^{n/n}$ mice were susceptible. $Fv-1^{n/n}$ mice not carrying multiple copies of C-type retrovirus in their genomes were not susceptible. Such resistant C-type virus-deficient mice ($Fv-1^{n/n}$), however, became susceptible when crossed with C58 females. Maternal resistance effects typical (Melief et al., 1975) of those found in retrovirus transmission studies were demonstrable. The virtual absolute restriction of susceptibility by the $Fv-1^b$ allele indicated that retrovirus expression was required for susceptibility. The paradox here is that two classes of viruses that are ubiquitous in mice, and that ordinarily do not cause disease, appeared to act together to cause an age-dependent motor neuron disease in a genetically susceptible host. These results suggest the possibility that some age-dependent human neurologic diseases of suspected viral etiology may result from coinfection by a common human environmental virus and human endogenous retroviruses. For example, in multiple sclerosis it may be worthwhile to consider (ter Meulen, 1977; Koprowski, 1977) that more than one type of virus common to the environment may serve to trigger the disease in a genetically susceptible individual. It has not been possible to date (Viola et al., 1975), however, to implicate silent retrovirus infection in such human neurologic diseases.

In analyzing the protective response of C58 mice to paralytic LDV infection we have found consistently (Duffey et al., 1976; Murphy et al., 1980) that, as mice age, they lose a 350R resistant T cell subpopulation of key importance in the efferent response. Such a loss appears to correlate (Murphy et al., 1980) with the inability of susceptible mice to clear LDV from their tissues. These findings suggest a defect in their neutralizing antibody response to LDV. In this report we describe a reconstitution model designed to analyze the afferent response. Using the described model it now should be possible, by the use of the appropriate monoclonal Lyt antisera, to define quantitatively how T-cell subpopulations change as a function of age, and how this affects the neutralizing antibody response to LDV.

On the basis of the work we have completed to date, and from related studies (Creighton et al., 1979; Zinkernagel and Dixon, 1974; Callard et al., 1980), there is good reason to believe that the immunologic deficiency that impairs the neutralizing antibody response is not necessarily restricted to T-cell subpopulations, but may involve macrophages as well, i.e., macrophages are key target cells for LDV infection (Lagwinska et al., 1975). The key point may be that in the immune-deficient host, virus multiplication in the brain may not be restricted (Thomsen et al., 1979) and neuron destruction occurs as a consequence. Thus, the type of antibody response and the rate of production appear to be of central importance. One also must consider that the immunologic defect may involve the neutralizing antibody response (Debré et al., 1980; Vlug et al., 1981) to the endogenous C-type viruses found in C58 mice. The failure to neutralize such viruses would permit progressive interactions to occur between LDV and the endogenous C-type retroviruses in mice, as they age.

The importance of the neutralizing antibody response has been emphasized because of its possible selective effects on neurovirulent LDV populations as mice age. The central problem here may be how changes in the population genetics of lymphocyte subpopulations affect the population genetics of LDV and C-type retroviruses. Some insights are provided from the data in Table IX, which show that old C58 mice selected for neurovirulent LDV populations. Selection appeared to be most pronounced in the animals (12-month-old X-irradiated) that were the least immunocompetent, i.e. such mice did not select against the neurovirulent variants in the wild W-LDV virus population. The converse experiment (Table X) provides evidence indicating that 9-month-old BALB mice rapidly selected against neurovirulent LDV populations. Selection was illustrated best in the 7-month-old indicator mice, i.e. the less immunocompetent 10-month-old indicator mice (see Fig. 1) were not suitable for demonstrating selection against neurovirulent LDV populations (were not sufficiently restrictive). The caveat here is that no information exists concerning LDV/C-type retrovirus virus population interactions that also might account for the described results. Putting aside this important qualification, the crucial immunologic events appear to be those that limit the neutralizing antibody response to the viral antigens important in eliciting a protective response (Narayan et al., 1981; Wechsler et al., 1979; Ihle and Lazar, 1977). In the age-related human diseases of suspected viral etiology, the occurrence of antiviral antibody and its titer may be less important than whether it is neutralizing antibody, i.e. whether such antibodies select against neurovirulent virus populations containing the corresponding protective antigens (Wechsler et al., 1979). The described model of age-dependent motor neuron disease provides the opportunity to analyze such phenomena in detail.

REFERENCES

Brinton-Darnell, M. and Plagemann, P.G.W. (1975) Structure and chemical–physical characteristics of lactate dehydrogenase-elevating virus and its RNA. *J. Virol.*, 16: 420–433.

Callard, R.E., Fazekas De St. Groth, B., Basten, A. and McKenzie, I.F.C. (1980) Immune function in aged mice. V. Role of suppressor cells. *J. Immunol.*, 124: 52–58.

Creighton, W.D., Katz, D.H. and Dixon, F.J. (1979) Antigen-specific immunocompetency, B cell function, and regulatory helper and suppressor T cell activities in spontaneously autoimmune mice. *J. Immunol.*, 123: 2627–2636.

Debré, P., Boyer, B., Gisselbrecht, S., Bismuth, A. and Levy, J.-P. (1980) Genetic control of sensitivity to Moloney leukemia virus in mice. III. The three H-2 linked RMV genes are immune response genes controlling the antiviral antibody response. *Europ. J. Immunol.*, 10: 914–918.

Duffey, P.S., Martinez, D., Abrams, G.D. and Murphy, W.H. (1976) Pathogenetic mechanisms in immune polioencephalomyelitis: induction of disease in immunosuppressed mice. *J. Immunol.*, 116: 475–481.

Duffey, P.S., Lukasewycz, O.A., Olson, D.S. and Murphy, W.H. (1978) Differential protective effects of immune lymphoid cells against transplanted line Ib leukemia and immune polioencephalomyelitis. *J. Immunol.*, 121: 2316–2321.

Heberman, R.B. and Ortaldo, J.R. (1981) Natural killer cells: their role in defenses against disease. *Science*, 214: 24–30.

Ihle, J.N. and Lazar, B. (1977) Natural immunity in mice to the envelope glycoprotein of endogenous ecotropic type C viruses: neutralization of virus infectivity. *J. Virol.*, 21: 974–980.

Koprowski, H. (1977) In search of the abominable snowman or "deine Viren, meine Viren" in multiple sclerosis. In V. ter Meulen and M. Katz (Eds.), *Slow Virus Infections of the Central Nervous System*, Springer, New York, pp. 152–158.

Lagwinska, E., Stewart, C.C., Adles, C. and Schlessinger, S. (1975) Replication of lactic dehydrogenase virus and Sinbis virus in mouse peritoneal cells. Induction of interferon and phenotypic mixing. *Virology*, 65: 204–214.

Martinez, D., Brinton, M.A., Tachovsky, T.G. and Phelps, A.H. (1980) Identification of lactate dehydrogenase-elevating virus as the etiological agent of genetically restricted, age-dependent, polioencephalomyelitis of mice. *Infect. Immun.*, 27: 979–987.

Melief, C.J.M., Louie, S. and Swartz, R.S. (1975) Ecotropic leukemia viruses in congenic C57BL mice: natural dissemination by milk borne infection. *J. nat. Cancer Inst.*, 55: 691–698.

Murphy, W.H., Pease, L.R. and Nawrocki, J.F. (1980) Aetiologic mechanisms in age-dependent murine motor neurone disease. In C.F. Rose and P.O. Behan (Eds.), *Animal Models of Neurological Diseases*, Pitman Medical, Tunbridge Wells, Kent, pp. 123–135.

Narayan, O., Clements, J.E., Griffin, D.E. and Wolinsky, J.S. (1981) Neutralizing antibody spectrum determines the antigenic profiles of emerging mutants of Visna virus. *Infect. Immun.*, 32: 1045–1050.

Nawrocki, J.F., Pease, L.R. and Murphy, W.H. (1980) Etiologic role of lactic dehydrogenase virus infection in an age-dependent neuroparalytic disease in C58 mice. *Virology*, 103: 259–264.

Notkins, A.L., Mahar, S., Scheele, C. and Goffman, J. (1966) Infectious virus-antibody complex in the blood of chronically infected mice. *J. exp. Med.*, 124: 81–97.

Oldstone, M.B.A. and Dixon, F.J. (1969) Pathogenesis of chronic disease associated with persistent lymphocytic choriomeningitis infection. I. Relationship of antibody production to disease in neonatally infected mice. *J. exp. Med.*, 129: 483–505.

Oldstone, M.B.A. and Dixon, F.J. (1971) Lactic dehydrogenase virus-induced immune complex type of glomerulonephritis. *J. Immunol.*, 106: 1260–1263.

Pease, L.R. and Murphy, W.H. (1980) Co-infection by lactic dehydrogenase virus and C-type retrovirus elicits neurological disease. *Nature (Lond.)*, 286: 398–400.

Pease, L.R., Abrams, G.D. and Murphy, W.H. (1982) Fv-1 restriction of age-dependent neuroparalytic lactic dehydrogenase virus infection. *Virology*, 117: 29–37.

Pilarski, L.M. and Cunningham, A.J. (1975) Host-derived antibody-forming cells in lethally irradiated mice. *J. Immunol.*, 114: 138–140.

Rowe, W.P. and Sato, H. (1973) Genetic mapping of the Fv-1 locus in mice. *Science*, 180: 640–641.

Rowson, K.E.K. and Mahy, B.W.J. (1975) *Lactic dehydrogenase virus. Virology Monographs, Vol. 13*, Springer, New York, pp. 1–121.

Steeves, R. and Lilly, F. (1977) Interactions between host and viral genomes in mouse leukemia. *Ann. Rev. Genet*, 11: 277–296.

Ter Meulen, V. (1977) Multiple sclerosis: a case for viral etiology. In V. ter Meulen and M. Katz (Eds.), *Slow Virus Infections of the Central Nervous System*, Springer, New York, pp. 143–151.

Thomsen, A.R., Volkert, M. and Marker, O. (1979) The timing of the immune response in relation to virus growth determines the outcome of the LCM infection. *Acta path. microbiol. scand.*, 87: 47–54.

Viola, M.V., Frazier, M., White, L., Brody, J. and Spiegelman, S. (1975) RNA-instructed DNA polymerase activity in a cytoplasmic particulate fraction in brains from Guamian patients. *J. exp. Med.*, 142: 483–494.

Vlug, A., Schoenmakers, H.J. and Meleif, J.M. (1981) Genes of the H-2 complex regulate the antibody response to murine leukemia virus. *J. Immunol.*, 126: 2355–2360.

Wechsler, S.J., Weiner, H.L. and Fields, B.N. (1979) Immune response in subacute sclerosing panencephalitis: reduced antibody response to the matrix protein of measles virus. *J. Immunol.*, 123: 884–889.

Zinkernagel, R.M. and Dixon, F.J. (1977) Comparison of T cell-mediated immune responsiveness of NZB, (NZB × NZW)F$_1$hybrid and other murine strains. *Clin. exp. Immunol.*, 29: 110–121.

Immunology of Nervous System Infections, Progress in Brain Research, Vol. 59, edited by P.O. Behan, V. ter Meulen and F. Clifford Rose

Pathogenetic Aspects of Demyelinating Lesions in Chronic Relapsing Experimental Allergic Encephalomyelitis: Possible Interaction of Cellular and Humoral Immune Mechanisms

H. LASSMANN, B. SCHWERER, K. KITZ, M. EGGHART and H. BERNHEIMER

Neurologisches Institut der Universität Wien, Schwarzspanierstr. 17, A-1090 Vienna (Austria)

INTRODUCTION

A major difference between acute and chronic experimental allergic encephalomyelitis (EAE) lesions is the extent of demyelination. Whereas acute EAE is a predominately inflammatory disease with little or no perivenous myelin destruction (Alvord, 1970; Lampert, 1965; Lampert and Kies, 1967), the formation of large demyelinated plaques is the leading event in pathology of chronic EAE (Raine et al., 1974; Wisniewski and Keith, 1977; Lassmann and Wisniewski, 1979). It is now well established that acute EAE is due to a cell-mediated immune reaction against myelin basic protein (MBP) (Waksman and Morrison, 1951; Paterson, 1960; Shaw et al., 1965; Kies et al., 1960; Roboz Einstein et al., 1962; Traugott and Raine, 1979). Also in chronic EAE, fluctuations of T-cell subpopulations have been noted with exacerbations of the disease (Traugott et al., 1979). Humoral immune responses against central nervous system (CNS) antigens play little or no role in the pathogenesis of acute EAE (Bernard 1976; Ortiz-Ortiz and Weigle, 1976).

A major difference in immunology between acute and chronic EAE is the appearance of a humoral immune response with chronicity of the disease characterized by increased γ-globulins in serum and cerebrospinal fluid (CSF) (Karcher et al., 1982) and increased IgG/albumin ratio as well as oligoclonal bands of IgG in brain extracts (Mehta et al., 1981).

The aim of the present study was to investigate whether the humoral immune response in chronic EAE is directed against autoantigens of the CNS and whether it may play a role in the pathogenesis of inflammatory demyelinating lesions in chronic relapsing EAE.

MATERIALS AND METHODS

Sensitization of animals

Hartley guinea pigs were sensitized for chronic relapsing EAE according to the method described by Wisniewski and Keith (1977). The animals were daily examined for neurological signs and sacrificed between 10 and 220 days after sensitization (dps). Blood was obtained by cardiac puncture under sterile conditions at the time of sacrifice and sera were frozen in multiple small vials at $-80°$C until further use. All animals were perfused via the aorta with either 4% freshly prepared paraformaldehyde solution or with a mixture of 0.5% paraformaldehyde and 1.5% glutaraldehyde. Multiple blocks of brain and spinal cord were embedded routinely for light and electron microscopy. The incidence of confluent demyelinated plaques in the brain and spinal cord was determined by dividing the plaque numbers counted in at least 15 complete cross-sections of the spinal cord and 6 coronal sections of the brain, by the number of examined sections. Thus a plaque incidence of 1 represents an average of one confluent demyelinated plaque per investigated section.

Fourteen control Hartley guinea pigs were sensitized either with complete Freund's adjuvant (CFA) to which 10 mg/ml heat inactivated mycobacterium (Difco H37Ra) had been added or with guinea pig liver tissue in CFA. Another 5 control Hartley guinea pigs were sensitized with 5 mg bovine serum albumin (BSA) in CFA.

For the induction of anti-ganglioside sera 3 rabbits were immunized with 5 mg of bovine brain gangliosides (BBG, Sigma) and 5 mg BSA in CFA with 0.5 mg/ml mycobacterium. Animals were boosted with 5 mg BBG + 5 mg BSA in incomplete Freund's adjuvant twice (3 weeks and 7 months after the initial immunization) and sera were obtained 14–40 days after the booster-injections. For control, one rabbit was immunized with 5 mg BSA in CFA.

Injection of EAE sera into the CSF of normal recipient rats

The injection procedure has been described in detail earlier (Lassmann et al., 1981). Briefly, 50 μl serum were slowly infused into the sacral subarachnoid space of normal 200 g Sprague–Dawley rats. Sera were either used undiluted or, when thawed and refrozen before injection, diluted 1:1 with normal fresh guinea pig serum as a source of complement. Anti-ganglioside sera which were raised in rabbits were diluted 1:1 with normal fresh rabbit serum. Recipient rats were sampled 48 h after serum injection by perfusion fixation. Multiple blocks of the spinal cord and pia mater preparations (Kitz et al., 1981) were examined for demyelination in the central and peripheral nervous system (Lassmann et al., 1981). The extent of demyelination in the recipient animals was determined by a semiquantitative assay as described in Fig. 2.

Demonstration of precipitating antibodies against CNS antigens

Eighteen EAE sera were tested for the presence of precipitating antibodies against the following antigens: a crude and a purified lipid fraction prepared from spinal cord tissue (Schwerer et al., 1981) and suspended according to Niedieck (1975); galactocerebroside (Sigma) and sulfatide (Sigma), suspended with lecithin (L) and cholesterol (C) in the proportions 1:0.5:1, per weight (Niedieck, 1975); and bovine brain gangliosides (Sigma) suspended with L and C in the proportions 1:2:10, per weight (Naiki et al., 1974). Precipitating antibodies were demonstrated using the "reversed" Mancini technique (Vaerman et al., 1969). The lipid antigens in 0.6% agarose gel (Behring) were used in at least 3 different concentrations in the following ranges (mg/ml gel): crude and purified lipid fractions: 0.35–0.035; galactocerebroside and sulfatide: 0.07–0.007; gangliosides: 0.028–0.007. Serum samples (10 μl each) were allowed to diffuse into the antigen-containing gel for 5 days at 4°C and precipitates were stained with Coomassie brilliant blue.

Sera from 3 rabbits immunized with bovine brain gangliosides were tested for precipitating antibodies against ganglioside G_{M1} as described above.

Demonstration of antibodies against myelin basic protein (MBP), galactocerebroside (CER) and ganglioside G_{M1} with the enzyme-linked immunosorbent assay (ELISA)

Thirty EAE sera were tested for antibodies against MBP as described by Groome (1980). Thirty-four EAE sera were tested for antibodies against CER and G_{M1} with an ELISA-technique as follows: polystyrol microtiter plates were coated with glycosphingolipid-LC-suspensions 1:2:10, per weight (Naiki et al., 1974) (2 μM CER or G_{M1}, respectively) followed by

0.5% human serum albumin, incubated with EAE sera in 1:2 dilution series and then with peroxidase-conjugated anti-guinea pig IgG (RAGp/IgG(H-L)/Po, Nordic) diluted 1/500. After incubation with ABTS (Böhringer) the extinction at 405 nm was measured using a Dynatech AM 120 microelisa autoreader. CER and G_{M1}-antibody titers represent the highest dilution of antiserum with an extinction above the control range.

Complement fixation

Rabbit antisera were tested for the presence of antibodies against gangliosides by a quantitative complement fixation assay according to the micromethod of Wassermann and Levine (1961). The optimal amount of antigen to be used was determined to be 20 ng bovine brain gangliosides, suspended with L and C in the proportions 1:2:10, per weight (Naiki et al., 1974). The titer represents the highest dilution of antiserum, leading to a 50% inhibition of haemolysis with ganglioside-LC-suspensions as compared to the reference haemolysis with LC-suspensions.

RESULTS

Pathology of Hartley guinea pigs suffering from chronic relapsing EAE

The neuropathology of guinea pigs suffering from chronic relapsing EAE has been described in detail earlier (Lassmann and Wisniewski 1978, 1979; Lassmann et al., 1980). During the acute stage of the disease (10–20 dps) numerous inflammatory infiltrates were found, localized around veins and venules in the meninges, white matter and less frequently in the grey matter of the CNS. Demyelination in this stage of the disease was restricted to single perivenous nerve fibers. Animals which suffered from active disease during the subacute stage of the disease (20–40 dps) showed, in addition to perivenous inflammation, small rims of perivenous demyelination. During the early and late chronic stage of the disease (40–220 dps),

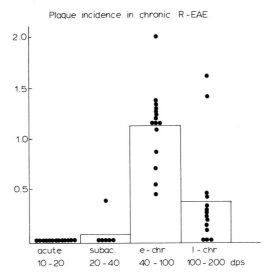

Fig. 1. Plaque incidence in the CNS of animals from different stages of chronic relapsing EAE. The incidence values only concern large confluent demyelinated plaques. Perivenous demyelination, especially noted during the acute and subacute stage of the disease is not included in the figure.

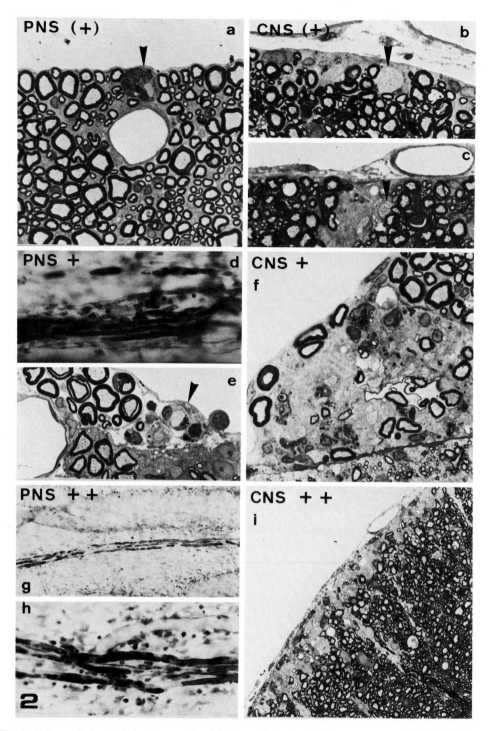

Fig. 2. Patterns of demyelination in normal recipient rats, following injection of chronic EAE sera into the cerebrospinal fluid. a: + positive in the PNS; a singular demyelinating fiber can be seen in the periphery of the root. Toluidine blue, × 999. b, c: + in the CNS. Singular demyelinating nerve fibers on the spinal cord surface. Toluidine blue, × 999, d: + positive in the PNS; root entry zone with multiple demyelinated nerve fibers. Isolated pia, SSB, × 250. e: cross-section of similar root as in d; several demyelinated nerve fibers in the root entry zone. Toluidine blue, × 999. f: + positive in the CNS; extensive demyelination in the central portion of a root. Toluidine blue, × 999. g: + + positive in the PNS; complete demyelination in a small caliber root. Isolated pia, SSB, × 64. h: higher magnification of g; shows segmental demyelination. × 250. i: + + positive in the CNS; a subpial rim of demyelination covering the whole circumference of the spinal cord. Toluidine blue, × 500.

large confluent demyelinated plaques were noted in the brain and spinal cord. The incidence of large confluent demyelinated lesions in chronic relapsing EAE is summarized in Fig. 1. The earliest appearance of confluent lesions was noted in an animal sampled 32 dps. The highest incidence of demyelinated plaques was observed during the early chronic stage of the disease. In animals sampled during the late chronic phase of chronic relapsing EAE the incidence of demyelinated confluent lesions was lower, the size of the individual lesions, however, was comparable to that found in the early chronic stage of the disease.

In vivo demyelinating activity of sera from animals with chronic relapsing EAE

Following injection into the lumbosacral subarachnoid space of normal recipient rats the majority of sera from animals with chronic relapsing EAE induced demyelination in the spinal cord white matter (central myelin) and (or) in the spinal roots (peripheral myelin) (Fig. 2). The ultrastructural patterns of myelin destruction were vesicular disruption of myelin and myelin stripping (Lassmann et al., 1981). The extent of demyelination induced in recipient animals by different EAE sera varied from singular scattered nerve fibers: (+), (Fig. 2a–c), demyelination of central and peripheral portions of the root entry zones: +, (Fig. 2d–f) to demyelination of the entire subpial spinal cord circumference or complete demyelination of small spinal roots: + +, (Fig. 2g–i). The incidence of demyelinating activity in sera from different stages of chronic relapsing EAE is summarized in Table I. Whereas only few sera from animals sampled during the acute and subacute stage of the disease induced demyelination in normal recipients, the incidence of demyelinating sera was high in animals sampled during the early and late chronic stage of the disease.

TABLE I

IN VIVO DEMYELINATING ACTIVITY OF CHRONIC EAE SERA (INCIDENCE)

Incidence of demyelinating activity of sera from animals sampled in different stages of chronic relapsing EAE and control animals

	CNS				PNS				CNS+PNS
	+ +	+	(+)	Total	+ +	+	(+)	Total	Total
Acute	0/5	0/5	0/5	0/5	0/5	0/5	1/5	1/5	1/5
Subacute	0/5	2/5	0/5	2/5	0/5	2/5	1/5	3/5	3/5
e-chr.	2/15	5/15	3/15	10/15	1/15	6/15	6/15	13/15	13/15
l-chr.	2/14	1/14	2/14	5/14	1/14	6/14	4/14	11/14	11/14
Total	4/39	8/39	5/39	17/39	2/39	14/39	12/39	28/39	28/39
Controls	0/14	0/14	0/14	0/14	0/14	0/14	0/14	0/14	0/14

Serum antibodies against CNS antigens in chronic relapsing EAE

Precipitating antibodies against one or more CNS antigens were present in 6/18 animals with chronic relapsing EAE (Table II) (Schwerer et al., 1983). These antibodies were directed against the crude lipid fraction, the purified lipid fraction, galactocerebroside, sulfatide and gangliosides. With the more sensitive ELISA technique (Table III), a higher incidence of glycosphingolipid antibodies in EAE sera was found (cerebroside: incidence 13/34, titers 1:20–1:2560; G_{M1}: incidence 10/34, titers 1:20–1:160). Antibodies against MBP (incidence

23/30) were detected as well. All sera from EAE animals sampled during the chronic stage of the disease contained antibodies directed against at least one of the tested CNS antigens. In contrast, only one animal sampled during the acute-subacute stage of the disease (10–40 dps) revealed a humoral immune response against one of the tested antigens (MBP).

TABLE II

INCIDENCE OF PRECIPITATING ANTIBODIES AGAINST CNS ANTIGENS IN CHRONIC EAE SERA

Demonstration of precipitating antibodies against CNS antigens by the "reversed" Mancini technique as described in Materials and Methods.

Crude lipid fraction	Purified lipid fraction	Cerebroside	Sulfatide	Gangliosides	One or more CNS-antigens
6/17	4/16	3/16	2/16	1/18	6/18

TABLE III

INCIDENCE OF SERUM ANTIBODIES AGAINST CNS ANTIGENS (ELISA TECHNIQUE) IN CHRONIC RELAPSING EAE

Demonstration of serum antibodies against myelin basic protein, galactocerebroside and ganglioside G_{M1} with ELISA techniques as described in Materials and Methods.

	Acute-subacute 10–40 dps	Early chronic 40–100 dps	Late chronic 100–200 dps	Total
MBP	1/5	10/11	12/14	23/30
Cerebroside	0/8	6/14	7/12	13/34
G_{M1}	0/8	6/14	5/12	10/34
Cer. or G_{M1}	0/8	9/14	9/12	18/34
MBP, Cer. or G_{M1}	1/5	14/14	12/12	27/31

TABLE IV

ANTIBODIES AGAINST GLYCOSPHINGOLIPIDS (GALACTOCEREBROSIDE AND G_{M1}) AND IN VIVO DEMYELINATING ACTIVITY OF EAE SERA

Demonstration of a statistically significant coincidence of antibodies against glycosphingolipids and demyelinating activity in EAE sera. $\chi^2 = 4.636$; $p < 0.05$.

Serum antibodies	Demyelinating activity		Total
	+	−	
+	16	2	18
−	9	7	16
Total	25	9	34

Relation between glycosphingolipid antibodies and in vivo demyelinating activity of chronic relapsing EAE sera

There was a significantly higher incidence of in vivo demyelinating activity in sera with glycosphingolipid antibodies as compared with the other EAE sera (Table IV). Two sera with glycosphingolipid antibodies (titers 1:80) were devoid of demyelinating activity but demyelination was always induced by sera with antibody titers > 1/160 (data not shown). On the other hand, there was a relatively large proportion of chronic EAE sera (9/34) which induced demyelination in vivo without any detectable antibodies against cerebroside or G_{MI} being present in those sera.

In vivo demyelinating activity of anti-ganglioside sera

When injected into the cerebrospinal fluid of normal recipient rats, sera from rabbits sensitized against gangliosides were able to induce demyelination in the central and peripheral nervous system of normal recipient rats (Table V). Differences in antibody titers were apparently reflected by the extent of demyelination (Table V).

TABLE V

DEMYELINATING ACTIVITY OF ANTI-GANGLIOSIDE SERA

Demyelinating activity and antibody titers in sera of rabbits sensitized against gangliosides and normal rabbit serum from an unsensitized animal. Precipitating: test performed with G_{MI} as antigen by "reversed" Mancini technique (see Materials and Methods). Complement fixing: test performed with bovine brain gangliosides as antigen; n.d., not determined.

Serum	Ganglioside antibodies		DM activity	
	Precipitating	*Complement fixing*	*CNS*	*PNS*
452	+	1/250	+	+
451	+	1/150	−	(+)
453	(+)	n.d.	−	−
336CO	−	n.d.	−	−

DISCUSSION

Sera from EAE animals and multiple sclerosis patients were shown to induce demyelination in vitro in organotypic tissue cultures (Bornstein and Appel, 1961; Bornstein and Appel, 1965; Lumsden, 1971). Demyelination in this system is induced by immunoglobulins and is dependent on the presence of complement (Grundke-Iqbal et al., 1979, 1981). The high amounts of immunoglobulins in brain extracts and CSF in both diseases (Tourtellotte, 1970; Mehta et al., 1981; Karcher et al., 1982) have been regarded as indicating that humoral immune mechanisms may play a role in the pathogenesis of inflammatory demyelinating lesion. In our present study we were able to show that the incidence of demyelinated plaques in chronic relapsing EAE correlates well with the appearance of a humoral immune response against several CNS antigens in the sera of affected animals. Beyond that, these sera induced demyelination in the central and peripheral nervous system when injected into the cerebrospinal fluid of normal recipient animals. These findings further support the concept that antibodies are involved in demyelination in EAE.

There are several possible mechanisms to explain how antibodies may play a role in the pathogenesis of demyelination in vivo (Lassmann et al., 1981). Demyelination may be induced by a direct complement-dependent destruction of myelin, similar to that described in vitro (Appel and Bornstein, 1964; Grundke-Iqbal et al., 1981). On the other hand, an interaction of specific antibodies with activated macrophages, as described by Brosnan et al. (1977), may lead to a cooperation of cellular and humoral immune mechanisms in the induction of demyelination. Furthermore, complement may augment antibody-dependent cellular cytotoxicity (Perlmann et al., 1981).

Although the presence of antibodies and demyelinating activity in the serum does not prove that they are equally present in the CNS compartment, it has to be considered that in chronic EAE lesions the blood–brain barrier is damaged (Kristensson and Wisniewski, 1977). Further studies, however, will have to be directed towards the antibody-reaction and specificity in the CNS in chronic relapsing EAE.

One major question concerns the antigens responsible for the induction of demyelinating antibodies in chronic relapsing EAE. Antibodies against MBP, myelin-associated glycoprotein and proteolipid protein have been reported to be ineffective (Seil et al., 1968, 1980, 1981). In contrast, it has been shown that antibodies directed against galactocerebrosides may induce demyelination in vitro (Dubois-Dalq et al., 1970; Fry et al., 1974; Dorfman et al., 1978) and in vivo after injection into peripheral nerves (Saida et al., 1979). In our present investigation we found demyelinating activity in vivo induced by antibodies against gangliosides. There was a statistically significant higher incidence of demyelinating activity in sera with antibodies against cerebroside and G_{M1} as compared with other EAE sera. However, demyelinating activity was also noted in a certain number of EAE sera without antibodies against these two glycosphingolipids. These findings indicate that demyelinating activity of EAE sera may be due to antibodies against cerebroside and gangliosides, respectively. Our results demonstrate, on the other hand, that demyelinating activity need not necessarily be associated with antibodies against these glycosphingolipids. It may be concluded from our findings that antibodies against other myelin antigens might be responsible as well for the demyelinating activity of an EAE serum. This possibility is supported by the findings of Lebar et al. (1976, 1979) and Saida et al. (1977) who showed that myelin and oligodendrocyte antigens, other than galactocerebroside, may induce demyelinating antibodies.

It is now well established that for the induction of EAE a cell-mediated immune response against MBP is required (Bernard, 1976; Ortiz-Ortiz and Weigle, 1976). Sensitization with MBP alone leads only to an acute or eventually chronic inflammatory disease of the central nervous system (Panitch and Ciccone, 1981). Our findings lend support to the view that demyelinating antibodies directed against various surface antigens of the myelin sheath may convert the predominately inflammatory process induced by MBP into the inflammatory demyelinating type of pathology characteristic of chronic relapsing EAE.

SUMMARY

In contrast to acute EAE, demyelination is the dominating feature in the pathology of chronic relapsing EAE in guinea pigs. The results of our present study indicate that humoral immune mechanisms may play a role in the pathogenesis of demyelination in this model.

(1) Antibodies against myelin basic protein, galactocerebroside, ganglioside (G_{M1}) and sulfatide were found in the majority of sera from animals sampled during the chronic stage of chronic relapsing EAE.

(2) A high percentage of chronic EAE sera induced demyelination in central and peripheral nerve fibers when injected into the cerebrospinal fluid of normal recipient rats.

(3) In the chronic stage of the disease there was an obvious coincidence of demyelinated plaques in donor animals, serum antibodies agains CNS antigens and serum demyelinating activity in vivo. Furthermore, there was a statistically significant connection between serum antibodies against glycosphingolipids and demyelinating activity of EAE sera.

(4) Sera from rabbits sensitized against gangliosides were shown to induce demyelination in vivo in normal recipient rats.

(5) Demyelinating activity was also observed in a certain number of EAE sera without antibodies against cerebroside and G_{M1}.

It is concluded that several different myelin surface antigens may induce demyelinating antibodies and that these antibodies may be important in the pathogenesis of demyelination in chronic relapsing EAE.

ACKNOWLEDGEMENTS

The excellent technical assistance (Angela Cervenka, Ursula Juszczak and Silvia Zimmermann) and secretarial assistance (Friderun Friedrich) is gratefully acknowledged. The study was supported by Fonds zur Förderung der Wissenschaftlichen Forschung, Austria, Projects S-25/04 and S-25/07.

REFERENCES

Alvord, E.C. (1970) Acute disseminated encephalomyelitis and "allergic" neuroencephalopathies. In P.J. Vinken, G.W. Bruyn (Eds), *Handbook of Clinical Neurology, Vol. 9*. North-Holland, Amsterdam, pp. 500–571.

Appel, S.H. and Bornstein, M.B. (1964) The application of tissue culture to the study of experimental allergic encephalomyelitis. II. Serum factors, responsible for demyelination. *J. exp. Med.*, 119: 303–312.

Bernard, C.C.A. (1976) Experimental autoimmune encephalomyelitis in mice. Genetic control of susceptibility. *J. Immunogenet.*, 3: 263–274.

Bornstein, M.B. and Appel, S.H. (1961) The application of tissue culture to the study of experimental "allergic" encephalomyelitis. I. Patterns of demyelination. *J. Neuropath. exp. Neurol.* 20: 141–147.

Bornstein, M.B. and Appel, S.H. (1965) Tissue culture studies of demyelination. *Ann. N.Y. Acad. Sci.*, 122: 280–286.

Brosnan, C.F., Stoner, G.L., Bloom, B.R. and Wisniewski, H.M. (1977) Studies on demyelination by activated lymphocytes in the rabbit eye. II. Antibody dependent cell mediated demyelination. *J. Immunol.*, 118: 2103–2110.

Dorfman, S.H., Fry, J.M., Silberberg, D.H., Grose, C. and Manning, M.C. (1978) Cerebroside antibody titers in antisera capable of myelination inhibition and demyelination. *Brain Res.*, 147: 410–415.

Dubois-Dalcq, M., Niedieck, B. and Buyse, M. (1970) Action of anti-cerebroside sera on myelinated nervous tissue cultures. *Pathol. Europ.*, 5: 331–347.

Fry, J.M., Weissbarth, S., Lehrer, G.M. and Bornstein, M.B. (1974) Cerebroside antibody inhibits sulfatide synthesis and myelination and demyelinates in cord tissue cultures. *Science*, 183: 540–542.

Groome, N.P. (1980) Enzyme-linked immunosorbent assays for myelin basic protein and antibodies to myelin basic protein. *J. Neurochem.*, 35: 1409–1417.

Grundke-Iqbal, I., Raine, C.S., Johnson, A.B., Brosnan, C.F. and Bornstein, M.B. (1981) Experimental allergic encephalomyelitis: characterization of serum demyelinating factors. *J. neurol. Sci.*, 50: 63–79.

Grundke-Iqbal, I. and Bornstein, M.B. (1979) Multiple sclerosis: immunological studies on the demyelinating serum factors. *Brain Res.* 160: 489–503.

314

Karcher, D., Lassmann, H., Lowenthal, A., Kitz, K. and Wisniewski, H.M. (1982) Antibodies-restricted heterogeneity in serum and cerebrospinal fluid of chronic relapsing experimental allergic encephalomyelitis. *J.
Neuroimmunol.*, 2: 93–106.

Kies, M.W., Murphy, J.B. and Alvord, E.C. (1960) Fractionation of guinea pig brain proteins with encephalitogenic
activity. *Fed. Proc.*, 19: 207.

Kitz, K., Lassmann, H. and Wisniewski, H.M. (1981) Isolated leptomeninges of the spinal cord: an ideal tool to study
inflammatory reaction in EAE. *Acta Neuropath.*, Suppl. 7: 179–181.

Kristensson, K. and Wisniewski, H.M. (1977) Chronic relapsing experimental allergic encephalomyelitis. Studies in
vascular permeability changes. *Acta Neuropath.*, 39: 189–194.

Lampert, P.W. (1965) Demyelination and remyelination in experimental allergic encephalomyelitis. *J. Neuropath.
exp. Neurol.*, 24: 371–385.

Lampert, P.W. and Kies, M.W. (1967) Mechanism of demyelination in allergic encephalomyelitis of guinea pigs. An
electron microscopic study. *Exp. Neurol.*, 18: 210–223.

Lassmann, H. and Wisniewski, H.M. (1978) Chronic relapsing EAE. Time course of neurological symptoms and
pathology. *Acta Neuropath.*, 43: 35–42.

Lassmann, H. and Wisniewski, H.M. (1979) Chronic relapsing experimental allergic encephalomyelitis. Clinicopa-
thological comparison with multiple sclerosis. *Arch. Neurol.*, 36: 490–497.

Lassmann, H., Kitz, K. and Wisniewski, H.M. (1980) Structural variability of demyelinating lesions in different
models of subacute and chronic experimental allergic encephalomyelitis. *Acta Neuropath.*, 51: 191–201.

Lassmann, H., Kitz, K. and Wisniewski, H.M. (1981) In vivo effect of sera from animals with chronic relapsing
experimental allergic encephalomyelitis on central and peripheral myelin. *Acta Neuropath.*, in press.

Lebar, R., Boutry, J.M., Vincent, C., Robineaux, F. and Voisin, G.A. (1976) Studies on autoimmune encephalomyelitis in the guinea pig. II. An in vitro investigation on the nature, properties, and specificity of the
serum-demyelinating factor. *J. Immunol.*, 116: 1439–1446.

Lebar, R., Vincent, C., Fischer-Le Boubennec, E. (1979) Studies on autoimmune encephalomyelitis in the guinea
pig. III. A comparative study of two autoantigens of central nervous system myelin. *J. Neurochem.*, 32:
1451–1460.

Lumsden, C.E. (1971) The immunogenesis of the multiple sclerosis plaque. *Brain Res.*, 28: 365–390.

Mehta, P.D., Lassmann, H. and Wisniewski, H.M. (1981) Immunologic studies of chronic relapsing EAE in guinea
pigs: similarities to multiple sclerosis. *J. Immunol.*, 127: 334–338.

Naiki, M., Marcus, D.M. and Ledeen, R. (1974) Properties of antisera to Ganglioside G_{M1} and Asialo G_{M1}. *J.
Immunol.*, 113: 84–93.

Niedieck, B. (1975) On a glycolipid hapten of myelin. *Progr. Allergy*, 18: 353–422.

Ortiz-Ortiz, L. and Weigle, W.O. (1976) Cellular events in the induction of experimental allergic encephalomyelitis
in rats. *J. exp. Med.*, 144: 604–616.

Panitch, H. and Ciccone, C. (1981) Induction of recurrent experimental allergic encephalomyelitis with myelin basic
protein. *Ann. Neurol.*, 9: 433–438.

Paterson, P.Y. (1960) Transfer of allergic encephalomyelitis in rats by means of lymph node cells. *J. exp. Med.*, 111:
119–135.

Perlmann, H., Perlmann, P., Schreiber, R.D. and Müller-Eberhard, H.J. (1981) Interaction of target cell bound C 3 bi
and C 3 d with human lymphocyte receptors. Enhancement of antibody mediated cellular cytotoxicity. *J. exp.
Med.*, 153: 1592–1603.

Raine, C.S., Snyder, D.H., Valsamis, M.P. and Stone, S.H. (1974) Chronic experimental allergic encephalomyelitis
in inbred guinea pigs. An ultrastructural study. *Lab. Invest.*, 31: 369–380.

Roboz Einstein, E., Robertson, D.M., DiCaprio, J.M. and Moore, W. (1962) The isolation from bovine spinal cord of
a homogeneous protein with encephalitogenic activity. *J. Neurochem.*, 9: 353–361.

Saida, T., Abramsky, O., Silberberg, D.H., Pleasure, D., Lisak, R.P. and Manning, M. (1977) Antioligodendrocyte
serum demyelinates cultured CNS tissue. *Neurosci. Abstr.* 3: 527.

Saida, K., Saida, T., Brown, M.J. and Silberberg, D.H. (1979) In vivo demyelination induced by intraneural injection
of anti-galactocerebroside serum. A morphologic study. *Amer. J. Pathol.*, 95: 99–116.

Schwerer, B., Lassmann, H., Kitz, K., Bernheimer, H. and Wisniewski, H.M. (1981) Fractionation of spinal cord
tissue affects its activity to induce chronic relapsing experimental encephalomyelitis. *Acta Neuropath.*, Suppl.
VII: 165–168.

Seil, F.J., Falk, G.A., Kies, M.W. and Alvord, E.C. (1968) The in vitro demyelinating activity of sera from guinea
pigs sensitized with whole CNS and with purified encephalitogen. *Exp. Neurol.*, 22: 545–555.

Seil, F.J. and Agrawal, H.C. (1980) Myelin-proteolipid protein does not induce demyelinating or myelination
inhibiting antibodies. *Brain Res.*, 194: 273–277.

Seil, F.J., Quarles, R.H., Johnson, D. and Brady, R.O. (1981) Immunisation with purified myelin-associated
glycoprotein does not evoke myelination-inhibiting or demyelinating antibodies. *Brain Res.*, 209: 470–475.

Shaw, C.M., Alvord, E.C., Kaku, J. and Kies, M.W. (1965) Correlation of experimental allergic encephalomyelitis with delayed type skin sensitivity to specific homologous encephalitogen. *Ann. N.Y. Acad. Sci.,* 122: 318–331.

Tourtellotte, W. (1970) On cerebrospinal fluid immunoglobulin G (IgG) quotients in multiple sclerosis and other diseases. *J. Neurol. Sci.,* 10: 279–304.

Traugott, U. and Raine, C.S. (1979) Acute experimental allergic encephalomyelitis: myelin basic protein reactive T-cells in the circulation and in meningeal infiltrates. *J. neurol. Sci.,* 42: 331–336.

Traugott, U., Stone, S.H. and Raine, C.S. (1979) Chronic relapsing experimental allergic encephalomyelitis. Correlation of circulating lymphocyte fluctuations with disease activity in suppressed and unsuppressed animals. *J. neurol. Sci.,* 41: 17–29.

Vaerman, J.P., Lebacq-Verheyden, A.M., Scolari, L. and Heremans, J.F. (1969) Further studies on single radial immunodiffusion. II. The reversed system: diffusion of antibodies in antigen-containing gels. *Immunochemistry,* 6: 287–293.

Waksman, B.H. and Morrison, L.R. (1951) Tuberkulin type sensitivity to spinal cord antigen in rabbits with isoallergic encephalomyelitis. *J. Immunol.,* 66: 421–444.

Wassermann, E. and Levine L. (1961) Quantitative micro-complement fixation and its use in the study of antigenic structure by specific antigen-antibody inhibition. *J. Immunol.,* 87: 290–295.

Wisniewski, H.M. and Keith, A.B. (1977) Chronic relapsing experimental allergic encephalomyelitis — an experimental model of multiple sclerosis. *Ann. Neurol.,* 1: 144–148.

Immunology of Nervous System Infections, Progress in Brain Research, Vol. 59, edited by P.O. Behan, V. ter Meulen and F. Clifford Rose

Characterization by Acid α-Naphthyl Acetate Esterase Staining of the Spinal Cord Cellular Infiltrate in the Acute and Relapse Phases of Chronic Relapsing Experimental Allergic Encephalomyelitis

A.J. SUCKLING, J.A. KIRBY and M.G. RUMSBY

Department of Biology, University of York, Heslington, York YO1 5DD (U.K.)

INTRODUCTION

Several years ago, Wisniewski and Keith (1977) described a procedure for inducing a chronic relapsing variant of experimental allergic encephalomyelitis (EAE). Whilst classical acute EAE is essentially monophasic, primarily inflammatory, and often fatal, the chronic relapsing disease in guinea pigs displays a relapsing and remitting course together with the development of demyelinating plaques. The nature of the cellular infiltrates has been extensively studied over many years in the acute disease. Morphological studies have shown that lymphocytes and monocytes form the bulk of the infiltrate (Traugott et al., 1978; Allsopp et al., 1980). Allsopp et al. (1980) have also characterized isolated meningeal cells in terms of their ability to form E, EA, and EAC rosettes.

There are few studies relating to the chronic relapsing disease. A histopathological examination of the central nervous sytem (CNS) at different stages of the chronic relapsing model has shown variations in the inflammatory reaction (Lassmann et al., 1981). The infiltrates are largely meningeal in the acute phase, becoming parenchymal and associated with demyelinating plaques during established relapses. Lymphocytes, macrophages and plasma cells have been described in these lesions by morphological criteria. In this chapter we describe the characterization of guinea pig lymphocytes and macrophages by histochemical means. Studies on human lymphocytes have shown staining for acid α-naphthyl acetate esterase (ANAE) to be specific for a large proportion of T-lymphocytes (Knowles et al., 1978; Ranki et al., 1976). Monocytes (macrophages) also stain, but their esterase activity is inhibited by the addition of 10 mM fluoride ion (F^-) to the staining medium. B-cells have been shown in man not to stain for ANAE.

MATERIALS AND METHODS

Animals

Chronic relapsing EAE was induced in strain 13 guinea pigs from the colony maintained at the University of York. Juveniles (18–22 days old) were sensitized with an emulsion of 1 part incomplete Freund's adjuvant containing 10 mg/ml mycobacterium tuberculosis H37Ra (Difco) and 1 part 50% whole spinal cord homogenate. Inoculations of 0.1 ml were made in each hind foot dorsum. Before sampling CNS tissue for analysis the animals were anesthetized with Sagatal (May and Baker) and perfused with 250 ml phosphate-buffered saline at 4°C via the left ventricle. The grades of clinical illness, which appear in figure legends, were scored according to the system of Wisniewski and Keith (1977).

[317]

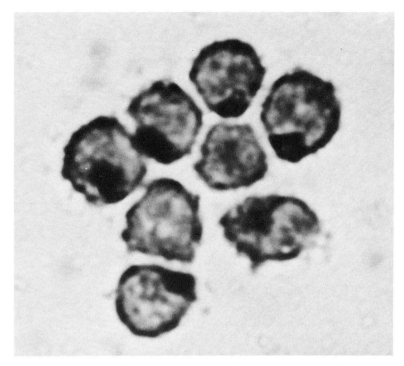

Fig. 1. Stained lymphocytes from peripheral blood. Six cells show a discrete single area of reaction product and are regarded as ANAE-positive. The remaining two cells show no staining. × 5000.

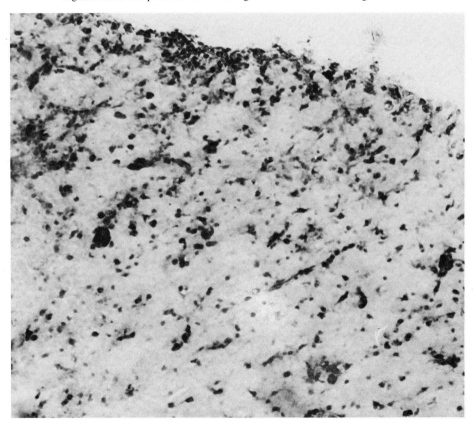

Fig. 2. Acute phase lesion from thoracic spinal cord of guinea pig 132/81 (grade 5, 14 days after inoculation). Fluoride-inhibited staining showing lymphocytes located mainly in the meninges. × 175.

ANAE histochemistry

The technique was performed by the method of Mueller et al. (1975) based on the detection of α-naphthate released from α-naphthyl acetate by esterase hydrolysis. Coupling of α-naphthate to hexazotised pararosaniline then yields a highly chromophoric, insoluble brown dye. Activity of ANAE in formalin fixed samples was detected by incubation in a medium consisting of 40 ml 0.067 M phosphate buffer, pH 5.0, 2.4 ml hexazotised pararosaniline and 10 mg α-naphthyl acetate (Sigma, London) dissolved in 0.4 ml acetone. The mixture was then adjusted to pH 5.8 by the addition of 2 M NaOH.

Spinal cord sections, 1 cm in length, were taken from animals at various stages of the chronic relapsing disease and were immersion-fixed in buffered formol-sucrose, pH 6.8 at 4°C for 24 h. The tissue was then transferred to Holt's gum sucrose at 4°C for a further 24 h before 12 μm sections were cut using a cryostat at -25°C. These sections were air-dried onto slides before staining and after staining were dehydrated and mounted in DPX. In some staining reactions sodium fluoride (NaF) was added to a final concentration of 10 mM. This addition reduced background staining, particularly of neuronal cells bodies in the gray matter, and eliminated monocyte staining in buffy coat smears.

Staining specificity

The specificity of the procedure for various types of guinea pig mononuclear cells was verified by staining isolated T- and T-cell-depleted lymphocyte smears. Cell preparations were separated by Ficoll-Paque (Pharmacia) density gradient centrifugation after the formation of late (total T-cell) E rosettes. Late E rosettes were prepared by mixing at a ratio of 1:30 isolated peripheral blood lymphocytes suspended in medium 199 with 2-aminoethylisothiouronium bromide hydrobromide-treated rabbit erythrocytes suspended in Alsever's solution. This mixture was centrifuged at 250 g for 5 min and the pellet incubated at 4°C for 2 h before resuspension and application to the gradient. Cell smears were air-dried, fixed in Baker's formol calcium, pH 6.7, at 4°C for 10 min and washed in water at room temperature for 20 min before staining.

RESULTS

Validation of ANAE staining specificity

Guinea pig peripheral blood lymphocytes from 3 animals were separated into T- and B-cell fractions by E rosetting as described earlier. ANAE staining was then performed on both fractions. For each fraction 200 cells were counted and of the T-cell fraction a mean of 86% stained with ANAE, whilst 29% of the B-cell fraction was positive. These results were comparable with those obtained for human peripheral blood lymphocytes by Ranki (1978). The appearance of ANAE-positive and ANAE-negative cells is shown in Fig. 1.

A longitudinal study of T-cell percentages in blood, as defined by ANAE activity, in two control animals gave a mean value of 65%.

Staining characteristics of spinal cord sections

Figs. 2–5 demonstrate the appearance of sections from animals in the acute and first relapse phases of the chronic relapsing disease.

320

One of the major areas of interest in the pathogenesis of chronic relapsing EAE must be the circumstances surrounding the generation of the relapse. Lassmann et al. (1981) have described the pathological changes occurring in the CNS during different stages of the disease and documented changes in the distribution and intensity of the monocytic infiltration. During the initiating period of a first relapse lesion, a gradual increase in the presence of monocytic inflammatory cells was noted. Their distribution developed from focal meningeal sites to an association in the parenchyma with demyelination in plaque-forming areas. It is often difficult, however, to distinguish by light microscopy between different types of mononuclear cells in tissue sections. ANAE staining does allow fast detection of T-cells and macrophages within such sections.

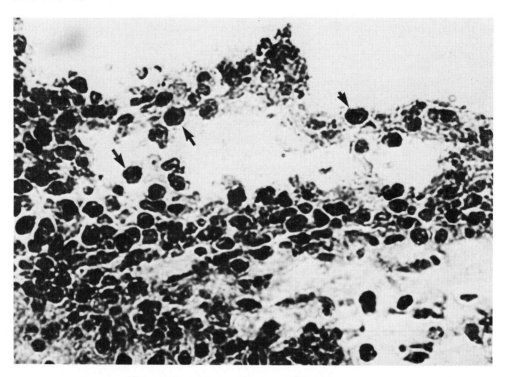

Fig. 3. Acute phase lesion from thoracic spinal cord of guinea pig 66/81 (grade 4, day 14). The majority of cells show discrete areas of reaction product characteristic of T-lymphocytes (arrowed). × 700.

Acute phase lesions appear in Figs. 2 and 3 and are characterized by mainly meningeal and closely perivascular infiltrates, a large percentage of which show the staining characteristics of T-lymphocytes. In contrast, the lesions in the plaque areas of an animal in first relapse (Fig. 4) stain intensely for ANAE, but the majority of the staining reaction is abrogated by the addition of fluoride (F⁻) (Fig. 5) implying a much larger contribution to the staining reaction by macrophages. It should be emphasized, however, that the sections presented here are from an established plaque where it is almost certain that macrophages will be the most numerous cell type present because of the secondary response to tissue damage. Plaques formed earlier will have a different response to ANAE staining.

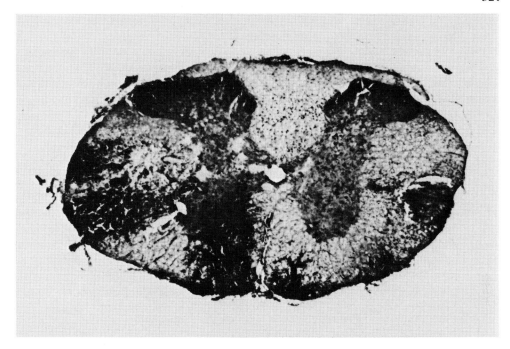

Fig. 4. First relapse lesion from spinal cord of animal 105/81 (grade 4, day 84). Several plaque areas can be seen in the ventral and lateral aspects of the cord. Dark areas in the white matter indicate regions of intense ANAE activity. Note also staining of gray matter areas. × 40.

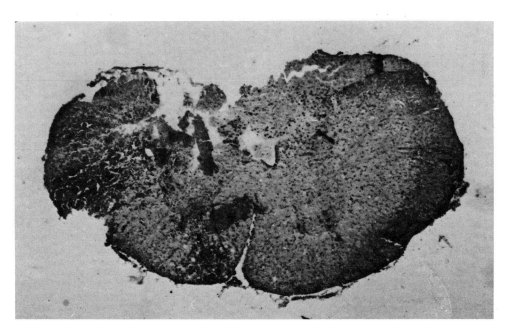

Fig. 5. As Fig. 4, but the staining reaction has been fluoride-inhibited. Note marked reduction in plaque area staining and inhibition of background gray matter staining. × 40.

Whilst the illustrations in this paper provide qualitative data on cellular distribution, as do other non-histochemical stains, an increase in discrimination between cell types could be achieved by using thinner, embedded sections or by using meningeal stretch preparations as described by Lassmann et al. (1981). These techniques will allow a quantitative assessment of lymphocytes and macrophages within tissue sections. This work is in progress and will demonstrate which cell populations change first during the important transition from remission to the commencement of relapse phases in chronic relapsing EAE.

ACKNOWLEDGEMENTS

We gratefully acknowledge the financial support of this work by the Multiple Sclerosis Society of Great Britain and Northern Ireland.

REFERENCES

Allsopp, G., Roters, S. and Turk, J.L. (1980) Isolation and characterisation of the inflammatory infiltrate in the central nervous system of the guinea pig with experimental allergic encephalomyelitis. *Neuropath. appl. Neurobiol.*, 6: 109–118.

Knowles, D.M., Hoffman, T., Ferrarini, M. and Kunkel, H.G. (1978) The demonstration of acid α-naphthyl acetate esterase activity in human lymphocytes: usefulness as a T-cell marker. *Cell Immunol.*, 35: 112–123.

Lassmann, H., Kitz, K. and Wisniewski, H.M. (1981) Histogenesis of demyelinating lesions in the spinal cord of guinea pigs with chronic relapsing experimental allergic encephalomyelitis. *J. neurol. Sci.*, 50: 109–121.

Mueller, J., Brun del Re, G., Buerki, H., Keller, H.-U., Hess, M.W. and Cottier, H. (1975) Nonspecific acid esterase activity: a criterion for differentiation of T and B lymphocytes in mouse lymph nodes. *Europ. J. Immunol.*, 5: 270–274.

Ranki, A. (1978) Nonspecific esterase activity in human lymphocytes: histochemical characterisation and distribution among major lymphocyte subclasses. *Clin. Immunol. Immunopath.*, 10: 47–58.

Ranki, A., Totterman, T.H. and Hayry, P. (1976) Identification of resting human T and B lymphocytes by acid α-naphthyl acetate esterase staining combined with rosette formation with *S.aureus* strain Cowan 1. *Scand. J. Immunol.*, 5: 1129–1138.

Traugott, U., Stone, S.H. and Raine, C.S. (1978) Experimental allergic encephalomyelitis: migration of early T cells from the circulation into the CNS. *J. neurol. Sci.*, 36: 55–61.

Wisniewski, H.M. and Keith, A.B. (1977) Chronic relapsing experimental allergic encephalomyelitis — an experimental model of multiple sclerosis. *Ann. Neurol.*, 1: 144–148.

Immunology of Nervous System Infections, Progress in Brain Research, Vol. 59, edited by P.O. Behan, V. ter Meulen and F. Clifford Rose
© *1983 Elsevier Science Publishers B.V.*

Immunological Behaviour of Meningeal Exudate Cells in Experimental Allergic Encephalomyelitis

GRETA ALLSOPP and J.L. TURK

Department of Pathology, Royal College of Surgeons of England, Lincoln's Inn Fields, London, WC2A 3PN (U.K.)

INTRODUCTION

Experimental allergic encephalomyelitis (EAE) is a cell-mediated autoimmune disease of the central nervous system induced in laboratory animals by the injection of emulsified spinal cord in Freund's incomplete adjuvant (FIA) with added mycobacterium tuberculosis. EAE induced in adult Hartley strain guinea pigs develops as an acute disease with symptoms occurring 11 days after immunization, and usually results in death by 14 days. In contrast, a chronic relapsing form of EAE can be induced using the same protocol for the induction of EAE, but with juvenile guinea pigs (Stone and Lerner, 1965). It was shown in 1949 that guinea pigs injected with brain tissue emulsified in Freund's adjuvant without mycobacteria not only failed to develop EAE but were resistant to subsequent injections of encephalitogenic material (Ferraro and Cazzullo, 1949). This protection of animals against EAE has been subsequently confirmed in a number of laboratory animals using both whole CNS tissue or the purified antigen myelin basic protein (MBP) (Alvord et al., 1965; Einstein et al., 1968; Swanborg, 1973). In early studies of acute EAE the inflammatory infiltrate was found by light microscopy to be composed of cells of the mononuclear phagocyte series (Waksman and Adams, 1962). Subsequently, Lampert (1965) and Lampert and Carpenter (1965) have demonstrated myelin laden macrophages by electron microscopy and more recently Raine et al. (1974) have described macrophages to be the constant component of all affected areas in chronic EAE and to be the predominant feature of the perivascular cuff. Traugott et al. (1978) have attempted to extract cells of the inflammatory infiltrate by ultrasonication of the brain and spinal cord of guinea pigs with EAE. They showed that a high level of early T-lymphocytes in the CNS coincided with a decrease of this cell population in the peripheral blood. Allsopp et al. (1980) found the meningeal inflammatory cells isolated from the brains of guinea pigs with acute EAE to be composed of 60 % lymphocytes, the majority of which were T-cells, 30 % cells of the mononuclear phagocyte series and 5 % neutrophils. The meningeal exudate cells of guinea pigs with acute EAE have been counted and compared with counts made from guinea pigs showing no signs of disease. A significant increase in cells has been found in guinea pigs showing signs of EAE when compared: (i) with animals protected by injection with spinal cord in FIA before sensitization; (ii) with animals at a time prior to the first signs of EAE; and (iii) with control guinea pigs (Allsopp et al., 1981). Similar numbers of inflammatory cells were isolated from guinea pig brains of animals with chronic relapsing EAE as from those with acute EAE (Allsopp and Turk, 1982).

It has been postulated that animals might be protected from developing clinical signs of

EAE, when pretreated with spinal cord in FIA, by the recruitment of suppressor cells (Coates et al., 1974; Welch et al., 1978). As immunological tolerance to contact sensitization can be reversed by cyclophosphamide (CY) (Polak and Turk, 1974; Turk et al., 1976), it was suggested that CY might break tolerance by inhibition of suppressor cells. We therefore decided to see whether the administration of CY would reverse tolerance in animals protected against EAE (Allsopp et al., 1982). Two doses of CY (300 mg/kg and 20 mg/kg) were given either before the protective dose of spinal cord, to try to eliminate the suppressor cell precursors, or before immunization to eliminate the suppressor cells. No clinical signs of EAE developed in these guinea pigs. Changes were, however, found in the meningeal cell infiltrate. The number of cells isolated from animals treated with CY (300 mg/kg), when the protective dose of spinal cord in FIA was given one week before immunization, was found to be as great as the number of meningeal inflammatory cells obtained from animals showing clinical signs of EAE, and significantly higher than protected animals not treated with CY.

The second question asked was whether CY given prior to immunization (FCA/SC) would increase the intensity of clinical signs of EAE and increase the inflammatory cell numbers. In addition, would clinical signs develop earlier after immunization? No apparent change in the course of the disease was found in animals treated with CY. Previous studies have not demonstrated whether the cells surrounding the brain in the inflammatory infiltrate are recruited specifically or attracted non-specifically to the site of inflammation. It has been shown in delayed hypersensitivity in the guinea pig (Turk, 1962) that, after passive transfer, equal numbers of labeled lymphoid cells from specifically sensitized donors may be found at non-specific as well as specific skin test sites. The immunological specificity of cells in the inflammatory infiltrate in EAE was therefore studied (Allsopp et al., 1981, 1982; Allsopp and Turk, 1982). The inflammatory cells isolated from the brains of EAE guinea pigs were assayed by the lymphocyte transformation test to determine if these cells would respond by proliferation when in contact with a specific brain antigen (myelin basic protein, MBP), tuberculin (PPD) or with the mitogen concanavalin A (Con A). The inflammatory cell population of meningeal origin was compared with a similar population from the peritoneal cavity. Meningeal exudate cells from animals with acute EAE only proliferated in the presence of the mitogen Con A, although PECs from the same animals responded to MBP, PPD and Con A. Meningeal exudate cells from guinea pigs with chronic relapsing EAE and guinea pigs protected against EAE did not proliferate in the presence of either antigens or mitogen whereas their PEC's did proliferate in the presence of tuberculin and Con A but not to MBP.

ISOLATION AND CHARACTERIZATION OF THE MENINGEAL EXUDATE CELLS

Histological sections of the central nervous system of guinea pigs with EAE showed the meninges to be heavily infiltrated with inflammatory cells. When the brain is removed and an impression smear made from the ventral surface of the brainstem, inflammatory cells are found to adhere to the slide and can be stained and examined microscopically. Sixty percent of the cells may be identified as lymphocytes, 30 % as cells of the mononuclear phagocyte series, and 5 % as neutrophils; the occasional plasma cell and eosinophil were also identified (Fig. 1). Inflammatory cell suspensions were obtained by washing the brain surface and the closely adhering meninges with medium (Allsopp et al., 1980). The inflammatory cells were then examined by E, EA and EAC rosette techniques, the Nigrosin test for phagocytic cells and by transmission and scanning electron microscopy. Using these methods, 43.5 % of the cells were positively identified as T-lymphocytes (this is similar to that found by Traugott et al., 1978),

35.4 % had receptors for Fc and C3 and 28 % of the cells were actively phagocytic. A similar analysis has been made of the composition of the meningeal exudate cells: (i) from animals protected against clinical signs of EAE; (ii) from animals protected and then treated with CY;

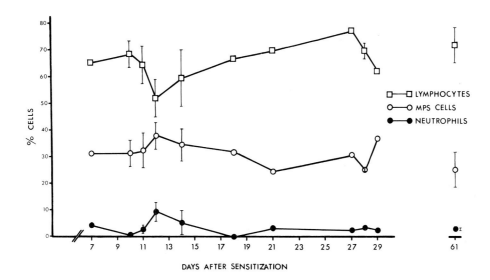

Fig. 1. Percentage of cell counts (± S.E.M.) made from imprints of the basal surface of the EAE guinea pig brain with days after sensitization.

and (iii) from animals with chronic relapsing EAE (Table I). The percentage of T-lymphocytes was found to be similar in all 3 cases, but there was a significant fall in the percentage of phagocytic cells (Allsopp and Turk, 1982; Allsopp et al., 1982).

TABLE I

THE PERCENTAGE OF T-LYMPHOCYTES AND PHAGOCYTIC CELLS IN THE MENINGEAL INFLAMMATORY INFILTRATE

Results expressed as mean ± standard deviation.

Day					%T-cells	Phagocytic cells	Day killed
−10	−7	0					
		Acute EAE	FCA/SC		43.5 ± 16.8	28.3 ± 12.3	11–15
		CREAE	FCA/SC		n.d.	5.3 ± 3.0*	46–207
	FIA/SC		FCA/SC		31.0 ± 14.1	3.6 ± 5.4**	27–32
CY(300)	FIA/SC		FCA/SC		36.4 ± 11.5	12.9 ± 11.8***	27–32

* $P < 0.001$ as compared to acute EAE.
** $P < 0.001$ as compared to acute EAE.
*** $P < 0.005$ as compared to acute EAE.

QUANTITATION OF THE MENINGEAL EXUDATE CELLS

Total cell counts have been made of the inflammatory cells washed from the surface of the brain (Allsopp et al., 1981, 1982; Allsopp and Turk, 1982). Significantly high numbers of cells (mean 8×10^6) (Fig. 2) were found after washing the brains of guinea pigs showing clinical signs of disease. As clinical signs of EAE began with weight loss at day 9 after immunization cell counts were made prior to this time, at day 7. A mean of 1.5×10^6 cells was found in contrast to 6 times this number a few days later when guinea pigs showed clinical signs of disease ($P < 0.001$). Animals which had been strongly sensitized with a non-encephalitogenic protein and normal guinea pigs were used as controls and as can be seen from Fig. 2, no increase in cell counts was detected (mean 1.0×10^6 and 0.8×10^6 cells were counted respectively; $P < 0.001$ for both when compared with FCA/spinal cord counts).

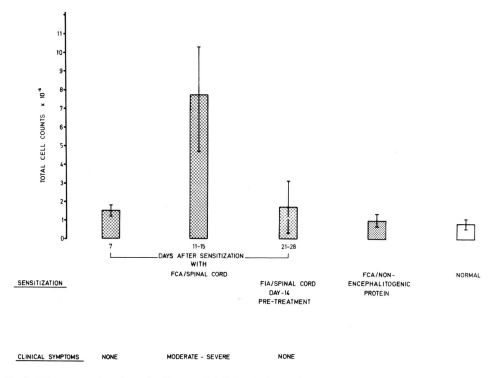

Fig. 2. Histogram to show the total cell counts ($\pm$ S.D.) made from cells recovered from the meninges of guinea pig brains.

Animals exposed to spinal cord or myelin basic protein (MBP) in Freund's incomplete adjuvant (FIA) prior to immunization are prevented from developing clinical signs of EAE (Alvord et al., 1965). Guinea pigs pretreated 14 days before immunization showed no signs of EAE. When the animals were killed the number of meningeal exudate cells obtained was low (Fig. 2). A mean of 1.7×10^6 cells was found, the difference being statistically significant ($P < 0.001$) when compared to animals sick from EAE. If, however, the protective inoculum (FIA/SC) was given only 7 days before immunization (FCA/SC) to protect the guinea pigs against EAE, a large number (mean 4.7×10^6) of meningeal inflammatory cells could be isolated and the number of cells further significantly increased when the animals received CY,

TABLE II

A COMPARISON OF MENINGEAL INFLAMMATORY CELLS FROM GUINEA PIGS WITH CLINICAL SIGNS OF EAE AND FROM GUINEA PIGS PROTECTED AGAINST EAE

All groups were immunized with FCA/SC at day 0. Doses of CY expressed in mg/kg body weight.

Pretreatment (days)					Day killed	Number of animals	Clinical disease	Meningeal inflammatory cells $\times 10^{-6}$
−17	−14	−10	−7	−3				
					Acute EAE — 11 → 15	22	+	8.0 ± 3.2
					CREAE — 46 → 207	9	+	6.2 ± 1.3
	FCA/saline				11 → 15	6	+	8.8 ± 1.7
				CY(300)	11 → 15	7	+	6.8 ± 2.6
				CY(20)	11 → 15	7	+	8.0 ± 2.4
	FIA/SC				22 → 26	11	−	1.7 ± 1.4
	FIA/SC			CY(300)	21	7	−	1.4 ± 0.4
	FIA/SC			CY(20)	26	6	−	2.8 ± 0.5
CY(300)	FIA/SC				27	7	−	2.0 ± 1.1
CY(20)	FIA/SC				27	7	−	1.7 ± 0.5
			FIA/SC		28 → 32	20	−	4.7 ± 2.1
			FIA/SC	CY(300)	28 → 32	21	−	7.2 ± 3.1*
		CY(300)	FIA/SC		28 → 32	21	−	10.1 ± 5.4**
			FIA/SC	FIA/SC	28 → 32	10	−	5.4 ± 1.7

* $P < 0.01$ as compared with results shown in italics.
** $P < 0.001$ as compared with results shown in italics.

either before FIA/SC (mean 10.1×10^6) or before FCA/SC (mean 7.2×10^6) (Table II). It has been postulated that the animals might be protected by the recruitment of suppressor cells (Coates et al., 1974; Welch et al., 1978). CY has been shown to reverse immunological tolerance to contact sensitization (Polak and Turk, 1974; Turk et al., 1976) by eliminating a population of suppressor cells, induced by the tolerizing injection. Recently, Lando et al. (1979) have shown that mice may be protected against EAE by injection of either mouse spinal cord homogenate, mouse myelin basic protein or Copolymer I (the synthetic polypeptide that cross-reacts with MBP (Teitelbaum et al., 1971) in FIA given before EAE induction. This protection was abrogated by a low dose of CY (20 mg/kg) given 2 days before the encephalito-genic challenge. They found higher and lower doses of CY did not break the protection against EAE. Allsopp et al. (1982), attempted to eliminate suppressor cell precursors by giving CY prior to the protective inoculum and to eliminate the suppressor cells themselves by giving CY before immunization. Although no clinical signs of EAE developed in any of these groups, there was a large increase in the number of meningeal exudate cells obtained, and this was of a similar order of magnitude to the number of cells obtained from animals with clinical signs of EAE. The numbers of meningeal inflammatory cells obtained from guinea pigs with chronic relapsing EAE (6.2×10^6) were also similar to those of animals with acute EAE (Allsopp and Turk, 1982).

THE SPECIFICITY OF IMMUNOLOGICAL REACTIVITY OF CELLS DERIVED FROM MENINGEAL EXUDATES

The reactivity of the inflammatory cells washed from the meninges was assessed by the lymphocyte transformation test to see whether these cells would react directly with specific antigen. Myelin basic protein (MBP) is highly encephalitogenic when incorporated in Freund's complete adjuvant containing mycobacterium tuberculosis. Therefore, this antigen (MBP), tuberculin (PPD) and the mitogen concanavalin A (Con A) were used in the assay. The proliferation of the meningeal exudate cells was compared with that of the peritoneal exudate cells (PECs) which were selected to represent a population of lymphoid cells derived from the circulation as a result of a non-specific inflammatory stimulus (Allsopp et al., 1982; Allsopp and Turk, 1982). A highly significant difference was found in the stimulation indices of these two cell populations (Table III). The PECs from animals with acute EAE responded to both MBP and PPD as well as Con A, whereas meningeal exudate cells responded to the non-speci-fic mitogen Con A, but did not respond to the two antigens. This responsiveness was compared with similar cell populations obtained from animals with chronic relapsing EAE (Allsopp and Turk, 1982), with animals protected against EAE with animals protected against EAE and treated with CY (Allsopp et al., 1982). In all these cases the meningeal exudate cells failed to proliferate in the presence of antigen and mitogen. Although the PECs did respond to tuberculin (PPD) and mitogen they did not respond to the brain antigen MBP. CY treatment of the animals had no apparent effect on the lymphocyte proliferative responses either of the meningeal inflammatory cells or of the PECs. The viability of the cells was good after the three day culture period and, therefore, the lack of response to the mitogen was not due to cell death.

The percentage of T-lymphocytes in the meningeal inflammatory infiltrate of protected guinea pigs was found to be similar to that of animals showing acute signs of EAE. The background counts, showing the uptake of tritiated thymidine in the control cultures, were markedly increased for the meningeal inflammatory cells obtained from CY-pretreated guinea pigs protected against clinical signs of EAE and from guinea pigs with chronic relapsing EAE.

TABLE III

COMPARISON OF LYMPHOCYTE PROLIFERATION OF THE MENINGEAL INFLAMMATORY CELLS AND OF THE PERITONEAL EXUDATE CELLS

All groups were immunized with FCA/SC at day 0. Results expressed as mean ± standard deviation.

Pretreatment days			Day killed	Meningeal inflammatory cells				Peritoneal exudate cells			
−10	−7	−3		Stimulation index			Background counts	Stimulation index			Background counts
				MBP	PPD	Con A		MBP	PPD	Con A	
			Acute EAE 11 → 15	1.3±0.4	1.5±0.7	11.4±7.9	657±341	5.6±3.1	4.6±2.4	15.8± 8.7	582±282
			CREAE 46 → 207	1.3±0.5	2.0±1.3	3.0±2.8	1700±1020	2.8±1.9	8.7±7.4	20.6±28.3	460±249
	FIA/SC		30	1.4±0.6	1.9±1.3	2.6±1.8	2293± 995	2.6±0.7	12.2±6.1	15.4± 8.4	697± 91
		FIA/SC	30	1.1±0.3	1.0±0.2	1.4±0.4	1887± 860	2.0±1.2	5.7±4.3	9.2± 5.6	947±581
	FIA/SC	CY(300)	30	1.2±0.3	1.0±0.2	1.2±0.5	4118±2102	1.3±0.4	6.2±6.6	9.0± 5.7	973±465
CY(300)	FIA/SC		30	1.2±0.3	1.0±0.3	1.4±1.0	5526±2658	1.4±0.6	5.5±2.6	10.7± 7.1	1078±682

These counts were very high when compared with those made from: (a) the meningeal inflammatory cells obtained from guinea pigs showing clinical signs of acute EAE; and (b) the PECs from the same guinea pig. One might have been able to demonstrate a response to both mitogen and antigen if the background counts had been lower, of the same order as those from acute EAE guinea pigs. The high background counts would appear to indicate that these cells are turning over more rapidly. Tosca et al. (1981), studying the effect of a delayed hypersensitivity skin reaction on the in vitro parameters of cell-mediated immunity in the guinea pig, found an increase in background counts of unstimulated cultures (hence a depression of the stimulation indices) of guinea pigs which had been skin tested. They found some evidence for mitogenic activity in the sera from these skin-tested animals and postulated that circulating lymphokines might be producing this effect. In our study the PECs from the same groups of pretreated guinea pigs and those with CREAE did not show a significant elevation in background counts. Therefore, if the increase is due to the action of a mitogenic factor, this must have been released locally.

The small number of phagocytic cells (macrophages) present might be responsible for a depression in the proliferative response of the meningeal exudate cells to antigen and mitogen, but would not account for a lack of responsiveness and the elevation in the backgrounds counts.

SUMMARY

The inflammatory infiltrate in the central nervous system of guinea pigs with experimental allergic encephalomyelitis (EAE) has been characterized and quantitated. Inflammatory cells found over the surface of the brain and within the leptomeninges have been isolated by washing, and subsequently identified and their immunological specificity determined. By light microscopy approximately 60% were lymphocytes, 30% were cells of the mononuclear phagocyte series and 5% were neutrophils. E, EA and EAC rosetting techniques were used to determine the proportions of T-lymphocytes and cells with Fc and C3 receptors respectively. The percentage of phagocytic cells in the meningeal exudate was also determined. A mean of 8.0×10^6 cells were recovered from the brains of guinea pigs showing clinical signs of acute EAE in contrast to only 1.5×10^6 cells in the controls. A similar high number of cells were isolated from the brains of guinea pigs with chronic relapsing EAE. Guinea pigs were found to be fully protected against the clinical signs of EAE when they were given a protective inoculum of spinal cord in Freund's incomplete adjuvant either 3, 7 or 14 days before immunization with spinal cord in Freund's complete adjuvant. CY at 300 mg/kg and 20 mg/kg was given either before the protective inoculum to try to eliminate suppressor cell precursors, or before immunization to eliminate the suppressor cells themselves. No clinical signs of EAE developed in any of these groups of guinea pigs. It was found, however, that large numbers of meningeal inflammatory cells could be isolated from the brains of guinea pigs protected from EAE when the protective inoculum was given only one week before immunization. These cell numbers were further significantly increased by giving CY in addition to the protective inoculum, although the animals still did not develop any clinical signs of the disease.

The immunological specificity of the meningeal inflammatory cells was determined using the lymphocyte transformation test and compared with another inflammatory cell population from the same animal derived from an oil-induced peritoneal exudate. The meningeal exudate cells from animals with acute EAE responded only to the mitogen concanavalin A (Con A) and not to the antigens myelin basic protein (MBP) and tuberculin (PPD). In contrast the PECs proliferated in the presence of both antigens and the mitogen. The meningeal inflammatory cells from guinea pigs with CREAE and from those protected against EAE did not respond, in the lymphocyte transformation test, either to the specific antigens or to the mitogen. PECs from these animals did, however, respond to tuberculin and to the mitogen but not to the brain antigen (MBP).

REFERENCES

Allsopp, G., Roters, S. and Turk, J.L. (1980) Isolation and characterization of the inflammatory infiltrate in the central nervous system of the guinea-pig with experimental allergic encephalomyelitis. *Neuropathol. appl. Neurobiol.*, 6: 109–118.

Allsopp, G., Parker, D., Hinrichs, D.J. and Turk, J.L. (1981) Quantitation in vitro analysis of the inflammatory cells in experimental allergic encephalomyelitis in the guinea pig. *Neuropathol. appl. Neurobiol.*, 7: 127–134.

Allsopp, G., Parker, D. and Turk, J.L. (1982) The effect of protecting guinea-pigs against EAE on the meningeal inflammatory cell infiltrate. *Neuropathol. appl. Neurobiol.*, 7: 477–487.

Allsopp, G. and Turk, J.L. (1982) Chronic relapsing experimental allergic encephalomyelitis in the guinea-pig: in vitro analysis of meningeal inflammatory cells. *Neuropathol. appl. Neurobiol.*, 8: 63–70.

Alvord, E.C., Shaw, C.M., Hruby, S. and Kies, M.W. (1965) Encephalitogen-induced inhibition of experimental allergic encephalomyelitis: prevention, suppression and therapy. *Ann. N.Y. Acad. Sci.*, 122: 333–345.

Coates, A., Mackay, I.R. and Crawford, M. (1974) Immune protection against experimental autoimmune encephalomyelitis: optimal conditions and analysis of mechanism. *Cell. Immunol.*, 12: 370–381.

Einstein, E.R., Csejtey, J. and Davies, W.J. (1968) Protective action of the encephalitogen and other basic proteins in experimental allergic encephalomyelitis. *Immunochemistry*, 5: 567–575.

Ferraro, A. and Cazzullo, C.L. (1949) Prevention of allergic encephalomyelitis in guinea pigs (a preliminary report). *J. Neuropathol. exp. Neurol.*, 8: 61–69.

Lampert, P.W. (1965) Demyelination and remyelination in EAE. Further electron microscope observations. *J. Neuropathol. exp. Neurol.*, 24: 371–385.

Lampert, P.W. and Carpenter, S. (1965) Electron microscope studies on the vascular permeability and mechanism of demyelination in EAE. *J. Neuropathol. exp. Neurol.*, 24: 11–24.

Lando, Z., Teitelbaum, D. and Arnon, R. (1979) Effect of cyclophosphamide on suppressor cell activity in mice unresponsive to EAE. *J. Immunol.*, 123: 2156–2160.

Polak, L. and Turk, J.L. (1974) Reversal of immunological tolerance by cyclophosphamide through inhibition of suppressor cell activity. *Nature (Lond.)*, 249: 654–656.

Raine, C.S., Snyder, D.H., Valsamis, M.P. and Stone, S.H. (1974) Chronic experimental allergic encephalomyelitis in inbred guinea pigs. An ultrastructural study. *Lab. Invest.*, 31: 369–380.

Stone, S.H. and Lerner, E.M. (1965) Chronic disseminated allergic encephalomyelitis in guinea pigs. *Ann. N.Y. Acad. Sci.*, 122: 227–241.

Swanborg, R.H. (1973) Antigen-induced inhibition of experimental allergic encephalomyelitis. II. Studies in guinea pigs with the small rat myelin basic protein. *J. Immunol.*, 111: 1067–1070.

Teitelbaum, D., Meshorer, A., Hirshfeld, T., Arnon, R. and Sela, M. (1971) Suppression of experimental allergic encephalomyelitis by a synthetic polypeptide. *Europ. J. Immunol.*, 1: 242–248.

Tosca, N., Parker, D. and Turk, J.L. (1981) The effect of a delayed hypersensitivity skin reaction on in vitro parameters of cell mediated immunity. *Cell. Immunol.*, 62: 28–37.

Traugott, U., Stone, S.H. and Raine, C.S. (1978) Experimental allergic encephalomyelitis — migration of early T cells from the circulation into the central nervous system. *J. neurol. Sci.*, 36: 55–61.

Turk, J.L. (1962) The passive transfer of delayed hypersensitivity in guinea pigs by the transfusion of isotopically-labelled lymphoid cells. *Immunology*, 5: 478–488.

Turk, J.L., Polak, L. and Parker, D. (1976) Control mechanisms in delayed-type hypersensitivity. *Brit. Med. Bull.*, 32: 165–170.

Waksman, B.H. and Adams, R.D. (1962) A histological study of the early lesion in EAE in the guinea pig and rabbit. *Amer. J. Pathol.*, 41: 135–162.

Welch, A.M., Swierkosz, J.E. and Swanborg, R.H. (1978) Regulation of self tolerance in experimental allergic encephalomyelitis. I. Differences between lymph node and spleen suppressor cells. *J. Immunol.*, 121: 1701–1705.

Immunology of Nervous System Infections, Progress in Brain Research, Vol. 59, edited by P.O. Behan, V. ter Meulen and F. Clifford Rose
© *1983 Elsevier Science Publishers B.V.*

Monitoring Changes in the Blood of Patients with Multiple Sclerosis

R. JONES, R. CAPILDEO, A.W. PREECE, N.P. LUCKMAN and F. CLIFFORD ROSE

Charing Cross Hospital, Department of Neurology, Fulham Palace Road, London W6 8RF (U.K.)

INTRODUCTION

Despite numerous studies on the immunological status of patients with multiple sclerosis (MS), the precise nature of the involvement of the immune system remains open to question. Although much is known about the distribution (Kam-Hansen, 1979, 1980) and activity of lymphocytes in different phases of the disease (Antel et al., 1978; Huddleston and Oldstone, 1979; Reinherz et al., 1980), there is, as yet, no conclusive evidence regarding the initial challenge to the immune system (see Lisak, 1980).

We have adopted a different approach in an attempt to monitor changes in the blood of patients with MS. It has been found that the electrophoretic mobility (EPM) of erythrocytes from patients with MS, when challenged with linoleic acid (LA), differs from that of control subjects (Field and Joyce, 1976; Field et al., 1977). It was proposed that this difference in EPM was related to abnormalities in cell membrane structure and that it might therefore reflect the presence of abnormalities in glial cell membranes. Field's test uses fresh erythrocytes in culture medium, and some laboratories have failed to reproduce Field's results (Stoof et al., 1977; Forrester and Smith, 1977; Hawkins and Millar, 1979; Cuypers and Reddemann, 1980). Zukoski et al. (1979), however, introduced the use of glutaraldehyde-fixed erythrocytes, thus enabling the test to be run in simple physiological salines with consequent ease of challenge with different concentrations of LA. It is this modification of the test that we have adopted here to examine the erythrocytes of patients with MS, their close family members and non-related control subjects, as well as some patients with other neurological disorders.

METHODS AND MATERIALS

Collection and preparation of blood samples

Morning venous blood samples were obtained from patients and control subjects asked to fast overnight. After centrifugation, separated erythrocytes were washed in modified phosphate-buffered saline (PBS) (NaCl: 0.145 M, Na_2HPO_4 7.7×10^{-3} M, $NaH_2 PO_4$: 2.3×10^3 M) and fixed in 1% glutaraldehyde (ESCO, EM grade in PBS) at pH 7.3. Plasma was recentrifuged and stored at $-30°C$. Fixed samples of erythrocytes were stored and examined in matched groups comprising patients and control subjects.

[333]

334

Experimental procedure

Fixed cells were washed 3 times in and finally resuspended in PBS at a concentration of $1-3 \times 10^7$ cells/ml. The initial mobility of cells was measured in a laser cytopherometer (Preece and Luckman, 1981a, b). Each cell suspension was then mixed with sol containing 80 μg/ml LA in the ratio 1:4 or 2:1 sol to cell suspension, and, after incubation for 6 min, introduced into the cytopherometer chamber to obtain a second mobility value. All mobility values following challenge with LA were expressed as percentage change over the initial mobility. A single control sample was tested repeatedly to monitor cytopherometer performance (see Jones et al., 1981).

RESULTS

Twenty-eight patients, in whom the diagnosis of MS satisfied MRC criteria, ranged in age from 18 to 68 and included subjects with different levels of severity of illness ranging from those with minimal neurological impairment to those wheelchair-bound or bed-ridden. Each time blood was taken, a full neurological examination was carried out and, using a standard proforma, the condition of the patients recorded (Capildeo et al., in preparation). Controls were grouped into subjects with no family connection with MS and spouses of patients, other close family members (parents, children, siblings) or patients with other neurological diseases (two with Guillain–Barre syndrome and two with motor neuron disease).

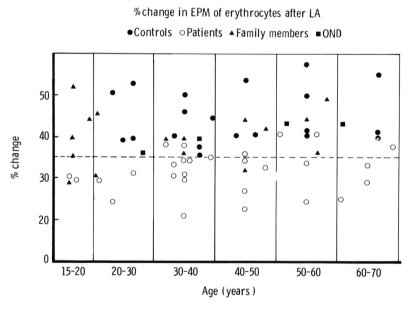

Fig. 1. Scattergram showing the percentage change in mobility of erythrocytes following challenge with linoleic acid sol in the ratio 1 ml sol to 4 ml cells: samples were patients with MS, control subjects, close family members, and patients with other neurological disorders.

The scattergram in Fig. 1 shows the accumulated results for all blood samples. Subjects are grouped according to age, and mobility of erythrocytes after challenge with LA is plotted as percent change over initial mobility. A dotted line drawn at 35% indicates the level below which none of the non-related controls fell. The distribution of points around this arbitrary division shows that in all but 6 cases erythrocytes from patients with MS had a slower mobility following challenge with LA than did non-related controls. This is in agreement with the findings of Zukoski et al. (1979). The erythrocytes of 3 of the family members (two daughters and one mother) also had mobilities below the control values. Field and Joyce (1977) first noted that some close family members of patients had erythrocytes showing slow mobility in the presence of LA. The blood of patients with other neurological disorders (OND) fell within the control range.

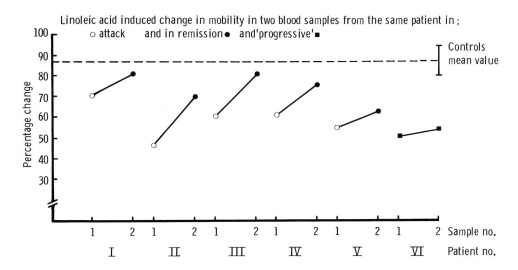

Fig. 2. Mobility changes in blood samples from 5 patients with MS taken during relapse and remission and one patient thought to have a progressive form of the disease. The cells were mixed with linoleic acid sol in the ratio 1 ml cells to 2 ml sol. The dotted line represents the mean value for sex and age-matched controls (n = 6) with standard deviation indicated as a vertical bar.

We were interested in the wide scatter of values from patients with MS and, in particular, the occasional samples which fell within the control sector. It appeared that slower mobility was obtained when blood was taken while patients were in a relapse. We studied this more closely by comparing blood samples taken during both relapse and remission in 5 patients and in one patient with the "progressive" form of the disease. The results of these studies are illustrated in Fig. 2. Samples were taken at intervals of between two months and one year and in every case the sample taken during relapse had a slower mobility than that taken in remission; the patient with the progressive form of the disease showed little difference between the two blood samples but these were taken only 3 months apart. The dotted line in Fig. 2 represents the mean change in mobility for 6 age- and sex-matched controls, with standard deviation indicated as the vertical bar. Samples from some of the patients taken during remission fall within this value and this may partially explain the "grey" area (the MS cases above the line) obtained in Fig. 1.

336

DISCUSSION

The electrophoretic mobility test for MS, first proposed by Field (Field and Joyce, 1976) infers that the surface charge on erythrocytes from patients with MS differs from that of control subjects. Field interpreted this as indicating a difference in membrane construction perhaps related to the mishandling of essential fatty acids (see Thompson, 1966). Such an abnormality might, if present in oligodendrocytes, make them liable to degenerative changes which may, in turn, give rise to an autoimmune reaction. Alternatively, abnormal membranes may be more vulnerable to attack by cells sensitized to other agents.

The suggestion that there is a membrane abnormality expressed in erythrocytes is supported by findings that in patients with MS these cells are more fragile (Caspary et al., 1967; Stasiw et al., 1977; Schauf et al., 1980) and larger (Plum and Fog, 1954; Prineas, 1968). It has also been noted that membrane fatty acid content differs in MS (Homa et al., 1979). How these differences are related to the observed changes in electrophoretic mobility is not known, but studies are in progress to examine this further.

Many laboratories failed to confirm Field's initial findings with fresh cells, but Bisaccia et al. (1977) and Tamblyn et al. (1980) found that the mobility of fresh cells from patients with MS had a slower mobility than controls after challenge with LA. Tamblyn et al. (1980) found that there was some overlap between patient and control groups and, in order to try and overcome this problem, the use of glutaraldehyde-fixed erythrocytes was introduced (Zukoski et al., 1979). The advantages of using fixed cells are numerous; they can be stored and re-examined in the same or different laboratories but, more importantly, mobility can be measured in simple electrolyte solutions, allowing more flexibility in the concentrations of LA used and simplifying interpretation of the findings.

In the present experiments, we have combined the advantages of using fixed erythrocytes with laser cytopherometry which permits rapid measurements and automatic recording of mobility changes (see Preece and Luckman, 1981a, b; Jones et al., 1981). These factors combine to provide an excellent system for objective testing of erythrocyte mobility. We have confirmed that the mobility of erythrocytes from most patients with MS was slower than that of control subjects, the only controls showing slow mobility being 3 close relatives of patients; this is in accordance with Field's and Seaman's findings (Field et al., 1977; Tamblyn et al., 1979).

A more interesting result was the finding that in 5 patients, blood samples taken during relapse had a slower mobility than those taken during remission although, in all but one case, remission samples remained in the MS sector and did not overlap with the controls. This finding suggests the possibility that during attacks a further factor influences erythrocyte membranes, exaggerating the surface phenomenon already present, and this factor could be related to the immunological changes taking place during relapse (see Antel et al., 1978; Vandenbark et al., 1979; Huddlestone and Oldstone, 1979; Reinherz et al., 1980).

Support for this suggestion comes from recent findings of Seaman et al. (1979) showing that incubation of red cells from control subjects with MS plasma converts their electrophoretic mobility to values similar to those found in cells from MS patients. This finding is being explored further in the hope that it will be possible to explain the observed changes in red cell mobility in remission and attack, thus providing a simple test for monitoring blood in patients with MS and improving the value of the test as a diagnostic aid.

ACKNOWLEDGEMENTS

This work was supported by ARMS (Action for Research into Multiple Sclerosis). We are grateful to Dr. G.D. Perkin for allowing us to examine his patients.

REFERENCES

Antel, J.P., Richman, D.P., Medof, M.E. and Arnason, B. (1978) Lymphocyte function and the role of regulator cells in multiple sclerosis. *Neurology*, 28: 106–110.

Bisaccia, G., Caputo, D. and Zibetti, A. (1977) E-UFA test in multiple sclerosis. *Boll. Ist. sieroter. milan.*, 56: 583–588.

Caspary, E.A., Sewell, F. and Field, E.J. (1967) Red blood cell fragility in multiple sclerosis. *Brit. Med. J.*, 11: 610–611.

Cuypers, J. and Reddemann, H. (1980) Evaluation of the erythrocyte (E-UFA) mobility test for the diagnosis of multiple sclerosis. *J. Neurol. Neurosurg. Psychiat.*, 43: 995–998.

Field, E.J. and Joyce, G. (1976) Simplified laboratory test for multiple sclerosis. *Lancet*, ii: 367–368.

Field, E.J., Joyce, G. and Smith, B.M. (1977) Erythrocyte-UFA (EUFA) mobility test for multiple sclerosis: implications for pathogenesis and handling of the disease. *J. Neurol.*, 214: 113–127.

Forrester, J.A. and Smith, W.J. (1977) Screening of children at risk of multiple sclerosis. *Lancet*, ii: 453–454.

Hawkins, S.A. and Millar, J.H.D. (1979) Erythrocyte electrophoretic mobility test for multiple sclerosis. *Lancet*, i: 165–166.

Homa, S.T., Belin, J., Smith, A.D., Monro, J.A. and Zilkha, K.J. (1979) Levels of linoleate and anachidonate in red blood cells of healthy individuals and patients with multiple sclerosis. *J. Neurol. Neurosurg. Psychiat.*, 43: 106–110.

Huddlestone, J.R. and Oldstone, M.B.A. (1979) T Suppressor (Tg) Lymphocytes fluctuate in parallel with changes in the clinical course of patients with multiple sclerosis. *J. Immunol.*, 123: 1615–1618.

Jones, R., Capildeo, R., Clifford Rose, F., Forrester, J.A., Luckman, N.P. and Preece, A.W. (1981) A diagnostic test for multiple sclerosis using glutataldehyde fixed erythrocytes and laser cytopherometry. A.W. Preece and P.A. Light (Eds.), *Cell Electrophoresis in Cancer and other Clinical Research*, Elsevier, North-Holland Biomedical Press, Amsterdam, pp. 189–195.

Kam-Hansen, S. (1979) Reduced number of active T cells in cerebrospinal fluid in multiple sclerosis. *Neurology*, 29: 897–899.

Kam-Hansen, S. (1980) Distribution and function of lymphocytes from the cerebrospinal fluid and blood in patients with multiple sclerosis. *Acta neurol. scand.*, 62. Suppl. 75.

Lisak, R.P. (1980) Multiple sclerosis: evidence for immunopathogenesis. *Neurology*, 30: 99–105.

Plum, C.M. and Fog, T. (1959) Studies in multiple sclerosis, *Acta neurol. scand.*, 34. Suppl. 128.

Preece, A.W. and Luckman, N.P. (1981) A laser doppler cytopherometer for measurement of electrophoretic mobility of bioparticles. *Phys. Med. Biol.*, 26: 11–18.

Preece, A.W. and Luckman, N.P. (1981) Differential doppler microelectrophoresis. In A.W. Preece and P.A. Light (Eds.), *Cell Electrophoresis in Cancer and other Clinical Research*, Elsevier/North - Holland Biomedical Press, Amsterdam, pp. 295–298.

Prineas, J. (1968) Red blood cell size in multiple sclerosis. *Acta neurol. scand.*, 44: 81–90.

Reinherz, E.L., Weiner, H.L., Hauser, S.L., Cohen, J.A., Distaso, J.A. and Schlossman, S.F. (1980) Loss of suppressor T cells in active multiple sclerosis. *New Engl. J. Med.*, 303: 125–129.

Schauf, C.L., Frischer, M. and Davis, F.A. (1980) Mechanical fragility of erythrocytes in multiple sclerosis. *Neurology*, 30: 323–324.

Seaman, G.V.F., Swank, R.L. and Zukoski, C.F. (1979) Red cell membrane differences in multiple sclerosis are acquired from plasma. *Lancet*, i: 1139.

Stasiw, D.M., Rosato, S. and Mazza, J. (1977) Quantitative osmotic fragility and disease states: a preliminary study. *J. Lab. clin. Med.*, 89: 409–413.

Stoof, J.C., Vrijmoed de Vries, M.C., Koetsier, J.C. and Langevoort, H.L. (1977) Evaluation of the red blood cell cytopherometric test for the diagnosis of multiple sclerosis. *Acta neurol. scand.*, 56: 170–176.

Tamblyn, C.H., Swank, R.L., Seaman, G.V.F. and Zukoski, C.F. (1980) Red cell electrophoretic mobility test for early diagnosis of multiple sclerosis. *Neurol. Res.*, 2: 69–83

Thompson, R.H.S. (1966) A biochemical approach to the problem of multiple sclerosis. *Proc. roy. Soc. Med.*, 59: 269–276.

338

Vandenbark, A.A., Hallum, J.V., Swank, R.L., Tong, A. and Burger, D.R. (1979) Myelin basic protein binding cells in active multiple sclerosis. *Ann. Neurol.*, 6: 8–12.

Zukoski, C.F., Tamblyn, C.H., Swank, R.L. and Seaman, G.V.F. (1979) The basis for the unsaturated fatty acid red cell electrophoretic mobility test for multiple sclerosis. In A.W. Preece and D. Sabolovic (Eds.), *Cell Electrophoresis: Clinical Application and Methodology*, Elsevier/North-Holland Biomedical Press, Amsterdam, pp. 303–312.

Immunology of Nervous System Infections, Progress in Brain Research, Vol. 59, edited by P.O. Behan, V. ter Meulen and F. Clifford Rose

Immunoregulation in Multiple Sclerosis

HOWARD L. WEINER and STEPHEN L. HAUSER

Department of Neuroscience, Children's Hospital Medical Center and Department of Medicine, Section of Neurology, Brigham and Women's Hospital, Boston, MA 02115 (U.S.A.)

INTRODUCTION

A large body of evidence suggests that multiple sclerosis (MS) is an autoimmune disease that in some way may be related to a viral infection (Weiner, 1978).

To determine whether abnormalities of immunoregulatory T-cells were associated with multiple sclerosis, we characterized peripheral lymphocytes in 33 patients with untreated MS and compared them with 42 normal persons and 29 age-matched control subjects who had other neurological diseases (Reinherz et al., 1980). For this analysis, we used monoclonal antibodies to the surface antigens of helper (T4) and suppressor (T5) T-cell subsets and to a common T-cell antigen (T3). In contrast to normal persons and the controls with other neurologic diseases, the patients with MS had a reduced percentage of T3-positive (T3$^+$) cells ($P < 0.05$). More importantly, there was a selective decrease in T5-positive (T5$^+$) cells in 11 of 15 patients with active MS, but in only one of 18 patients with inactive MS and in none of the normal persons or controls with neurologic disease ($P < 0.00001$). Serial analysis of 5 patients with MS showed a correlation between the absence of the T5$^+$ subset and disease activity. Thus, there is loss of peripheral suppressor cells in many patients with active MS, suggesting that immunoregulatory abnormalities may contribute to the pathogenesis of the disease.

MATERIALS AND METHODS

Following these initial studies, a major question related to the precise relationship between suppressor cell abnormalities and disease activity. For this study we performed serial analysis of T-cell subsets in 4 ambulatory MS patients chosen specifically because they had relapsing remitting disease with a minimum of two attacks within the previous year. Four age-matched healthy controls were studied concurrently (Hauser et al., 1983). Weekly analysis of T-cell subsets was performed for a 6-month period in both patients and controls. Each MS patient underwent a detailed neurological examination at the onset of the study, was interviewed weekly at the time blood was drawn, and when appropriate, neurological examination was repeated. Interpretation of T-cell subset data was done without knowledge of the patient's clinical status. Results were expressed as a T4:T8 ratio, which represents the ratio of helper cells to suppressor/cytotoxic cells. (The T8 monoclonal has replaced the T5 monoclonal as a marker of the suppressor/cytotoxic cell).

In the 4 control subjects this ratio ranged between 1.4 and 3 and was less than 4 on every occasion. Based on a large number of normals and patients studied, a T4:T8 ratio less than 4 is considered normal (Weiner and Hauser, 1982). Flu-like viral illnesses or menstrual periods were not associated with changes in subset ratios. The first MS patient, a 24-year-old woman, was neurologically stable during the study period and had no abnormalities of T-cell subsets. Patient 2, a 36-year-old woman, had abnormalities of T-cell subsets associated with fatigue and numbness of the right upper extremity, and then normal subset ratios until one week prior to an attack, at which time an abnormal ratio was found. Patient 3, a 22-year-old man, had multiple clinical symptoms during the study, although subsets ratios were abnormal on only 3 occasions, twice associated with fatigue, and once preceding a major attack. Of note is that many of the symptoms that the patient reported were signs and symptoms that he had experienced previously. The fourth patient was the most seriously ill patient, who, during the 6 month period, had multiple attacks and suffered severe deterioration of functional status. During this period, his T4:T8 ratio was elevated on 12 of 27 occasions and fluctuated widely, more than in any other patient or control.

RESULTS

In summary then, this study demonstrates that episodic elevations of T4:T8 ratios were present in multiple sclerosis patients and not in controls. Although not correlating 100% with each attack in every patient, the frequency of these elevations correlated well with clinical disease activity and, in some instances, preceded attacks by 1.5–7 days. On no occasion did subset changes precede an exacerbation by more than one week. These results suggest that an elevated ratio may appear during the preclinical phase of an acute attack and suggests that subset changes may be linked to the earliest events in the pathogenesis of new MS lesions.

Although speculative, it is possible to interpret the T-cell subset correlations we observed in the context of current knowledge of the pathophysiology of MS. One patient had developed a variety of symptoms without T4:T8 elevations. It is well known that new symptoms in a patient with established MS do not always imply new white matter lesions, but may be due to physiologic changes in conduction across a region of old demyelination. The absence of changes of immunoregulatory cells in this patient is consistent with the hypothesis that changes in conduction, rather than new foci of disease, were responsible for these short-lived, relatively minor worsenings. In two instances an elevated ratio was associated primarily with fatigue. Fatigue is a well-known symptom in MS and has never been adequately explained. Our data suggest the possibility that fatigue may reflect an immunologically active state. The finding of fatigue with T-cell subset changes in patients with MS may relate to subclinical foci of demyelination in silent regions of the neuraxis. Finally, it is possible that the mechanism of immune damage in multiple sclerosis may not be the same in all patients, involving changes in suppressor cells that can be measured in the peripheral blood in some patients, while in others involving a yet undefined mechanism.

Suppressor cells in childhood MS

We have recently studied 3 children with multiple sclerosis beginning at 4, 10 and 3 years of age (Hauser et al., 1982a). Clinical symptoms included a relapsing brainstem syndrome in the first, Devic's syndrome and recurrent optic neuritis in the second, and multiple attacks with accumulating neurological deficits in the third child. Two of these children represent the youngest cases of MS yet reported. In each child, circulating suppressor/cytotoxic cells as measured by monoclonal antibodies were reduced or absent during acute exacerbations of disease. Following disease stabilization, there was a return of suppressor/cytotoxic cells and a normalization of the T4:T8 ratio. No changes in T-cell subsets were seen in a group of age-matched healthy children or children suffering from other neurological diseases. Our findings that young children with active MS have an identical pattern of T-cell abnormalities as adult patients suggests that the same pathophysiological process which causes MS in adults may occur in young children as well.

TABLE I

ANALYSIS OF T-CELL SUBSETS IN NEUROLOGIC DISEASE

Results are expressed as mean +S.E.M. The T4:T5/8 ratio reflects the relative numbers of helper to suppressor T-cells in the peripheral blood. In normal individuals, the T4:T5/8 ratio is less than 4. Active MS = 17 patients in acute relapse and 40 patients with chronic progressive MS. Other neurological diseases: includes vascular, inflammatory, infectious, degenerative and malignant diseases.

Patient group	% Reactivity with monoclonal antibodies			T4:T5/8 ratio	
	T3	T4	T5/8	<4	>4
Normals (n = 40)	67 ± 3	41 ± 2	20 ± 5	42	0
Active multiple sclerosis (n = 57)	46 ± 4*	35 ± 3	11 ± 2**	24	33***
Acute Guillain–Barre (n = 12)	64 ± 4	47 ± 5	20 ± 2	12	0
Acute myasthenia gravis (n = 12)	50 ± 5	35 ± 5	19 ± 2	11	1
Other neurological diseases (n = 26)	53 ± 4	34 ± 2	17 ± 2	26	0

* $P = <0.05$ between MS and normal controls.
** $P = <0.00001$ (Fisher's exact test) between MS and normal controls.
*** 14 of 17 patients in acute relapse and 19 of 40 patients with chronic progressive disease had abnormal T4:T5/8 ratios.

Immunoregulatory T-cell changes in other disease processes

The changes in immunoregulatory T-cells that we and other investigators (Antel et al., 1979; Huddlestone and Oldstone, 1979; Bach et al., 1980) have observed are the first immune aberrations in MS to be so clearly linked to disease activity. The aberration can be measured in the peripheral blood and may ultimately provide an insight into the pathogenesis of the disease. Reduced numbers of circulating suppressor cells are not seen in a variety of other neurological diseases (malignant, infectious, vascular) and thus far we have not found them in two other presumably autoimmune diseases of the nervous system, myasthenia gravis and acute inflammatory polyneuritis (Guillain–Barre syndrome) (see Table I). Similar changes are seen, however, in systemic lupus erythematosus, graft vs host disease, acute renal graft rejection, and hemolytic anemia, demonstrating that these changes are common to a number of autoimmune diseases which do not affect the nervous system (reviewed in Weiner and Hauser, 1982).

DISCUSSION

What do changes in suppressor cells in the peripheral blood of MS patients mean?

The loss of suppressor cells with disease activity in MS cannot itself explain the specificity of white matter injury. An entire subset of regulatory T-cells is decreased, representing thousands of clones, each with a unique idiotype and clonally restricted specificity. If T-cell subset changes play a primary role in the pathogenesis of MS (something as yet unproven), one possible explanation for the specificity of injury is that the loss of suppressor influence on the immune system allows previously primed cells which have specificity for CNS white matter to escape immune regulation, migrate to the CNS, and cause injury. The specific immune mechanisms which are activated following a loss of T-suppressor cells may be determined by a combination of prior environmental exposure and an individual's immune response genes. This may explain why a loss of suppressor cells might result in MS in some people and lupus in others.

Where do the suppressor cells go and what does their loss mean? One possibility is that they are destroyed. In lupus, autoantibodies exist which react with the T5/8 subset. Lymphocyto-toxic antibodies exist in MS (Schocket et al., 1977), and a variety of white matter-specific autoantibodies have been reported as well (Weiner, 1978), although their significance is not clear. We have been unable to find antibodies in MS sera that react with isolated T-cell subsets in vitro. There is no evidence at this time that autoantibodies against suppressor cells play a pathophysiological role in the loss of suppressor cells from the blood of MS patients. A second possibility is that the suppressor cells migrate to the CNS where they are effector cells for the autoimmune response. Although it has thus far not been possible to characterize T-cell subsets in acute MS plaques, evaluation of CSF from patients with active MS has failed to show large numbers of T5/8 cells. (Hauser et al., in press). Recent data suggest, however, that in some disease processes, one or another T-cell subset may selectively accumulate in target organs, although these changes as yet show no consistent pattern. Two examples are as follows: (1) in pulmonary sarcoidosis a decrease in T4+ inducer cells in peripheral blood is associated with sequestration of activated T4+ cells in the lung (Hunninghake and Crystal, 1981); and (2) a young woman with an acute demyelinative encephalomyelitis who had normal peripheral blood T-cell subsets was found to have a perivascular CNS infiltrate consisting primarily of T8 cells (Weiner, unpublished observations). In two children with dermatomyositis, on the other hand, a loss of circulating T8 cells was associated with a mixed T-cell subset infiltrate in muscle, suggesting that in this disease, T8-cells were not selectively sequestered (Bresnan et al., 1981). Our current hypothesis is that in active MS, T5/8 cells may be sequestered in an extravascular site, perhaps in lymphoid tissue.

In summary, the mechanism by which immunoregulatory cells change in the peripheral blood of patients with certain autoimmune diseases and their role in the pathogenesis of these diseases, remain major biological questions. It is probable that these changes are secondary phenomena in some diseases and primarily linked to the genesis of the autoimmune response in others.

ACKNOWLEDGEMENTS

Supported by Grant NSI7182 from the NIH; S.L.H. is a fellow of the National Multiple Sclerosis Society.

REFERENCES

Antel, J.P., Arnason, B.G.W. and Medof, M.E. (1979) Suppressor cell function in multiple sclerosis: correlation with disease activity. *Ann. Neurol.,* 5: 338–43.

Bach, M.A., Phan-Dinh-Toy, F., Tournier, E., Chatenoud, L. and Bach, J.F. (1980) Deficit of suppressor T cells in active multiple sclerosis. *Lancet,* 2: 1221–1223.

Bresnan, M.B., Hauser, S.L., Weiner, H.L., Reinherz, E.L., Borel, Y. and Bhan, A. (1981) Characterization of T lymphocyte subsets in peripheral blood and muscle in childhood dermatomyositis. *Ann. Neurol.,* 10: 283 (Abstr.).

Hauser, S.L., Bresnan, M.J., Reinherz, E.L. and Weiner, H.L. (1982a) Childhood multiple sclerosis; clinical features and demonstration of T-cell subset changes with disease activity. *Ann. Neurol.,* 11: 463–468.

Hauser, S.L., Reinherz, E.L., Hoban, C.J., Schlossman, S.F. and Weiner, H.L. (1982b) Analysis of CSF mononuclear cells in multiple sclerosis using monoclonal antibodies: correlation with disease activity and peripheral blood T cell subset changes. *Neurology,* in press.

Hauser, S.L., Reinherz, E.L. and Weiner, H.L. (1981) Serial studies of immunoregulatory abnormalities in active multiple sclerosis. *Ann. Neurol.,* in press.

Huddlestone, J.R. and Oldstone, M.B.A. (1979) T suppressor (T_G) lymphocytes fluctuate in parallel with changes in the clinical course of patients with multiple sclerosis. *J. Immunol.,* 123: 1615–18.

Hunninghake, G.W. and Crystal, R.G.K. (1981) Pulmonary sarcoidosis. A disorder mediated by excess helper T lymphocyte activity at sites of disease activity. *New Engl. J. Med.,* 305: 429–39.

Schocket, A.L., Weiner, H.L., Walker, J. et al. (1977) Lymphocytotoxic antibodies in multiple sclerosis. *Clin. Immun. Immunopathol.,* 7: 15–23.

Weiner, H.L. (1978) Multiple sclerosis. In H.R. Tyler and D.M. Dawson (Eds.) *Current Neurology,* Houghton-Mifflin, Boston, pp. 53–85.

Weiner, H.L. and Hauser, S.L. (1982) Neuroimmunology I. Immunoregulation in neurologic disease. *Ann. Neurol.,* 11: 437–449.

Immunology of Nervous System Infections, Progress in Brain Research, Vol. 59, edited by P.O. Behan, V. ter Meulen and F. Clifford Rose

Humoral and Cellular Immune Responses to Staphylococcal Lipoteichoic Acid in Multiple Sclerosis Patients

HARALD NYLAND and PER AASJORD

Department of Neurology, Broegelmann Research Laboratory for Microbiology and Department of Microbiology and Immunology, The Gade Institute, University of Bergen, Bergen (Norway)

INTRODUCTION

The possibility that multiple sclerosis is due to an infectious agent has been the subject of numerous studies over the years. Pierre Marie (1884) first emphasized the relationship to infectious diseases, especially enteric fever. Almost all classes of micro-organisms have been suggested as causative at one time or another, including protozoa, spirochetes, rickettsia, bacteria and viruses (Prineas, 1970). The precipitating agent(s) in multiple sclerosis is still not known. Epidemiological evidence including the geographical distribution, the data on migrating populations and the age-of-onset curve strongly suggest involvement of one or more infectious agents in the initiation of the disease process. The causative agent(s) may be widespread and exposure may occur in childhood with a long asymptomatic period before clinical onset (Prineas, 1970).

The tissue lesions in multiple sclerosis seem to be of an autoimmune type, with activated macrophages and infiltrating T-lymphocytes (Nyland et al., 1981b). The immunopathological response in the central nervous system (CNS) may be caused by a remote microbial infection (Dumonde, 1979). McAlpine and Compston (1952) have demonstrated a statistically significant incidence of skin infections preceding attacks of multiple sclerosis. Poskanzer (1965) found that a group of multiple sclerosis patients had had tonsillectomies more often than their siblings. Multiple sclerosis is associated with disordered immune regulation as revealed by peripheral blood T-lymphocytopenia (Nyland and Naess, 1978), fluctuating T-suppressor cell

TABLE I

MODULATION OF IMMUNE RESPONSES BY BACTERIAL PRODUCTS

Polyclonal B-cell activators
Staphylococcus aureus
protein A
peptidoglycan
Escherichia coli
Lipopolysaccharide (LPS)
Purified protein derivative of tuberculin (PPD)
T-cell mitogen
Lipoteichoic acid (LTA)

levels (Arnason and Antel, 1978), increased numbers of cerebrospinal fluid (CSF) T-helper cells (Oger et al., 1981) and local synthesis of IgG with a number of antibody specificities (Vandvik et al., 1976; Vartdal et al., 1980; Salmi et al., 1981). Experimental evidence obtained during the last 10 years has revealed that a number of bacterial products are potent modulators of immune responses (Raziuddin et al., 1981; Rindgén et al., 1979) (Table I). They may both enhance and suppress antibody production, and in addition, they may serve as immunological nonspecific mitogens, as B- and/or T-cell activators.

During our work on lipoteichoic acid (LTA) from staphylococcus aureus bacteria, it appeared that LTA could be a possible candidate for the explanation of the disordered immune regulation which is observed in multiple sclerosis patients.

LTA OF GRAM-POSITIVE BACTERIA

Lipoteichoic acids (LTA) are a group pf phosphate-containing polymers associated with the plasma membranes of Gram-positive bacteria (Wicken and Knox, 1975). LTA are amphipathic molecules characterized by both a hydrophilic and a hydrophobic region. They consist of phosphodiester-linked chains of 25–30 glycerol phosphate residues substituted with glucosyl and D-alanyl ester groups (Wicken and Knox, 1975). The lipid moiety is a glycolipid. LTA have a number of potential antigenic determinants; the glycerolphosphate backbone, the carbohydrate and D-alanyl substituents, and the glycolipid. Antibodies directed against the glycolipid have not been found, but glycolipids seem to be necessary for the immune response of the molecule. LTA is released from the bacteria during rapid growth (Alkan and Beachey, 1978). Thus humans may be exposed continuously to LTA released from the normal streptococcal and staphylococcal flora. In addition, LTA also has other biological properties. LTA can activate the alternative pathway of complement, participate in bone resorption, suppress the immune responses in mice, stimulate carbon clearance by the reticular endothelial system, and stimulate the release of lysosomal enzymes from macrophages (Courtney et al., 1981; Miller et al., 1976). The biological activities of LTA seem to be dependent on their membrane-binding properties via the lipid part of the molecule.

STAPHYLOCOCCAL LTA

In our experiments staphylococcal aureus strain Cowan I (NCTC 8530) was used for the preparation of LTA. The isolation and chemical characterization was carried out as described by Aasjord and Grov (1978a). This LTA had both glucosyl and alanyl substituents. The major fatty acid present was a C-15. Antisera to LTA were raised in New Zealand white rabbits and tested in the double diffusion in agar and by indirect haemagglutination (Aasjord and Grov, 1978a). Only IgM antibodies were formed when the antigen was introduced to rabbits.

ENCEPHALITIS IN RABBITS IMMUNIZED WITH STAPHYLOCOCCAL LTA

During our immunization programme with staphylococcal LTA in Freund's adjuvant, 2 of 5 rabbits developed clinical signs of encephalitis (Aasjord et al., 1980). The first effects appeared after the fourth injection (6 weeks), when the rabbits showed minor clinical symptoms with decreased motor activity and unsteadiness of the head with slow, turning movements. After the sixth injection (10 weeks) additional symptoms appeared, such as nystagmus, ataxia and dragging of the hind legs. Coronal sections of the brain showed patchy inflammatory infiltrates in the leptomeninges and around brain vessels, consisting of small lymphocytes and plasma cells, but without demyelination. It has been reported that inflammatory lesions within the brain can be induced by non-brain antigens as a so-called bystander effect. Recently, immunization with extracts from human glioma lacking myelin basic protein, has been shown to induce an inflammatory encephalitis in rabbits (Bigner et al., 1981). After the conclusion of our studies, it was found that some of our laboratory animals were sero-positive for encephalitozoon cuniculi. However, the rabbits had no histopathological organ lesions which might indicate a generalized protozoal infection. Nevertheless, the immunization procedure may have altered the immune responsiveness of the animals and activated a latent protozoal infection.

ANTIBODIES TO STAPHYLOCOCCAL LTA IN HUMAN SERUM AND CEREBROSPINAL FLUID

A group of patients with definite multiple sclerosis and a group of normal individuals were examined serologically (Aasjord and Nyland, 1981). In the Agar precipitation test, 48 out of 94 control sera (51%) produced a line against LTA, while 11 out of 74 (15%) multiple sclerosis sera did so. Gel filtration showed that only immunoglobulins of the IgG class were involved in the precipitation test. $F(ab')_2$ fragments of IgG prepared from positive multiple sclerosis serum precipitated with LTA, indicating an antigen–antibody reaction. An indirect haemagglutination assay (IHA) was performed with sheep erythrocytes sensitized with LTA, and antibodies were determined in sera and in unconcentrated cerebrospinal fluid (CSF) using a microtitration technique (Fossan, 1976). Titers in 20 control sera ranged from 160 to 10,240, while the titers in sera from 20 multiple sclerosis patients ranged from 160 to 2560 (Table II).

TABEL II

INDIRECT HAEMAGGLUTINATION OF LTA-SENSITIZED SHEEP ERYTHROCYTES BY HUMAN SERA: DISTRIBUTION OF NUMBER OF SERA ACCORDING TO TITERS

Serum from	Titers in indirect haemagglutination test						
	160	320	640	1280	2560	5120	10,240
MS patients	4	4	6	5	1	0	0
Controls	1	2	4	3	4	3	3

The demonstration of a reduced frequency of precipitating antibodies to LTA and a higher incidence of low antibody titers in the IHA in sera from multiple sclerosis patients, is in good accordance with the results reported by Uyeda et al. (1966). Significantly lower anti-beta-haemolysin titers were observed in patients with multiple sclerosis as compared to patients with other neurological disorders. Uyeda et al. (1966) and Sibley and Foley (1966) found antistreptolysin titers in multiple sclerosis to be within the normal range indicating that the patients do not have a generalized immunological incompetence. The findings may indicate that multiple sclerosis patients are incapable of making an adequate antibody response to staphylococcal antigens.

TABLE III

INDIRECT HAEMAGGLUTINATION OF LTA-SENSITIZED SHEEP ERYTHROCYTES BY HUMAN CSF:
DISTRIBUTION OF NUMBER OF CSFs ACCORDING TO TITERS

CSF from	Titers in indirect haemagglutination test								
	<0.25	0.25	0.5	1	2	4	8	16	32
MS patients	0	0	1	1	4	6	5	2	1
Controls	2	3	1	2	12	0	0	0	0

All the unconcentrated multiple sclerosis CSF samples contained detectable antibodies to LTA in the IHA, with titers varying from 0.5 to 32. Of the 20 control CSF, 18 contained detectable antibodies with titers varying from 0.25 to 2 (Table III). Naturally occurring antibodies to rabbit erythrocytes were used as marker proteins for the blood–brain barrier function (Fossan, 1976). The multiple sclerosis patients had normal ratios of serum to CSF for antibodies to rabbit erythrocytes, indicating an intact blood–brain barrier. The ratio of serum to CSF for anti-LTA antibodies was then calculated for each of the multiple sclerosis patients. A 4-fold or greater difference was found in 7 out of 20 multiple sclerosis patients, suggesting local synthesis within the CNS of anti-LTA antibodies. Vartdal et al. (1980) and Salmi et al. (1981) have demonstrated local synthesis of antibodies to other bacterial antigens in CNS of some multiple sclerosis patients. The demonstration of local antibody synthesis does not necessarily reflect an etiological relationship between the respective infectious agent and the disease. The antibody production may be a co-phenomenon of a humoral immune response localized to CNS, which in turn could be the result of a polyclonal activation induced by ligands acting non-specifically on T- and/or B-lymphocytes (Möller et al., 1980).

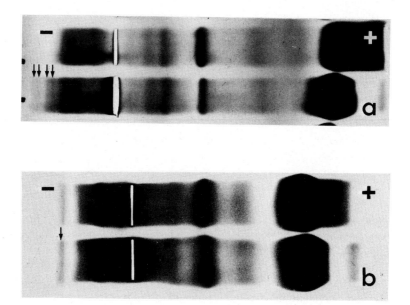

Fig. 1. Agarose electrophoresis of two CSF samples containing oligoclonal IgG bands (arrows) before and after (upper a and b) absorption with LTA. a: CSF sample from an MS patient. b: CSF sample from a patient with serous meningitis of presumed viral etiology.

Absorption of multiple sclerosis CSF was carried out according to the method of Vandvik et al. (1976). LTA was mixed with the CSF, and after incubation the mixture was centrifuged and the supernatant concentrated to 10–20 mg IgG/ml, and then studied by agarose electrophoresis (Aasjord and Nyland, 1982). Control CSF was treated in the same way. Electrophoresis showed that the most cathodic oligoclonal bands from the multiple sclerosis CSF samples had been removed (Fig. 1a). Oligoclonal bands in CSF samples from 4 control patients, 2 with the diagnosis of serous meningitis, one with neurosyphilis and one with chronic polyneuritis showed no change after the absorption (Fig. 1b). Determination of IgG in the 7 multiple sclerosis CSF samples showed a reduction of 13–25% after absorption. The titers of agglutinating antibodies to LTA in these samples ranged from 4 to 32. CSF from 3 patients were available for IHA titration after absorption. One showed a reduction in titer from 32 to 0.25, and 2 from 16 to 2. Together the results indicated that locally synthesized antibodies to LTA are associated with oligoclonal CSF IgG. The possibility exists, however, that the oligoclonal IgG are adsorbed non-specifically to LTA due to the high negative charge of this molecule (Wicken and Knox, 1975). The antibody specificities of the major IgG bands have not been identified, although a small fraction of the locally produced IgG carries antibody activities against several different viruses (Vandvik et al., 1976; Vartdal et al., 1980). Tourtelotte et al. (1981) have recently reported an absorption in the range of 3–45% of multiple sclerosis CSF IgG by a homogenate of multiple sclerosis brain, while no more than 3% absorption was obtained with control brain. These results have been interpreted as presence of a specific multiple sclerosis antigen.

CELL-MEDIATED IMMUNITY TO STAPHYLOCOCCAL LTA

Lipoteichoic acid binds to a variety of animal cells (Ofek et al., 1975; Beachey et al., 1977; Beachey et al., 1979b; Courtney et al., 1981). Beachey et al. (1979b) have recently shown that streptococcal LTA binds to human lymphocytes and has a mitogenic effect on T-lymphocytes. We have studied the interaction of staphylococcal LTA with peripheral blood lymphocytes isolated from multiple sclerosis patients, patients with other neurological diseases (OND) and normal controls (Nyland et al., 1981a). Mononuclear cells were separated from heparinized peripheral blood by Ficoll–Isopaque gradient centrifugation. Lymphocytes bearing receptors for sheep erythrocytes (E) were determined using rosette procedures. The number of active (early) T-lymphocytes was determined as described by Wybran and Fudenberg (1973). The active E-rosette test (AER) was performed as described by Felsburg and Edelman (1977). This test is a sensitive in vitro substitute for the conventional skin test for cell-mediated immunity. Fcγ-receptor and complement receptor-positive cells were enumerated with rosette assays as described by Matre et al. (1977). The mononuclear cells were stimulated in vitro with the mitogens phytohaemagglutinin (PHA), concanavalin A (Con A), pokeweed mitogen (PWM), and staphylococcal aureus (SA) in various concentrations using a microculture system as described by Steel and Creasey (1976).

The binding of LTA to the lymphocyte was studied by preincubating cells from normal individuals with LTA in the concentration of 10 and 100 μg/ml, and performing rosette tests before and after the incubation. E-receptors were almost completely blocked, showing a reduction in the number of rosette-forming cells from 40% to 5%. Similarly, LTA blocked the complement receptors and the Fcγ receptors, but not to the same extent. The percentage of rosette-forming cells was reduced from 25% to 16% and from 32% to 12%, respectively. The

350

TABLE IV

MITOGENIC RESPONSE OF LYMPHOID CELLS TO PHYTOHAEMAGGLUTININ (PHA), POKEWEED MITOGEN (PWM), CONCANAVALIN A (Con A), STAPHYLOCOCCUS AUREUS (SA) AND STAPHYLOCOCCAL LIPOTEICHOIC ACID (LTA) (COUNTS/MIN, INCREMENT)

		MS		OND		Normals	
		Mean value	Range	Mean value	Range	Mean value	Range
PHA	2.5 μg/ml	10,836	(2272–25,839)	9610	(1937–15,139)	6986	(3692–22,434)
PWM	6.0 μg/ml	4454	(2422–6434)	2687	(687–4132)	3269	(536–5245)
Con A	25.0 μg/ml	5500	(1881–12,568)	3043	(812–10,241)	3710	(637–12,985)
SA	1/256	1777	(81–4543)	1027	(97–3241)	1692	(137–5134)
LTA	0.001 μg/ml	3223	(730–6508)	1387	(72–2670)	2886	(305–4127)

data give evidence for the binding of LTA to both B- and T-lymphocytes, and correspond well to the data obtained with radiolabeled streptococcal LTA (Beachey et al., 1979a).

We then studied the mitogenic effect of LTA on human lymphocytes. LTA was mitogenic at a concentration as low as 0.0001 μg/microculture. Maximal stimulation was obtained with 0.001 μg (Table IV). Experiments were also performed with separated B- and T-lymphocytes. Only T-lymphocytes in the presence of monocytes were stimulated to a mitogenic response, while B-lymphocytes gave no detectable response. The selective stimulation of T-lymphocytes indicates the presence of distinct membrane receptors for LTA (Beachey et al., 1979b). When the multiple sclerosis patients were compared with OND patients and with the normal individuals, only minor differences were recorded (Table IV). Slightly higher stimulation by LTA occurred in the multiple sclerosis patients, but this difference was also observed using the mitogens PHA, Con A, PWM and SA. The data correspond well with other studies (McCrea et al., 1979; Platz et al., 1976) showing normal responses of peripheral blood lymphocytes from multiple sclerosis patients to mitogens.

The multiple sclerosis patients had significantly reduced numbers of active (early) T-cells as compared to the two control groups, $31.4 \pm 3.5\%$ vs $40.2 \pm 5.3\%$ for the OND group and $39.7 \pm 4.6\%$ for the normal individuals. This is in line with previous reports (Traugott et al., 1981). In our experiments the AER test was performed by incubating isolated mononuclear cells with 0.001, 0.01, 0.1 and 1 μg/ml of LTA, a homogenate of multiple sclerosis brain and a homogenate of normal brain (Offner et al., 1979). The lymphocytes were incubated for 4 h at 37°C. Responsiveness of lymphocytes to the antigens was indicated when there was an increase in the percentage of active (early) T-cells of at least 25% when compared to the percentage of active T-cells without antigen. Seven out of 14 multiple sclerosis patients showed a cellular sensitization to LTA, while none of the controls responded (Fig. 2).

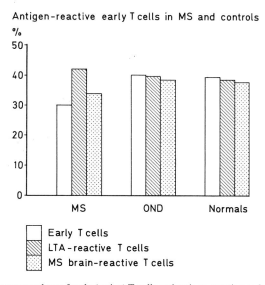

Fig. 2. Histogram showing mean values of early (active) T-cells and antigen-reactive early T-cells from patients with multiple sclerosis (MS) and other neurological diseases (OND), and from normal controls.

Dose–response curves showed that the optimal antigen dose was 0.001 μg. In addition, 3 of the multiple sclerosis patients showed a response to the multiple sclerosis brain homogenate, but not to normal brain homogenate. Using the AER test, Offner et al. (1979) found that multiple sclerosis lymphocytes were stimulated by multiple sclerosis brain homogenate, myelin basic protein, isolated brain cerebrosides and gangliosides from multiple sclerosis brains. Traugott et al. (1981) showed that multiple sclerosis lymphocytes responded to oligodendrocytes. However, a small number of the control patients in both of these studies reacted similarly to the antigens. An acidic extract from multiple sclerosis myelin appears to stimulate the multiple sclerosis lymphocytes specifically (Offner et al., 1979). They postulate the presence of a multiple sclerosis specific antigen which is responsible for this reaction. The reaction observed with the other brain antigens could represent an epiphenomenon associated with white matter destruction.

CONCLUSION

The possibility that a microbial infection could initiate the multiple sclerosis disease process has received considerable attention. The persistence of micro-organisms and/or the presence of their products causing immunological responses, may represent precipitating factors (Dumonde, 1979). Bacteria have not been likely candidates as infectious agents, but experimental studies in recent years have shown that bacterial products are potent modulators of immune responses.

During our studies of the immunobiological properties of LTA isolated from staphylococcal aureus, we observed that clinical and pathological signs of encephalitis developed in rabbits (Aasjord et al., 1980). The possibility that similar reactions may occur in humans led us to investigate the possible role of LTA in the pathogenesis of multiple sclerosis. In vitro experiments have shown that LTA is released from Gram-positive bacteria during growth, and over the years humans may be exposed to LTA from both the normal and the pathological streptococcal and staphylococcal flora. A number of immunobiological properties have been described for LTA (Wicken and Knox, 1975). Injection of LTA into the periodontal tissue of rats gave an intense inflammatory reaction (Bab et al., 1979), and hyperimmunization of rabbits with streptococcal LTA-induced nephritis (Fiedel and Jackson, 1979). Ofek et al. (1979) showed that LTA reacts with myelin basic protein isolated from bovine brain.

Our studies have shown that multiple sclerosis patients have an impaired humoral immune response to LTA. In addition, some of the patients showed cellular immunity to LTA by the active E-rosette test (Nyland et al., 1981b). LTA stimulated peripheral blood lymphocytes and appeared to be a T-lymphocyte mitogen. Multiple sclerosis is associated with increased numbers of CSF T-lymphocytes and locally synthesized oligoclonal IgG. Both phenomena could be explained by the stimulation of a T-lymphocyte mitogen which gives a secondary polyclonal B-lymphocyte activation (Bird et al., 1981; Möller et al., 1980). Together with the described local synthesis of anti-LTA antibodies (Aasjord and Nyland, 1981), this may indicate that LTA acts as a combined mitogen and immunogen in the multiple sclerosis CNS.

There is little clinical evidence that Gram-positive bacteria are the initiating infectious agents in multiple sclerosis. However, the geographic distribution of rheumatic fever and multiple sclerosis do show similarities, suggesting common pathogenetic mechanisms (Barlow, 1968). Furthermore, dental caries have epidemiological features in common with multiple sclerosis (Craelius, 1978). Several etiological factors are involved in dental caries, but LTA from Gram-positive oral bacteria probably play an important role for the initiation of the process (Rölla, 1977). Our investigations have focused on the possible relationship between LTA and multiple sclerosis. Naturally, further studies are needed before any conclusion can be drawn.

REFERENCES

Aasjord, P. and Grov, A. (1978a) Immunochemical studies on *Staphylococcus aureus* plasma membrane. 2. Antigenic properties. *Acta path. microbiol. scand.*, Sect. B, 86: 139–141.

Aasjord, P. and Grov, A. (1978b) Immunochemical studies on *Staphylococcus aureus* plasma membrane. 1. Isolation and chemical characterization. *Acta path. microbiol. scand.*, Sect. B, 86: 131–137.

Aasjord, P., Nyland, H. and Mörk, S. (1980) Encephalitis induced in rabbits by staphylococcal lipoteichoic acid. *Acta path. microbiol. scand.*, Sect. C, 88: 287–291.

Aasjord, P. and Nyland, H. (1982) Antibodies to staphylococcal lipoteichoic acid in serum and in cerebrospinal fluid from patients with multiple sclerosis. *Acta path. microbiol. scand.*, Sect. C, in press.

Arnason, B.G.W. and Antel, J. (1978) Suppressor cell function in multiple sclerosis. *Ann. Immunol.*, 129C: 159–170.

Alkan, M.L. and Beachey, E.H. (1978) Excretion of lipoteichoic acid by group A Streptococci. *J. clin. Invest.*, 61: 671–677.

Bab, I.A., Sela, M.N., Ginsburg, I. and Dishon, T. (1979) Inflammatory lesions and bone resorption induced in the rat periodontium by lipoteichoic acid of Streptococcus mutans. *Inflammation*, 3: 345–358.

Barlow, J.S. (1968) Comparative geography of rheumatic fever and rheumatic heart disease, multiple sclerosis, and rheumatoid arthritis. *J. chron. Dis.*, 21: 265–279.

Beachey, E.H., Chiang, T.J. Ofek, I. and Kang, A.H. (1977) Interaction of lipoteichoic acid of group A streptococci with human platelets. *Infect. Immun.*, 16: 649–654.

Beachey, E.H., Dale, J.B., Grebe, S., Ahmed, A., Simpson, A.W. and Ofek, I. (1979a) Lymphocyte binding and T cell mitogenic properties of group A streptococcal lipoteichoic acid. *J. Immunol.*, 122: 189–195.

Beachey, E.H., Dale, J.B., Simpson, W.A., Evans, J.D., Knox, W.K., Ofek, I. and Wicken, A.J. (1979b) Erythrocyte binding properties of streptococcal lipoteichoic acid. *Infect. Immun.*, 23: 618–625.

Bigner, D.D., Pitts, O.M. and Wikstrand, C.J. (1981) Induction of lethal experimental allergic encephalomyelitis in nonhuman primates and guinea pigs with human glioblastoma multiforme tissue. *J. Neurosurg.*, 55: 32–42.

Bird, A.G. Hammarstrøm, L., Smith, C.I.E. and Britton, S. (1981) Polyclonal human T lymphocyte activation results in the secondary functional activation of human B lymphocytes. *Clin. exp. Immunol.*, 43: 165–173.

Courtney, H., Ofek, I., Simpson, W.A. and Beachey, E.H. (1981) Characterization of lipoteichoic acid binding to polymorphonuclear leucocytes of human blood. *Infect. Immun.*, 32: 625–631.

Craelius, W. (1978) Comparative epidemiology of multiple sclerosis and dental caries. *J. Epid. Comm. Health*, 32: 155–165.

Dumonde, D.C. (1979) The paradox of immunity and infection in multiple sclerosis. In F.C. Rose (Ed.), *Clinical Neuroimmunology*, Blackwell Scientific Publications, Oxford, pp. 275–298.

Felsburg, P.J. and Edelman, R. (1977) The active E-rosette test: a sensitive in vitro correlate for human delayed-type hypersensitivity. *J. Immunol.*, 118: 62–66.

Fiedel, B.A. and Jackson, R.W. (1979) Nephropathy in the rabbit associated with immunization to a group A streptococcal lipoteichoic acid. *Med. Microbiol. Immunol.*, 167: 251–260.

Fossan, G.O. (1976) The transfer of IgG from serum to CSF, evaluated by means of a naturally occurring antibody. *Europ. Neurol.*, 15: 231–236.

Marie, P. (1884) Sclérose en plaque et maladie infectieuses. *Progr. méd.*, 12: 287–365.

Matre, R., Talstad, I. and Haugen, Å. (1977) Surface markers in non-phagocytic hairy cell leukemia. *Acta path. microbiol. scand.*, Sect. C, 85: 406–412.

McAlpine, D. and Compston, N. (1952) Some aspects of the natural history of disseminated sclerosis. *Quart. J. Med.*, 21: 135–167.

McCrea, S., Killen, M., Thompson, J., Fleming, W.A., McNeill, T.A. and Millar, J.H.D. (1979) Tests on peripheral blood cells in multiple sclerosis. *Ulster Med. J.*, 48: 83–90.

Miller, G.A., Urban, J. and Jackson, R.W. (1976) Effects of streptococcal lipoteichoic acid on host responses in mice. *Infect. Immun.*, 13: 1408–1417.

Möller, E., Ström, H. and Al-Balaghi, S. (1980) Role of polyclonal activation in specific immune responses. Relevance for findings of antibody activity in various diseases. *Scand. J. Immunol.*, 12: 177–182.

Nyland, H. and Naess, A. (1978) T lymphocytes in peripheral blood from patients with neurological diseases. *Acta neurol. scand.*, 58: 272–279.

Nyland, H., Aasjord, P. and Naess, A. (1981a) Lymphocyte responsiveness to staphylococcal lipoteichoic acid. *Acta path. microbiol. scand.*, Sect. C, in press.

Nyland, H., Matre, R. and Mörk, S. (1981b) Characterization of mononuclear cell infiltrates in the multiple sclerosis lesion. *Acta neurol. scand.*, 63: 141.

Ofek, I., Whitaker, J.N., Campbell, G.L. and Beachey, E.H. (1979) Interaction of group A streptococcal lipoteichoic acid with bovine myelin basic protein. *J. infect. Dis.*, 139: 93–96.

354

Offner, H., Rastogi, S.C., Konat, G. and Clausen, J. (1979) Stimulation of active E-rosette forming lymphocytes by myelin basic protein and specific antigens from multiple sclerosis brains. *J. neurol. Sci.*, 42: 349–355.

Offner, H. and Konat, G. (1980) Stimulation of active E-rosette forming lymphocytes from multiple sclerosis patients by gangliosides and cerebrosides. *J. neurol. Sci.*, 46: 101–104.

Oger, J.J.-F., Antel, J.P., Jackevicius, S., Noronha, A.B.C. and Arnason, B.G.W. (1981) Increased CSF T-helper cell subpopulation in active multiple sclerosis. In *Proceedings of the 12th World Congress of Neurology (Excerpta Medica International Congress Series, no. 548)*, Excerpta Medica, Amsterdam, p. 177.

Platz, P., Fog, T., Morling, N., Svejgaard, A., Sönderstrup, G., Ryder, L.P., Thomsen, M. and Jersild, C. (1976) Immunological in vitro parameters in patients with multiple sclerosis and normal individuals. *Acta path. microbiol. scand.*, Sect. C, 84: 501–510.

Poskanzer, D.C. (1965) Tonsillectomy and multiple sclerosis. *Lancet*, II: 1264–1266.

Prineas, J.W. (1970) Etiology of multiple sclerosis. In P.J. Vinken and G.W. Bruyn (Eds.), *Handbook of Clinical Neurology, Vol. 9*, North-Holland, Amsterdam, pp. 107–160.

Raziuddin, S., Kibler, R.F. and Morrison, D.C. (1981) Prevention of experimental allergic encephalomyelitis by bacterial lipopolysaccharides: inhibition of cell-mediated immunity. *J. Immunol.*, 127: 13–16.

Ringdén, O., Rynne-Dagö, B., Kunori, T., Smith, C.I.E., Hammarström, L., Freijd, A. and Möller, E. (1979) Induction of antibody synthesis in human B lymphocytes by different polyclonal B cell activators: evaluation by direct and indirect PFC assays. *Immunol. Rev.*, 45: 195–218.

Rölla, G. (1977) Formation of dental integuments — some basic chemical considerations. *Swed. Dent. J.*, 1: 241–251.

Salmi, A., Viljanen, M. and Reunanen, M. (1981) Intratechal synthesis of antibodies to diphtheria and tetamus toxoid in multiple sclerosis patients. *J. Neuroimmunol.*, 1: 333–341.

Sibley, W.A. and Foley, J.M. (1966) Infection and immunization in multiple sclerosis. *Ann. N. Y. Acad. Sci.*, 53: 457–468.

Steel, C.M. and Creasey, G.H. (1976) A micromethod for the activation of human blood lymphocytes in vitro. *Immunol. Commun.*, 5: 669–684.

Tourtelotte, W.W., Ma, B.I., Ingram, T.S., Cowan, T.M. and Potvin, A.R. (1981) Quantitative absorption of multiple sclerosis (MS) cerebrospinal fluid (CSF) IgG by MS plaque and periplaque tissue. In *Proceedings of the 12th World Congress of Neurology (Excerpta Medica International Congress Series no. 548)*, Excerpta Medica, Amsterdam, p. 127.

Traugott, U., Scheinberg, L.C. and Raine, C.S. (1981) Lymphocyte responsiveness to oligodendrocytes in multiple sclerosis. *J. Neuroimmunol.*, 1: 41–51.

Uyeda, C.T., Gerstl, B., Smith, J.K. and Carr, W.T. (1966) Anti-staphylococcal B-hemolysin antibodies in humans with neurological disease. *Proc. Soc. exp. Biol. (N.Y.)*, 123: 143–146.

Vandvik, B., Norrby, E., Nordal, H.J. and Degré, M. (1976) Oligoclonal measles virus-specific IgG antibodies isolated from cerebrospinal fluids, brain extracts, and sera from patients with subacute sclerosing panencephalitis and multiple sclerosis. *Scand. J. Immunol.*, 5: 979–992.

Vartdal, F., Vandvik, B. and Norrby, E. (1980) Viral and bacterial antibody responses in multiple sclerosis. *Ann. Neurol.*, 8: 248–255.

Wicken, A.J. and Knox, K.W. (1975) Lipoteichoic acids: new class of bacterial antigens. *Science*, 187: 1161–1167.

Wybran, J. and Fudenberg, H.H. (1973) Thymus-derived rosette-forming cells in various human disease states: cancer, lymphoma, bacterial and viral infections, and other diseases. *J. clin. Invest.*, 52: 1026–1032.

Immunology of Nervous System Infections, Progress in Brain Research, Vol. 59, edited by P.O. Behan, V. ter Meulen and F. Clifford Rose
© *1983 Elsevier Science Publishers B.V.*

Cell-Mediated Immunity in Multiple Sclerosis

J. MERTIN and S.C. KNIGHT

Clinical Research Centre, Watford Road, Harrow, Middlesex, HA1 3UJ (U.K.)

INTRODUCTION

There are striking similarities between experimental allergic encephalomyelitis (EAE) and multiple sclerosis (MS) in their clinical symptoms and histopathology. Since EAE is a cell-mediated autoimmune disease, it has been suggested that cell-mediated autoimmune reactions play an important role in the etiology and pathogenesis of MS. For some time this concept was challenged by those who, influenced by epidemiological data and the finding of increased concentrations in MS serum and cerebrospinal fluid (CSF) of antibodies against various viruses, held the view that immune deficiency, e.g. an inability of the immune system to eliminate a virus infecting the central nervous system (CNS), might be responsible for the cause and progression of the disease. We have since learned that autoimmunity and immune deficiency are not mutually exclusive, but may be interrelated in conditions where, for example, autoimmune reactions are brought about by a disturbance in the function of lymphocyte subpopulations involved in the regulation of the immune system (Moretta et al., 1979).

Studies of cell-mediated immune (CMI) responses in MS patients are usually directed towards solving two major problems: (1) the possibility that a global or circumscript functional abnormality may exist within the immune system; and (b) the search for one, or more, "MS antigen(s)", be it normal or altered self-components of the CNS or antigenic constituents of agents invading the CNS, such as viruses.

TABLE I

SOME METHODS FOR THE INVESTIGATION OF CMI RESPONSES

---

(1) Tests of delayed hypersensitivity (DH) reactions of the skin
    (a) established DH to common antigens
    (b) DH response to primary immunization

(2) In vitro lymphocyte response
    (a) proliferation stimulated by:
        (i) mitogens or soluble antigens (e.g. lymphocyte transformation tests)
        (ii) fixed antigens (e.g. mixed lymphocyte responses)
    (b) production of lymphokines by stimulated lymphocytes (e.g. macrophage or leukocyte migration inhibition tests)
    (c) lymphocyte cytotoxicity

(3) Identification of T-lymphocyte subpopulations and determination of their concentrations in blood or CSF
    (a) rosetting methods
    (b) by detection of surface markers (e.g. with monoclonal antibodies)

There are many in vivo and in vitro tests for the functional characterization of CMI, the screening for putative antigens, and the determination of the relative concentrations in blood and CSF of lymphocyte subsets within the two major families of B- and T-cells. The most widely used of these methods are listed in Table I.

DELAYED HYPERSENSITIVITY REACTIONS OF THE SKIN

Skin tests for established delayed hypersensitivity (DH) to various common antigens such as streptokinase-streptodornase or tuberculin have been found to be normal in MS patients. Tests with myelin or myelin basic protein were negative. The response resulting from primary immunization to keyhole limpet hemocyanin (KLH) was shown by Davis et al. (1972) to be absent or greatly reduced when compared to the reaction in healthy control subjects, indicating impairment of DH mechanisms in MS. In contrast, intradermal injection of autologous lymphocytes, which in healthy controls does not cause a skin reaction, gave a positive reaction in MS patients (Morariu and Böhm, 1973), a phenomenon known to occur also in patients with established autoimmune diseases such as systemic lupus erythematosus (Friedman et al., 1960) or chronic active hepatitis (Lebacq et al., 1970).

IN VITRO LYMPHOCYTE FUNCTION

There is a host of conflicting data suggesting reduced, normal or increased responsiveness of lymphocytes from MS patients to stimulation with T-cell mitogens. Some studies of lymphocyte transformation and macrophage (leucocyte) migration inhibition have shown lymphocyte sensitization to CNS or viral antigens, whereas other studies did not confirm this. Listing and discussing the results and various aspects of only the most relevant publications in this field would exceed the limitations of a review like this. The conclusion to be drawn from the confusing abundance of data is that there is, to date, no unequivocal evidence for a deficiency or hyperreactivity of the peripheral or CSF lymphocytes in MS. Neither has sensitization to one or more of the various CNS or viral antigens in question been shown to be convincingly different to that found in healthy individuals or patients with other neurological conditions. The question as to whether there may be cytotoxic cells with specific activity against CNS components in the blood of CSF of MS patients has also not yet been satisfactorily answered. This is due in part to methodological difficulties, such as the preparation of clean populations of CNS cells to be used as in vitro targets for cytotoxic cells. In this context, it is necessary that we remind ourselves of the current concept of immune recognition, according to which recognition of antigens by T-lymphocytes is restricted by products of the major histocompatibility complex (MHC) expressed on the surface of antigen-presenting cells. To date, little is known about the expression of such immune response-associated (Ia) antigens on the different cell types of human CNS tissue. In the mouse, Ia antigens have only recently been detected on intrafascicular oligodendrocytes (Ting et al., 1981), indicating that there may be a basis for the assumption that cytotoxic T-cells are able to attack and destroy CNS cells.

LYMPHOCYTE SUBPOPULATIONS

Immune responses are regulated by an intricate network of promoting and inhibiting factors, in which interaction between lymphocyte subpopulations has been given a prominent role. Functional aberration or simply reduction in the relative numbers of cells within such subpopulations may bring about miscarriage of immune regulation and thereby cause the upsurge of autoaggressive reactions (Moretta et al., 1979). In considering this concept, it is only too obvious that determination of the concentrations of cells in distinct T-cell subsets, studies on the possible correlation between changes in these concentrations and clinical disease activity, and studies on the function of the cells belonging to such subsets, have become of prime interest in present MS research. Using the sheep red blood cell rosetting method to determine the total number of peripheral T-cells in MS, no reproducible alteration was found when compared to healthy controls, and there was little variation with the course of the disease. However, the number of avid T-cells, i.e. cells binding 10 or more erythrocytes, was reduced in patients with clinically active disease (Oger et al., 1975). Antel et al. (1978) have reported diminished activity of Con A stimulated suppressor cells during clinical attacks, followed by an increase in activity above normal levels during the remission phase.

This observation has essentially been confirmed by other research groups using different techniques. Huddlestone and Oldstone (1979) showed a decrease in the concentration of T_G cells (which are regarded as having suppressor activity) in clinically active disease and a return to higher than normal values during remission. In more recent studies, monoclonal antibodies directed against T-cell surface markers were employed. Total T-cell numbers can be determined with the help of antibody OKT_3. A percentage of these can be detected by antibody OKT_4 and were shown in functional studies to possess ''helper'' function, whereas another subset recognized by OKT_5 showed cytotoxic as well as suppressor activity (Reinherz and Schlossman, 1980). During clinical attacks and in patients with a progressive course of MS, a reduction in total peripheral T-cell numbers but an even greater reduction in OKT_5-labeled cells was observed (Reinherz et al., 1980; Bach et al., 1980). It has been speculated that such a decrease in the number of suppressor cells may be instrumental in the precipitation of attacks.

These observations represent a major advance in MS research, and there is great hope that longitudinal studies on the fluctuation in the concentrations of T-cell subsets will provide important clues as to the pathogenetic mechanisms in MS. However, the possibility that the detected changes may not be causally related to the disease process, but merely represent an epiphenomenon have still to be excluded. Even if this was achieved there would remain many questions to be answered. There may, for example, still be a considerable degree of heterogeneity within the cell populations identified by OKT and similar antibodies. Another problem is posed by the difficulties encountered in defining the functional characteristics of T-cell subsets. Functional studies are carried out usually by lymphocyte stimulation in vitro. It has been pointed out by Knight (1982) that discrepancies in the results of such studies may be based on methodological differences between laboratories, and that the development of improved assay conditions is of utmost importance. Functional tests are usually carried out within a narrowly defined range of culture conditions. Knight, Farrant and co-workers (Knight and Farrant, 1978; Farrant and Knight, 1979; Knight et al., 1979; Farrant and Newton, 1981) have reported evidence showing that the growth of lymphocytes in culture is governed by a bell-shaped cell concentration curve similar to that established, for example, for the in vitro growth of cell lines. With increasing concentrations of lymphocytes, proliferation was shown first to increase and, after reaching a plateau, to decrease again. It appeared that lymphocyte growth was regulated by mechanisms mediated through cell–cell contacts resulting at higher

358

concentrations in contact inhibition. Thus, in vitro suppressor activity hitherto attributed to an intrinsic function of a discrete lymphocyte subset, may at times merely result from changes in relative cell concentrations. Therefore it has been proposed that future studies on the function of T-cell subsets should take into account the effect of varying cell concentrations on in vitro stimulation and their interaction with the dose of stimulant and duration of culture periods (Knight, 1981).

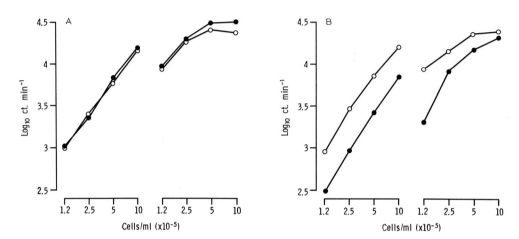

Fig. 1. Mean uptake into lymphocytes of [³H]thymidine in response to phytohaemagglutinin (for detailed methods see Knight et al., 1981). Different concentrations of cells from patients with multiple sclerosis were stimulated and the uptake measured on day 2 (right-side) and day 4 (left-side). A: the response in two groups of 4 patients before treatment (group 1, ○ ; group 2, ●). B: response in the two groups 4–8 months after start of the treatment. The patients in group 1 received immunosuppressive treatment (Mertin et al., 1980) with antilymphocyte globulin and azathioprine; those in group 2 received placebo treatment.

This new methodological approach should also be applied when responses of non-separated peripheral lymphocytes to mitogens or putative antigens are tested. We have recently shown that in MS, low lymphocyte responses to stimulation with mitogen or in mixed lymphocyte cultures may be due to changes in the number of cells required to generate a detectable reaction. With progression of the disease, or in clinical relapses, higher cell concentrations were required to produce comparable responses, suggesting an association between disease progression and a decrease in the proportion of peripheral lymphocytes able to respond to stimulation (Knight et al., 1980, 1982). This change in cell concentration requirement could possibly also explain the changed suppressor effects of cells from MS patients. The patients investigated in this study participated in a double-blind trial of immunosuppressive treatment (Mertin et al., 1980). In those undergoing immunosuppression, cell number requirement did not change when compared with pre-treatment values (Fig. 1A and B); this was in contrast to the cells from placebo-treated patients where more cells were required to produce responses (Knight et al., 1981). In the light of these observations it has become important to re-investigate the possible role of CNS and viral antigens using this new methodological approach, and it is hoped that this will provide more conclusive results than those reported in the past.

CONCLUSIONS

Although many observations have been reported indicating alterations in CMI responses in MS patients, the real importance of these often discrepant findings for MS etiology and pathogenesis, has remained unclear. Recent progress in the identification of lymphocyte subpopulations, and newly developed methods for studying the immune responsiveness of peripheral lymphocytes and defining the function of T-cell subsets, may represent a major step forward in the quest for the pathological mechanisms underlying MS.

REFERENCES

Antel, J.P., Arnason, B.G.W. and Medof, M.E. (1978) Suppressor cell function in multiple sclerosis — correlation with clinical disease activity. *Ann. Neurol.*, 5: 338–342.

Bach, M., Phan-Dinh-Tuy, F., Tournier, E., Chatenaud, L., Bach, J.-F., Martin, C. and Degos, J.-D. (1980) Deficit of suppressor T cells in active multiple sclerosis. *Lancet*, 2: 1221–1223.

Davis, L.E., Hersh, E.M., Curtis, J.E., Lynch, R.E., Ziegler, D.K., Neumann, J.W. and Chin, T.D.Y. (1972) Immune status of patients with multiple sclerosis. *Neurology*, 22: 989–997.

Farrant, J. and Knight, S.C. (1979) Help and suppression by lymphoid cells as a function of cellular concentration. *Proc. nat. Acad. Sci. U.S.A.*, 76: 3507–3510.

Farrant, J. and Newton, C. (1981) Relative ability to provide help: an explanation for Con A-induced suppression. *Clin. exp. Immunol.*, 45: 504–513.

Friedman, E.A., Bardawil, W.A., Merrill, J.P. and Hanau, C. (1960) "Delayed" cutaneous hypersensitivity to leucocytes in disseminated lupus erythematosus. *New Engl. J. Med.*, 262: 486–491.

Huddlestone, J.R. and Oldstone, M.B.A. (1979) T suppressor (T_G) lymphocytes fluctuate in parallel with changes in the clinical course of patients with multiple sclerosis. *J. Immunol.*, 123: 1615–1618.

Knight, S.C. and Farrant, J.F. (1978) Comparing stimulation of lymphocytes in different samples: separate effects of numbers of responding cells and their capacity to respond. *J. Immunol. Meth.*, 22: 63–71.

Knight, S.C., Harding, B., Burman, S., O'Brien, J. and Farrant, J. (1979) Clinical applications of leucocyte culture: the importance of cellular concentration. In J.G. Kaplan (Ed.), *The Molecular Basis of Immune Cell Function*, Elsevier/North-Holland Biomedical Press, Amsterdam, pp. 181–192.

Knight, S.C. (1982) Control of lymphocyte stimulation in vitro: "help" and "suppression" in the light of lymphoid population dynamics. *J. Immunol. Meth.*, 50: R51–R63.

Knight, S.C., Harding, B., Burman, S. and Mertin, J. (1981) Cell number requirement for lymphocyte stimulation in vitro: changes during the course of multiple sclerosis and the effects of immunosuppression. *Clin. exp. Immunol.*, 46: 61–69.

Lebacq, E., Smeets, F. and Desmet, V. (1970) Reaction cutanée aux lecocytes dans les cas d'hepatite chronique active. *Arch. Franc. Mal. Appl. Dig.*, 9: 601–607.

Mertin, J., Rudge, P., Knight, S.C., Thompson, E.J. and Healy, M.J.R. (1980) Double-blind, controlled trial of immunosuppression in treatment of multiple sclerosis. *Lancet*, 2: 949–951.

Mertin, J., Rudge, P., Kremer, M., Healey, M.J.R., Knight, S.C., Compston, A., Batchelor, J.R., Thompson, E.J., Halliday, A.M., Denman, M. and Medawar, P.B. (1982) Double-blind controlled trial of immunosuppression in the treatment of multiple sclerosis: final report. *Lancet*, 2: 351–354.

Morariu, M. and Böhm, T. (1973) Delayed dermal hypersensitivity to autologous lymphocytes in multiple sclerosis. *Neurology*, 23: 808–811.

Moretta, L., Mingari, M.C. and Moretta, A. (1979) Human T cell subpopulations in normal and pathological conditions. *Immunol. Rev.*, 45: 163–193.

Oger, J.F., Arnason, B.G.W., Wray, S.H. and Kistler, J.P. (1975) A study of B and T cells in multiple sclerosis. *Neurology*, 25: 444–447.

Reinherz, E.L. and Schlossman, S.F. (1980) The differentiation and function of human T lymphocytes. *Cell*, 19: 821–827.

Reinherz, E.L., Weiner, H.L., Hauser, S.L., Cohen, J.A., Distaso, J.A. and Schlossman, S.F. (1980) Loss of suppressor T cells in active multiple sclerosis. *New Engl. J. Med.*, 303: 125–129.

Ting, J.P.Y., Shigekawa, B.L., Linthicum, S., Weiner, L.P. and Frelinger, J.A. (1981) Expression and synthesis of murine immune response-associated (Ia) antigens by brain cells. *Proc. nat. Acad. Sci. U.S.A.*, 78: 3170–3174.

Immunology of Nervous System Infections, Progress in Brain Research, Vol. 59, edited by P.O. Behan, V. ter Meulen and F. Clifford Rose
© *1983 Elsevier Science Publishers B.V.*

In Vitro and In Vivo Effects of β-Endorphin and Met-Enkephalin on Leukocyte Locomotion

DENNIS E. VAN EPPS, LINDA SALAND, CECILLE TAYLOR and RALPH C. WILLIAMS, Jr.

Departments of Medicine, Microbiology, and Anatomy, University of New Mexico, Albuquerque, NM 87131 (U.S.A.)

INTRODUCTION

The 31 amino acid peptide, β-endorphin is derived from the precursor β-lipotropin peptide produced in the hypothalamus and pituitary. This peptide consists of amino acid residues 61–91 of the β-lipotropin precursor molecule and results from the direct cleavage of this peptide. Another 39 amino acid segment attached to the precursor β-lipotropin has been identified as adrenocorticotropic hormone (ACTH). This relationship has been recently reviewed by Krieger and Martin (1981). ACTH stimulates the adrenals to release hydrocortisone which has well known immunosuppressive properties. β-Endorphin, on the other hand, has been extensively studied with respect to its neurological effects, but only limited studies of its effects on the immune system have been performed. Indirect evidence of a role for both Met-enkephalin (a 5 amino acid segment of β-endorphin) and β-endorphin in modulation of the immune system, comes from studies showing that Met-enkephalin increases active T-lymphocyte rosettes (Wybran et al., 1979), and β-endorphin enhances lymphocyte proliferation in response to concanavalin A (Gilman et al., 1981). Both of the above effects are inhibited by naloxone, a competitive inhibitor of opiate receptor binding. In another study, β-endorphin has been shown to bind directly to cultured human lymphocytes; in this study, binding was not inhibited by naloxone or Met-enkephalin, and the authors speculate that a non-opiate receptor for β-endorphin exists on human lymphocytes (Hazum et al., 1979).

Over the past few years, several peptides have been described with chemotactic activity for neutrophils and monocytes. The one most widely studied has been formyl methionyl leucyl phenylalanine (f-MLP). This peptide is a potent chemotactic factor for both monocytes (Cianciolo and Snyderman, 1981) and neutrophils (Showell et al., 1976), and recent studies have demonstrated the presence of specific receptors for these peptides on human neutrophils (Williams et al., 1977), and monocytes (Weinberg et al., 1981). Although these peptides are potent chemotactic factors, there is no evidence that they are naturally produced by the host, although the production of similar agents by bacteria has been described (Schiffman et al., 1975). Recently the hypotensive, vasodilator and smooth muscle contracting peptide, substance P (Bury and Mashford, 1976; Von Euler and Gaddum, 1931) has been shown to stimulate rabbit neutrophil chemotaxis and lysosomal enzyme release (Marasco et al., 1981). This neuropeptide also blocks the binding of f-MLP to its receptor, and therefore may act through this receptor. Substance P has also been associated with pain transmission (Randic and Miletic, 1977). Other nervous system-produced peptides, such as amino and carboxyterminal substituent tetrapeptides of angiotension II, have been shown to be chemotactic for human monocytes (Goetzl et al., 1980), with lesser activity for neutrophils. Still other studies have shown that human mononuclear phagocytes specifically bind $[I^{125}]$8-L-arginine-vasopressin (Block et al., 1981), and that vasoactive intestinal polypeptides can be found in polymorphonuclear leukocytes (O'Dorisio et al., 1980). All of these studies indicate that cells of the immune system may be directly affected by products of the central nervous system.

Since immigration of leukocytes to a site of inflammation is a primary step in host defense, it is the purpose of this study to determine if β-endorphin or the 5 amino acid constituent of β-endorphin, Met-enkephalin, have any effect on monocyte, lymphocyte or neutrophil locomotor responses.

PROCEDURES

Cell preparation

Human neutrophils and mononuclear cells were isolated from normal adult peripheral blood by centrifugation over Ficoll–hypaque (Boyum, 1968). Mononuclear cells were removed from the plasma Ficoll–hypaque interface, washed 3 times, and adjusted to 5×10^6 cells/ml in minimal essential media (MEM) containing 0.1 % bovine serum albumin (BSA). These preparations contained from 18 to 30 % monocytes as determined by peroxidase staining (Yam et al., 1971). In some cases, monocytes were removed from the mononuclear cell preparation by adherence to glass wool (Sibbitt et al., 1978). This procedure results in a preparation of lymphocytes containing less than 2 % peroxidase-positive monocytes and is referred to here as monocyte depleted lymphocytes. In some cases, human T-cells were isolated by incubating lymphocytes (1×10^7/ml) with 2-aminoethylisothiouronium bromide (AET)-treated sheep erythrocytes (SRBC) as previously described (Kaplan and Clark, 1974). T-lymphocytes forming rosettes with SRBC were then separated from non-rosetting cells by Ficoll–hypaque centrifugation. T-cell rosettes which sedimented to the cell pellet were treated for 30 s with 4° C distilled water to lyse the SRBC. T-lymphocytes were then washed and resuspended in MEM-0.1 % BSA containing 10^{-8} M bacitracin to a concentration of 2×10^6/ml. Analysis of this cell preparation showed it to be greater than 95 % SRBC rosette forming cells and less than 1 % peroxidase-positive cells.

Neutrophils which sediment to the cell pellet with erythrocytes following the initial Ficoll–hypaque separation of peripheral blood were isolated as previously described (Van Epps et al., 1978). The erythrocyte-neutrophil pellet was resuspended to half the original volume with Hank's balanced salt solution (HBSS) and mixed with Plasmagel (HTI, Buffalo, NY) at a concentration of 1 cc Plasmagel/5 cc of cell suspension. Erythrocytes were allowed to sediment for 30 min at 37° C after which the neutrophil rich supernatant was removed, cells centrifuged and washed, and then resuspended in 0.1 % BSA-HBSS containing 10^{-8} M bacitracin at a final concentration of 5×10^6 cells/ml.

Chemotaxis assays

All cell locomotion assays were performed in modified Boyden type chemotaxis chambers. Assays of neutrophil and monocyte chemotaxis were performed using a $5 \mu m$ pore size membrane to separate the upper cell compartment from the lower compartment containing the test sample. In neutrophil assays, 0.2 ml of cells at 5×10^6/ml were added to the upper compartment and chambers were incubated for 30 min at 37° C and then fixed and stained with hematoxylin for analysis (Van Epps et al., 1978). Monocyte locomotion was evaluated similarly using 0.4 ml of a mononuclear cell preparation at 5×10^6 cells/ml in the upper compartment and a 1.5 h incubation period. Lymphocyte migration was assayed using an 8 μm pore size membrane to separate the upper and lower compartments and 3 h, 37° C incubation (El-Naggar et al., 1980). In this assay, 0.2 ml of a monocyte depleted lymphocyte preparation containing less than 2 % peroxidase-positive cells was added to the upper compartment of the chemotaxis chamber. In some instances, purified T-cells were used instead of monocyte-depleted lymphocytes. In all cases, after appropriate incubation times, membranes were fixed with formalin, stained with hematoxylin, and cleared with isopropyl alcohol and xylene (El-Naggar et al., 1980). Migration was assessed by the leading front technique (Zigmond and Hirsch, 1973) using the microscope micrometer to measure the distance that cells had penetrated into the membrane in response to the agent present in the lower compartment. Results are expressed as a "migration index", which is the difference between the response with the test sample present and that with control media alone. All chemotaxis assays were run in duplicate, counting 5 fields on each membrane and averaging results. Average migration in the absence of a stimulus was 38 ± 10 for neutrophils, 50 ± 13 for monocytes, and 65 ± 3 for lymphocytes.

Reagents

β-Endorphin and Met-enkephalin were purchased from Beckman (Palo Alto, CA) and made as 10^{-4} M stock solutions in dimethyl sulfoxide (DMSO). F-MLP was obtained from Sigma Chemicals (St. Louis, MO) and prepared as a stock at 10^{-2} M in DMSO. All stock samples were stored frozen and diluted in the assay media immediately before use. Casein (Fisher Scientific, Fairlawn, NJ) was prepared at 2 mg/ml stock concentration in MEM and diluted to 0.4 mg/ml just prior to use. Naloxone (Endo Laboratories, Garden City, NY) was prepared in media just prior to use.

In vivo assays of Met-enkephalin and β-endorphin

Ovine (camel, rat) β-endorphin (courtesy of Dr. N. Ling, The Salk Institute) or Met-enkephalin (20 μg in 15 μl of sterile saline) was infused into the right lateral cerebral ventricle of adult male Sprague–Dawley rats which had been previously implanted with a stainless-steel cannula. All animals were injected over 2–3 min while awake. Rats were lightly anesthesized with ether 45–60 min after injection, and perfused through the heart with 0.9 % sodium chloride followed by 1 % paraformaldehyde–2.5 % glutaraldehyde in 0.075 M cacodylate/HCl buffer at room temperature. Portions of the medial basal hypothalmus were then processed for scanning or transmission electron microscopy. Control animals were infused with sterile saline only.

RESULTS

Stimulation of human monocyte locomotion by β-endorphin and Met-enkephalin

Human neutrophils and monocytes were tested for responsiveness to varying concentrations of human β-endorphin or Met-enkephalin in Boyden chemotaxis chambers. As shown in Fig. 1A and B, locomotion assays using mononuclear cells and various β-endorphin or Met-enkephalin concentrations showed increasing migration in response to both agents with up to 10^{-8} M concentrations. Interestingly, the response appeared to be bimodal, with one peak in the range of 10^{-14}–10^{-12} M and a second peak occurring around 10^{-9}–10^{-8} M. This double peak response was a consistent finding although the amplitude of the response varied with

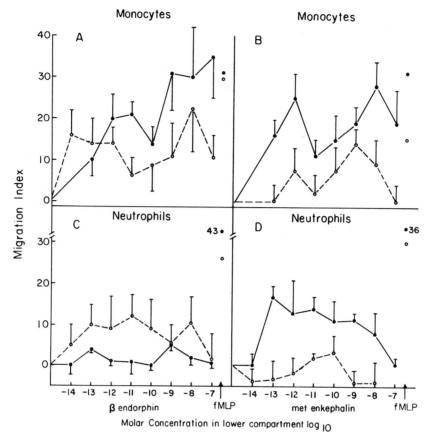

Fig. 1. Migration of human monocytes and neutrophils in response to β-endorphin (A and C) and Met-enkephalin (B and D). Two representative experiments with each cell type and stimulus are shown. The simultaneous response to f-MLP (10^{-8} M) is also indicated for comparison. Data are expressed as the mean migration index ± 1 S.D. at each concentration.

TABLE I

COMPARISON OF MONOCYTE RESPONSES TO MET-ENKEPHALIN AND β-ENDORPHIN

Experiment	Response as a migration index	
	β-endorphin	*Met-enkephalin*
1	32 ± 6	28 ± 6
2	30 ± 7	25 ± 5
3	31 ± 2	14 ± 2
4	70 ± 8	51 ± 5
5	8 ± 5	2 ± 3
6	25 ± 10	5 ± 3
7	22 ± 9	0 ± 4
8	21 ± 2	13 ± 9
9	8 ± 6	1 ± 3
Mean	27 ± 18	15 ± 17

different cell preparations. The response to an optimal concentration of f-MLP (10^{-8} M) is also included in Fig. 1 and shows that optimal monocyte migration in response to β-endorphin is similar in amplitude to the response to f-MLP. Although monocytes respond to both β-endorphin and Met-enkephalin, the response of different cell preparations to these two hormones was quite variable. Comparative responses of the same preparation of monocytes to 10^{-8} M β-endorphin and Met-enkephalin are shown in Table I. In general, although the degree of response to β-endorphin varied with respect to the source of cells in each experiment, the response to Met-enkephalin was always less than that observed with β-endorphin.

Aside from the morphologic appearance of migrating cells, experiments were conducted to assure that the observed responses were due to monocytes and not lymphocytes under these conditions. Mononuclear cell preparations containing monocytes were compared to monocyte depleted preparations (lymphocytes) under the same conditions. Migration of monocyte-depleted cells, in response to β-endorphin, the chemotactic stimuli casein or f-MLP, were far below the random locomotion control (medium alone) for monocyte containing preparations. Therefore, the observed response to the various agents tested in this system can be attributed to monocyte migration, since the migration index is the difference between migration with the test sample present and the random locomotion control. Examples of neutrophil responses are also shown in Fig. 1C and D and show that, although some response to β-endorphin and Met-enkephalin was observed with one of the two cell preparations in each case, comparison to the f-MLP response indicated that neutrophil responses to β-endorphin or Met-enkephalin were minimal. This comparison is also shown in the summary (Table II) which compares 10 different monocyte and neutrophil responses to β-endorphin with the response to f-MLP. As shown, monocyte responses to 10^{-8} M β-endorphin ranged from 47 to 120 % of the f-MLP response, with a mean of 79 %. Neutrophils, on the other hand, responded much more efficiently to f-MLP than to β-endorphin, with a β-endorphin range of 0–56 % and a mean response of only 30 % of that observed with f-MLP. Thus, by comparison to f-MLP, monocytes appeared to be much more responsive to β-endorphin than neutrophils.

TABLE II

COMPARISON OF β-ENDORPHIN (β) STIMULATED NEUTROPHIL AND MONOCYTE RESPONSES TO SIMULTANEOUS f-MLP RESPONSES

Experiment	Monocytes			Neutrophils		
	Migration index		% f-MLP response	Migration index		% f-MLP response
	10^{-8} β	10^{-8} f-MLP		10^{-8} β	10^{-8} f-MLP	
1	25	23	109	0	30	0
2	22	30	73	2	43	5
3	8	13	62	0	20	0
4	8	13	62	22	60	37
5	16	27	59	30	50	60
6	23	49	47	23	55	42
7	30	32	94	24	56	43
8	10	14	71	28	50	56
9	30	25	120	13	40	33
10	26	27	96	17	74	23
Mean ± 1 S.D.			79 ± 24			30 ± 22

Although many agents stimulate monocyte and neutrophil locomotion, they may be chemokinetic (stimulate random movement), chemotactic (stimulate directional movement in response to a chemotactic factor gradient) or both. Early studies of monocyte responses to β-endorphin indicated that monocytes elicited a chemotactic response to β-endorphin. This directional response is shown in Fig. 2, which depicts the response of monocytes to various concentrations of β-endorphin ranging from 10^{-10} M to 10^{-6} M in the upper cell compartment (negative gradient) the lower compartment (positive gradient) or equal concentrations in both compartments (no gradient). These data demonstrate that under these conditions, the response was greatest when a positive gradient exists, and β-endorphin was present in the lower compartment. This increased movement in response to the positive gradient of β-endorphin was indicative of chemotaxis.

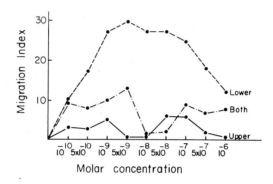

Fig. 2. Demonstration of directional locomotion of human monocytes in response to β-endorphin. Migration with various concentrations of β-endorphin in upper cell compartment, lower compartment, or equivalent concentrations in both compartments of the chemotaxis chamber are shown.

Naloxone blocking of monocyte migration in response to β-endorphin

Naloxone is a known antagonist of opiate receptor binding. To determine if β-endorphin might stimulate monocyte migration through interaction with an opiate receptor, monocytes were preincubated for 15 min in 10^{-7} M naloxone and the mixture was added to the upper compartment of the chemotaxis chamber with 10^{-8} M β-endorphin present in the lower compartment. As shown in Table III, the presence of naloxone markedly suppressed the monocyte response to β-endorphin, implying an opiate-like receptor interaction with β-endorphin. Naloxone itself had no adverse effects on random locomotion in the absence of

TABLE III

INHIBITION OF β-ENDORPHIN STIMULATED MONOCYTE MIGRATION BY NALOXONE

Experiment	Response to 10^{-8} M β-endorphin (migration index)		% Inhibition by Naloxone
	Control	10^{-7} M Naloxone present	
1	36 ± 7	4 ± 4	89 %
2	25 ± 9	1 ± 4	96 %

β-endorphin. Although these results indicated an opiate receptor interaction, other experiments showed that similar concentrations and treatment of monocytes with naloxone resulted in a suppression of monocyte responses to f-MLP. In 3 experiments, naloxone treatment reduced the f-MLP stimulated migration index by 12%, 61% and 67%. Thus, although naloxone suppressed β-endorphin stimulated monocyte migration without reducing random unstimulated migration, its effect on f-MLP stimulated responses made the data difficult to interpret.

Response of monocyte depleted lymphocytes and T-cells to β-endorphin

We have also used techniques for analyzing peripheral blood lymphocyte migration (El-Naggar et al., 1980) to determine if, like monocytes, lymphocytes respond to β-endorphin. In these assays both monocyte-depleted lymphocytes (T- and non-T-lymphocytes), as well as E-rosette-positive T-lymphocytes, were tested. As shown in Fig. 3, both populations of cells responded to β-endorphin with optimal migration again noted at 10^{-8} M. These studies also implied multiple peaks of activity, although the response was not as clearly bimodal as that observed with monocytes. In these studies, migration in response to β-endorphin was compared to that observed with casein. Casein was used for comparison in these studies since it is a potent migration stimulus for T-lymphocytes, whereas f-MLP has only low level activity in this system and stimulates primarily non-T-lymphocyte migration (El-Naggar et al., 1980). It was apparent that lymphocyte responses to β-endorphin approached that obtained with casein.

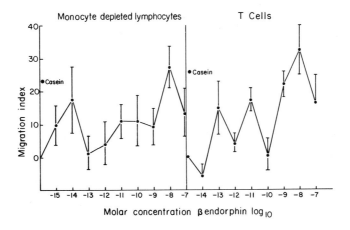

Fig. 3. Response of monocyte-depleted lymphocytes (left) and purified human T-cells to various concentrations of β-endorphin. The mean migration index $\pm$ 1 S.D. at each concentration is shown. The response of each lymphocyte preparation to casein is also shown for comparison.

The response to β-endorphin, as with monocytes, was blocked by a 15 min, 25° C, incubation of lymphocytes in 10^{-8} M naloxone. Again, although naloxone did not affect random migration, it did suppress the response of lymphocytes to casein.

368

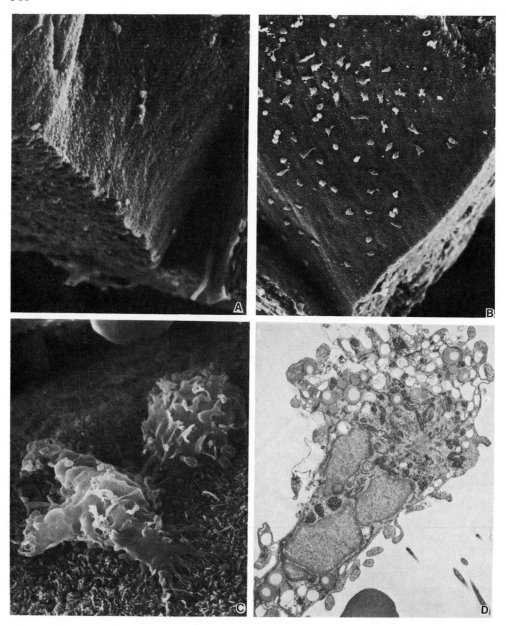

Fig. 4. A: Scanning electron micrograph (SEM) of control (saline-injected rat) median eminence. A small number of cells and fibers are present atop the ependyma. B: SEM of the median eminence of a rat injected with 20 µg β-endorphin 45–60 min prior to sacrifice. Numerous free supraependymal cells are visible above the ependyma. C: high magnification SEM of supraependymal cells from a β-endorphin-injected rat. Note the extensive "ruffling" of the cell membrane and pseudopod-like extensions onto surfaces of the ependymal region. D: transmission EM of a supraependymal cell after β-endorphin injection. Note the multilobular nucleus, extensive cell processes, and numerous inclusion bodies.

Macrophage response to β-endorphin and Met-enkephalin infused into the cerebral ventricle of adult rats

The role of β-endorphin as an in vivo stimulus of leukocyte migration was evaluated by infusing rat β-endorphin into the right lateral cerebral ventricle of adult rats. Under these conditions a focus of β-endorphin and a positive gradient of endorphin may be created. Following infusion, portions of the basal hypothalmus were then processed for scanning or transmission electron microscopy. Fig. 4 shows the results of these experiments. Control animals infused with saline alone showed only a few macrophage-like cells residing on the surface of the ventricle. In contrast, animals infused with β-endorphin showed a marked cellular infiltrate (Fig. 4B) with numerous cells adhering to the walls of the ventricle. Closer analysis of these cells (Fig. 4C) indicated that the majority appeared to have a motile configuration and resembled macrophages, with a high degree of membrane ruffling. Transmission electron microscopy, Fig. 4D, further indicated that most cells have macrophage morphology, showing multiple granules and vacuoles, high cytoplasmic to nuclear ratio, pseudopod-like properties and a lobular nucleus. Similar results were obtained with Met-enkephalin infusion, although the number of responding cells appeared to be qualitatively less. Occasional lymphocyte-like cells were also observed, but no neutrophils were seen. These in vivo results are consistent with the in vitro responsiveness of peripheral blood monocytes to β-endorphin and Met-enkephalin.

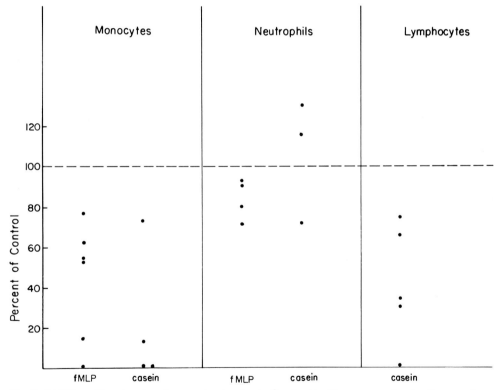

Fig. 5. Inhibition of lymphocyte and monocyte migration by β-endorphin. The response of each cell preparation to f-MLP or casein following a 15 min incubation at 25°C in 10^{-8} M β-endorphin is compared to the control response in the absence of β-endorphin. Data are expressed as the percent of the control migration index to each of the indicated factors. Random locomotion was not significantly decreased by the incubation in β-endorphin.

Effect of preincubation of leukocytes with β-endorphin on their response to other chemotactic stimuli

Since it was unlikely under normal conditions that high concentrations of β-endorphin may be diffusing from a single site in vivo, thereby creating a concentration gradient of endorphin, we have tested the effect of pre-exposure of leukocytes to β-endorphin on their locomotor response to f-MLP or casein. In this study, neutrophils, monocytes, and monocyte depleted lymphocytes were exposed to 10^{-8} M β-endorphin for 15 min at 25° C, and then added along with the β-endorphin to the upper compartment of the chemotaxis chamber. Assays for each cell type were performed and compared to controls incubated for the same time in media alone. As shown in Fig. 5, preincubation with β-endorphin markedly reduced the response of monocytes to both f-MLP and casein, as well as the lymphocyte response to casein. Little reduction in activity was observed with neutrophils to either f-MLP or casein. Although not shown, preincubation of monocytes in β-endorphin also inhibited their response to 10^{-8} M β-endorphin, implying down-regulation. Thus, when monocytes and lymphocytes were pre-exposed to β-endorphin, their response to other chemotactic stimuli appeared to be reduced.

DISCUSSION

β-Endorphin has been extensively studied with respect to its neurological effects and has been found to be a potent analgesic (Cox et al., 1976; Loh et al., 1976). β-Endorphin has been implicated in the mediation of the following activities: opioid activity on guinea pig ileum (Cox et al., 1976); minimizing the stress of chronic airway obstruction in individuals with chronic obstructive lung disease (Santiago et al., 1981); increased pain threshold during pregnancy (Gintzler, 1980); increased serum prolactin concentrations (Dupont et al., 1977; Rivier, et al., 1977); catatonic states and hypothermia in rats (Bloom et al., 1976); sedation and catalepsy (Bloom et al., 1976; Jacquet and Marks, 1976); and excessive grooming in rats (Gispen et al., 1976). In spite of all of the studies on the neurologic effects of β-endorphin, only recently have studies been performed on the possible effects of β-endorphin on the immune system. Most of these have concentrated on lymphocytes (Gilman et al., 1981; Hazum et al., 1979; Wybran et al., 1979). It is apparent from this study that monocytes, lymphocytes and possibly neutrophils, may all be affected by β-endorphin. These studies indicate that this hormone can interact with and stimulate leukocyte migration — in particular, monocyte and lymphocyte migration. Furthermore, in the case of monocytes, this stimulation of migration is directional, indicating that β-endorphin has chemotactic activity. From the data presented in Fig. 1 and Table II, it is apparent that β-endorphin is nearly as efficient as f-MLP in stimulating monocyte migration, although it is markedly less effective in stimulating neutrophil migration. This comparative difference is similar to that observed by Goetzl et al. (1980), with angiotension fragments which also showed a preference for stimulating monocyte locomotion and was found to be much less effective with neutrophils.

Another neuropeptide, substance P, has been shown to stimulate neutrophil chemotaxis and to block the binding of f-MLP (Marasco et al., 1981). Whether angiotension fragments, β-endorphin, substance P and f-MLP are all recognized by similar receptors is a question which remains to be answered. The unique bimodal response of monocytes was observed with β-endorphin and Met-enkephalin. Although there is currently no explanation for this bimodal effect, it may be due to the presence of more than one receptor, with each having a different affinity for these hormones. Alternatively, multiple subpopulations of monocytes responding optimally to different concentrations of β-endorphin or Met-enkephalin could also explain this phenomenon. The former has been implied for human lymphocytes where β-endorphin binding studies indicate the possible presence of multiple receptors with different affinities (Hazum et al., 1979). Some evidence for monocyte subpopulations also exists. Cianciolo and Snyderman (1981) have shown that the monocyte response to f-MLP reflects the response of certain monocyte subpopulations.

From the data in Fig. 1 and Table I, it can be seen that monocytes respond to both β-endorphin and Met-enkephalin, although within a given cell preparation, the response to 10^{-8} M β-endorphin exceeds that observed with a similar concentration of Met-enkephalin. These data indicate that Met-enkephalin is also recognized by monocytes. Since Met-enkephalin represents a 5 amino acid peptide sequence contained within the β-endorphin molecule, the implication is that this region may be responsible for at least some of the activity attributed to β-endorphin. Alternatively, the response to both β-endorphin and Met-enkephalin may also imply separate Met-enkephalin and β-endorphin receptors. The latter is consistent with studies on lymphocyte endorphin receptors showing that Met-enkephalin does not block β-endorphin binding (Hazum et al., 1979), whereas other studies show that Met-enkephalin increases active T-rosettes in human lymphocytes (Wybran et al., 1979), implying its interaction with lymphocytes.

The response of monocytes to a concentration gradient of β-endorphin is directional (Fig. 2), indicating that β-endorphin under the appropriate conditions is chemotactic for monocytes. Similar directional stimulation of monocytes by fragments of angiotensin (Goetzl et al., 1980), and of neutrophils by substance P (Marasco et al., 1981) have been reported. Although under normal conditions a concentration gradient of β-endorphin from a single site may not be expected in vivo, the recent use of intrathecal injection of β-endorphin to induce analgesia in obstetric patients at the time of delivery (Oyama et al., 1980) may produce such a condition. This artificial production of a concentration gradient in vivo may provide the necessary stimulus for directional locomotion in vivo. Indeed, as we have shown in Fig. 4, intraventricular injection in rats of β-endorphin does result in the migration of macrophage-like cells into the ventricle within 1 h. It is also notable that although Met-enkephalin stimulates a locomotor response in monocytes, by comparison at 10^{-8} M concentration, β-endorphin is more effective within a given cell preparation (Table I). This lesser activity is also consistent with our in vivo studies of Met-enkephalin in the rat model where qualitatively, the immigration of macrophages was less apparent than that observed when β-endorphin was injected (data not shown). Although lymphocytes also respond to β-endorphin in vitro (Fig. 3), they were observed infrequently in our in vivo studies. This may reflect the relatively short time (45 min to 1 h) between β-endorphin injection and termination of the experiment. Alternatively, the absence of lymphocytes may be due to the nature of the cell populations present in the region.

As mentioned previously, although β-endorphin shows monocyte chemotactic activity in vitro, generally, the formation of a β-endorphin concentration gradient in vivo is not likely to occur. It is likely, though, that peripheral blood leukocytes are exposed to β-endorphin in the circulation or at local sites where endorphin concentrations might be increased. Marked fluctuations in plasma β-endorphin concentrations have been shown to occur as the result of stress. In mice, foot pad shock stimulates a 6-fold increase in blood β-endorphin levels (Rossier et al., 1977). Similarly, strenuous running has been shown to elevate blood β-endorphin levels 3-fold from a mean of approximately 8 pg/ml to 28 pg/ml (Colt et al., 1981). β-Endorphin concentrations have also been shown to increase during pregnancy to a mean of 78 ± 7 pg/ml at the time of delivery (Genazzani et al., 1981). These shifts could provide a mechanism by which peripheral blood leukocytes may be exposed to higher concentrations of

β-endorphin when the host is stressed. The relationship of pre-exposure of leukocytes to β-endorphin and their responses to chemotactic stimuli is currently being studied. As shown in Fig. 5, we have determined that short-term exposure (15 min at 25°C) of lymphocytes and monocytes to 10^{-8}M concentrations of β-endorphin results in a depressed response of these cells to f-MLP and casein. This depression was most apparent with lymphocytes and monocytes. Studies to determine the effects of long-term exposure to lower concentrations of β-endorphin are currently in progress. Since single log shifts in β-endorphin concentrations can occur as the result of stress, β-endorphin may play a direct role in regulating one of the initial steps in the inflammatory process — the migration of leukocytes to a focus of inflammation. This may be particularly applicable to reactions involving lymphocytes and monocytes, since they appear to be more sensitive than neutrophils to the effects of β-endorphin.

This phenomenon of decreased chemotactic responsiveness following pre-exposure to chemotactic factor is not new and has been shown to occur in neutrophils with other chemotactic stimuli such as f-MLP (Nelson et al., 1978) or C5a (Skubitz and Craddock, 1981). Low concentrations of f-MLP have been shown specifically to depress neutrophil responsiveness to f-MLP but not to other factors, whereas high concentrations may deactivate neutrophils to multiple stimuli (Nelson et al., 1978). This phenomenon has also been shown to occur in vivo in patients on chronic hemodialysis (Skubitz and Craddock, 1981) where in vivo generation of C5a by the hemodialysis process results in decreased responsiveness of peripheral blood neutrophils to C5a. Whether the decreased locomotor responses of monocytes to f-MLP and casein, or of lymphocytes to casein following exposure to β-endorphin is specific to a single receptor which recognizes f-MLP, casein and β-endorphin, or is non-specific and represents a more general depression involving loss of chemotactic responsiveness to all stimuli regardless of receptor specificity, remains to be determined. A previous study by Shields and Wilkinson (1979) has shown that exposure of human lymphocytes to f-MLP does suppress their locomotion response to aggregated IgG, and thus demonstrates a similar type of depression of lymphocytes to a second chemotactic factor.

Some evidence also exists for a peptide region within β-casein which has opioid activity (Henschen et al., 1979), possibly inferring a common site of action between casein and hormones that react with opioid receptors. More information on the nature of β-endorphin receptors and receptors for f-MLP, casein and other chemotactic factors will have to be obtained before these questions can be resolved.

These studies show that the neurohormones β-endorphin and Met-enkephalin directly affect physiological activity of cells of the immune system and that this interaction can alter cell function. These studies provide a link between the central nervous system and the immune system, and may possibly explain such phenomena as stress-decreased tumor resistance in mice (Sklar and Anisman, 1979) or the psychosocial effects on the immune system (Stein et al., 1976).

ACKNOWLEDGEMENTS

We wish to thank Jeffrey Potter, S. Lori Brown and Ann Munger for their exceptional technical assistance and Sue Bonner for excellent secretarial assistance. This study was supported in part by USPH Grant CA20819 from the National Cancer Institute, DA-02269 from the National Institute on Drug Abuse, and the Kroc Foundation. D.E.V.E. is the recipient of a senior investigator award from the National Arthritis Foundation.

REFERENCES

Block, L.H., Locher, R., Tenschert, W., Siegenthaler, W., Hofmann, T., Mettler, R. and Vetter, W. (1981) ^{125}I-8-L-arginine vasopressin binding to human mononuclear phagocytes, *J. clin. Invest.*, 68: 374–381.

Bloom, F., Segal, D., Ling, N. and Guillemin, R. (1976) Endorphins: profound behavioral effects in rats suggest new etiological factors in mental illness. *Science*, 194: 630–632.

Böyum, A. (1968) A separation of leukocytes from blood and bone marrow. *Scand. J. clin. Invest.*, 21 (Suppl. 97): 7.

Bury, R.W. and Mashford, M.L. (1976) Interactions between local anesthetics and spasmogens on the guinea pig ileum. *J. Pharmacol. exp. Ther.*, 197: 633–640.

Cianciolo, G.J. and Snyderman, R. (1981) Monocyte responsiveness to chemotactic stimuli is a property of a subpopulation of cells that can respond to multiple attractants. *J. clin. Invest.*, 67: 60–68.

Colt, E.W., Wardlaw, S.L. and Frantz, A.G. (1981) The effect of running on plasma β-endorphin. *Life Sci.*, 28: 1637–1640.

Cox, B.M., Goldstein, A. and Li, C.H. (1976) Opioid activity of a peptide, β-lipotropin-(61-91), derived from β-lipotropin. *Proc. nat. Acad. Sci.*, 73: 1821–1823.

Dupont, A., Cusan, L., Labrie, F., Coy, D.H. and Li, C.H. (1977) Stimulation of prolactin release in the rat by intraventricular injection of β-endorphin and methionine-enkephalin. *Biochem. Biophys. Res. Commun.*, 75: 76–82.

El-Naggar, A.K., Van Epps, D.E. and Williams, R.C. Jr. (1980) Human B and T lymphocyte locomotion response to casein, C5a, and f-met-leu-phe. *Cell. Immunol.*, 56: 365–373.

Genazzani, A.R., Facchinetti, F. and Parrini, D. (1981) β-lipotropin and β-endorphin plasma levels during pregnancy. *Clin. Endocr.*, 14: 409–418.

Gilman, S.C., Jeffrey, M., Schwartz, R., Milner, J., Bloom, F.E. and Feldman, J.O. (1981) Enhancement of lymphocyte proliferative responses by β-endorphin. *Soc. Neurosci. Abstr.*, 7: 257.15.

Gintzler, A.R. (1980) Endorphin-mediated increases in pain threshold during pregnancy. *Science*, 210: 193–195.

Gispen, W.H., Wiegant, V.M., Bradbury, A.F., Hulme, E.C., Smyth, D.C., Snell, C.R. and de Wied, D. (1976) Induction of excessive grooming in the rat by fragments of lipotropin. *Nature (Lond.)*, 264: 794–795.

Goetzl, E.J., Klickstein, L.B., Watt, K.W.K. and Wintroub, B.U. (1980) The preferential human mononuclear leukocyte chemotactic activity of the substituent tetrapeptides of angiotensin. II. *Biochem. Biophys. Res. Commun.*, 97: 1097–1102.

Hazum, E., Chang, K.J. and Cuatrecasas, P. (1979) Specific nonopiate receptors for β-endorphin. *Science*, 205: 1033–1035.

Henschen, A., Lottspeich, F., Brantl, V. and Teschemarker, H. (1979) Novel opioid peptides derived from casein (β casomorphins). *Hoppe-Seylers Z. Physiol. Chem.*, 360: S1217–1224.

Jacquet, Y.F. and Marks, N. (1976) The C-fragment of β-lipotropin: an endogenous neuroleptic or antipsychotogen. *Science*, 194: 632–635.

Kaplan, M.E. and Clark, C. (1974) An improved rosetting assay for detection of human T-lymphocytes. *J. Immunol. Meth.*, 5: 131–135.

Krieger, D.T. and Martin, J.B. (1981) Brain peptides. *N. Engl. J. Med.*, 304: 876–885.

Loh, H.N., Tseng, L.F., Wei, E. and Li, C.H. (1976) β-Endorphin is a potent analgesic agent. *Proc. nat. Acad. Sci. U.S.A.*, 73: 2895–2898.

Marasco, W.A., Showell, H.J. and Becker, E.L. (1981) Substance P binds to the formylpeptide chemotaxis receptor on the rabbit neutrophil. *Biochem. Biophys. Res. Commun.*, 99: 1065–1072.

Nelson, R.D., McCormack, R.T., Fiegel, V.D. and Simmons, R.L. (1978) Chemotactic deactivation of human neutrophils: evidence for nonspecific and specific components. *Infect. Immun.*, 22: 441–444.

O'Dorisio, M.S., O'Dorisio, T.M., Cataland, S. and Bulcerzak, S.P. (1980) Vasoactive intestinal polypeptide as a biochemical marker for polymorphonuclear leukocytes. *J. Lab. clin. Med.*, 96: 666–672.

Oyama, T., Matsuki, A., Taneichi, T., Ling, N. and Guillemin, R. (1980) β-endorphin in obstetric analgesia. *Amer. J. Obstet. Gynecol.*, 137: 613–616.

Randic, M. and Miletic, V. (1977) Effect of substance P in cat dorsal horn neurones activated by noxious stimuli. *Brain Res.*, 128: 164–169.

Rivier, C., Vale, W., Ling, N., Brown, M. and Guillemin, R. (1977) Stimulation in vivo of the secretion of prolactin and growth hormone by β-endorphin. *Endocrinology*, 100: 238–241.

Rossier, J. French, E.D., Rivier, C., Ling, N., Guillemin, R. and Bloom, F.E. (1977) Foot shock induced stress increases β-endorphin levels in blood but not brain. *Nature (Lond.)*, 270: 618–620.

Santiago, T.V., Remolina, C., Scoles, V. and Edelman, W.H. (1981) Endorphins and the control of breathing. *New Engl. J. Med.*, 304: 1190–1194.

Schiffman, E., Showell, H.V., Corcoran, B.A., Ward, P.A., Smith, E. and Becker, E.L. (1975) The isolation and

374

partial characterization of neutrophil chemotactic factors from *Escherichia coli. J. Immunol.*, 114: 1831–1837.

Shields, J.M. and Wilkinson, P.C. (1979) Relation between Fc receptor function and locomotion in human lymphocytes. *Clin. exp. Immunol.*, 38: 598–608.

Showell, H.J., Freer, R.J., Zigmond, S.M., Schiffman, E., Aswanikumar, S., Corcoran, B. and Becker, E.L. (1976) The structure–activity relationship of synthetic peptides as chemotactic factors and inducers of lysosomal secretion for neutrophils. *J. exp. Med.*, 143: 1154–1169.

Sibbitt, W.C. Jr., Bankhurst, A.D. and Williams, R.C. Jr. (1978) Studies of cell subpopulations mediating mitogen hyporesponsiveness in patients with Hodgkins Disease. *J. clin. Invest.*, 61: 55–63.

Sklar, L.S. and Anisman, H. (1979) Stress and coping factors influence tumor growth. *Science*, 205: 513–515.

Skubitz, K.M. and Craddock, P.R. (1981) Reversal of hemodialysis granulocytopenia and pulmonary leukostasis. A clinical manifestation of down-regulation of granulocyte responses to C5a. *J. clin. Invest.*, 67: 1383–1391.

Stein, M., Schiavi, R. and Camerino, M. (1976) Influence of brain and behavior on the immune system. *Science*, 191: 435–440.

Van Epps, D.E., Wiik, A., Garcia, M.L. and Williams, R.C. Jr. (1978) Enhancement of human neutrophil migration by prostaglandin E_2. *Cell. Immunol.*, 37: 142–150.

Von Euler, U.S. and Gaddum, J.H. (1931) An unidentified depressor substance in certain tissue extracts. *J. Physiol. (Lond.)*, 72: 74–87.

Weinberg, J.B., Muscato, J.J. and Niedel, J.E. (1981) Monocyte chemotactic peptide receptor. Functional characteristics and ligand-induced regulation. *J. clin. Invest.*, 68: 621–630.

Williams, L.T., Snyderman, R., Pike, M.C. and Lefkowitz, R.J. (1977) Specific receptor sites for chemotactic peptides on human polymorphonuclear leukocytes. *Proc. nat. Acad. Sci. U.S.A.*, 74: 1204–1208.

Wybran, J., Appelborn, T., Famaey, J.P. and Govaerts, A. (1979) Suggestive evidence for receptors for morphine and methionine-enkephalin on normal human blood T lymphocytes. *J. Immunol.*, 123: 1068–1070.

Yam, L.T., Li, C.Y. and Crosby, W.H. (1971) Cytochemical identification of monocytes and granulocytes. *Amer. J. clin. Pathol.*, 55: 283–290.

Zigmond, S.H. and Hirsch, J.G. (1973) Leukocyte locomotion and chemotaxis: new methods for evaluation and demonstration of cell-derived chemotactic factor. *J. exp. Med.*, 137: 387–410.

Immunology of Nervous System Infections, Progress in Brain Research, Vol. 59, edited by P.O. Behan, V. ter Meulen and F. Clifford Rose

The Cerebrospinal Fluid in Subacute Sclerosing Panencephalitis and Multiple Sclerosis

R.W.H. WALKER and E.J. THOMPSON

The Institute of Neurology, The National Hospital, Queen Square, London WC1N 3BG (U.K.)

INTRODUCTION

Both subacute sclerosing panencephalitis (SSPE) and multiple sclerosis (MS) are characterized by intrathecal synthesis of immunoglobulin G (IgG) within the central nervous system (CNS), giving rise to qualitative and quantitative abnormalities of the cerebrospinal fluid (CSF) IgG. Whereas in the normal individual, polyclonal IgG reaches the CSF by transudation across the blood–CSF barrier, in pathological states an elevation of the amount of CSF IgG may indicate either an increase in the amount of transudation of polyclonal IgG or synthesis within the CNS or both. Synthesis of IgG within the CNS has been demonstrated in both MS (Frick and Scheid-Seydel, 1958) and SSPE (Cutler et al., 1968) by injecting radio-labeled gamma-globulin or IgG intravenously into patients and measuring the specific activity in simultaneous serial CSF and blood specimens.

A feature of both diseases is that electrophoresis of cerebrospinal fluid shows oligoclonal bands, i.e. bands of IgG of restricted heterogeneity, which are either not present in serum or are relatively less prominent. It should be noted that oligoclonal bands are seen in serum from SSPE patients in about 2/3 cases (Lowenthal et al., 1971; Peter et al., 1974), but bands are detected in CSF which are not seen in serum, or are relatively fainter. Faint bands are occasionally seen in serum from MS patients (Link, 1973; Olsson and Nilsson, 1979). The significance of oligoclonal bands is, firstly, that they provide good indirect evidence of local CNS production of IgG when they are present in CSF and not in serum, or are less conspicuous in serum relative to total gamma globulin than in CSF. Secondly, they indicate synthesis of IgG by a restricted number of B-cell clones, and therefore suggest a restricted number of antigenic determinants (see Siegelman and Capra, 1979). Moreover, oligoclonal responses can be generated experimentally by hyperimmunization with bacterial vaccines (Haber et al., 1979), and so the existence of oligoclonal bands may indicate prolonged antigenic exposure in some situations.

Because CNS IgG synthesis is such a feature of both SSPE and MS, comparisons of the CSF abnormalities, in particular the IgG, may highlight aspects of the pathology of each disease, especially since the etiological agent and the specificity of much of the IgG synthesized in SSPE is well established, while the etiology of MS remains obscure.

This chapter is a review of some of the literature concerning the CSF in SSPE and MS, particularly the immunoglobulins, and it incorporates some of our observations on CSF specimens from 14 SSPE patients.

THE WHITE CELLS

In SSPE, the white cell count is normal or slightly elevated (Booij, 1958; Dencker and Kolar, 1965; Liano, et al., 1971). The same is seen in our patients (Table I), only 2/11 having elevated cell counts. Patient no. 9 had 12 cells, which were all lymphocytes. Cytological examination of cells in the CSF collected by centrifugation showed 85% lymphocytes, 13% histiocytes and 2% reactive lymphocytes; a few plasma cells and polymorphs were seen. Zeman (1978) states that cytology reveals the presence of plasma cells in the majority of cases, even when the cell count is normal, but this has not been our experience in the small number of our patients whose CSF specimens have been examined by cytocentrifugation. Peter (1967) found plasma cells in only 6/30 cases.

By contrast, it is well known that in MS the CSF cell count is not infrequently elevated, being between 5 and 20 cells/mm^3 in 1/3 cases, but rarely higher (Tourtellotte, 1970a). Moreover, some but not all investigators have found correlations between the white cell count and clinical parameters of the disease. The white cell count tends to be higher in relation to relapses (reviewed by Tourtellotte, 1970a; Olsson and Link, 1973), although Tourtellotte himself (Tourtellotte, 1970a; Tourtellotte and Potvin, 1981) has not found this. There is a tendency for the white cell count to fall with increasing age and duration (Tourtellotte, 1970a; Schuller et al., 1973; Olsson et al., 1976). Even in cases where the white cell count is normal, cytological examination after centrifugation or sedimentation frequently reveals the presence of reactive lymphocytes or plasma cells (see Tourtellotte, 1970a; Thompson et al., 1979).

THE TOTAL PROTEIN CONCENTRATION

In SSPE, the CSF total protein concentration is normal or only slightly increased (Booij, 1958; Dencker and Kolar, 1965). Liano et al. (1971) studied 15 cases and concluded that there was a correlation between the total protein concentration and duration, 10 cases with a duration of less than 6 months having a mean total protein concentration of 35 mg/dl (range 14–97 mg/dl), with only 2 patients having protein concentrations greater than 40 mg/dl, while 5 cases with durations of 6 months or more had a mean total protein concentration of 48.2 mg/dl (range 28–62 mg/dl) with only 1 patient having a protein of less than 40 mg/dl. All patients with elevated total protein concentrations were thought to have evidence of impairment of the blood–CSF barrier (i.e. elevation of alpha-2-globulins). All the patients had elevated CSF gamma globulin levels, but these were particularly high in the patients with increased total protein concentrations.

Silva et al. (1981) reported a series of 30 cases of SSPE, and found that in their patients with raised CSF total protein concentrations the increase was attributable to gamma-globulin, and they found no evidence of impairment of the blood–CSF barrier.

In our series, 6 CSF specimens had elevated total protein concentrations (more than 40 mg/dl). There was no correlation with duration. Three CSF specimens showed transudates (i.e. elevation of high molecular weight haptoglobins, with or without elevation of group components), indicative of impairment of the blood–CSF barrier. Two of these specimens had elevated total protein concentrations. Thus it would appear that the blood–CSF barrier may be disturbed in some patients, but there are obvious difficulties in establishing definite correlations on the basis of 3 independent small series.

In multiple sclerosis, the total protein concentration may be elevated. In Tourtellotte's series (Tourtellotte, 1970a) 23% of patients had CSF protein concentrations greater than 55 mg/dl.

There was a close correlation between the total protein concentration and the albumin concentration, so that elevated total protein concentrations were assumed to be due to impaired blood–CSF barrier function rather than intrathecal IgG synthesis. Tourtellotte (1970a) did not find any correlation between the total protein concentration and whether patients were in relapse or remission. Olsson et al. (1976) also provided evidence that elevated total protein concentrations in MS reflected damage to the blood–CSF barrier. They found elevated total protein concentrations in patients with severe disability and a long duration of disease.

IgG CONCENTRATION

The majority of patients with SSPE have increased amounts of IgG in their CSF, whether it is measured as gamma-globulin by electrophoresis (Bücher et al., 1952; Bauer, 1956; Booij, 1958; Lowenthal et al., 1960; Liano et al., 1971; Peter et al., 1974; Silva et al., 1981) or as IgG (Link et al., 1973; Silva et al., 1981). The amount of IgG expressed as a percentage of total protein is generally higher in SSPE than in MS (Booij, 1958; Lowenthal et al., 1960). As mentioned (see Introduction), intrathecal synthesis of IgG has been demonstrated directly in a number of patients by Cutler et al. (1968; 1970). Using Tourtellotte's empirical formula for calculating the intrathecal IgG synththesis rate (Tourtellotte, 1970b), Ewan and Lachmann (1979) found elevated rates of synthesis in patients with SSPE, which were generally higher than in MS patients.

Liano et al. (1971) interpret their data as indicating that the amount of gamma-globulin increases as the disease progresses. Peter et al. (1974) in a series of 42 patients found that gross elevations of the amount of gamma-globulin correlated with the disease being progressive, whereas lower levels were found in those in whom the disease process was clinically static.

In our series IgG levels were not available for some of the patients whose CSF specimens were sent from other hospitals. IgG concentration expressed as a percentage of the total protein concentration was, however, raised in the majority of cases, but there was no correlation between the amount of cathodal gamma globulin, expressed as a ratio with the amount of transferrin (measured as areas on densitometric scans of polyacrylamide gels) and duration. It must be reiterated, however, that the series was small.

It is well known that relative elevation of CSF gamma-globulin levels is a frequent finding in patients with multiple sclerosis (see Tourtellotte, 1970a) and when measured as IgG concentration as a percentage of total protein concentration, levels higher than 15% are found in 2/3 patients. Higher percentages of patients are found to have abnormal levels when the IgG index (Tibbling et al., 1977) is calculated. This index is the quotient of the CSF: serum ratio of IgG and albumin, and its advantage is that it corrects for variations in serum albumin and IgG concentrations as well as for variations in the blood–CSF barrier, so that it represents synthesis of IgG within the CNS more accurately. Between 85 and 90% of MS patients have an abnormally elevated IgG index (Olsson and Petterson, 1976; Link and Tibbling, 1977; Hershey and Trotter, 1980). Tourtellotte derived an "empirical formula" for estimating the intrathecal IgG synthesis rate, and showed that this is abnormally elevated in a high percentage of patients (between about 80 and 90%) (Tourtellotte, 1970b; Tourtellotte and Ma, 1978; Hershey and Trotter, 1979). As already mentioned (see Introduction), intrathecal synthesis of gamma-globulin was demonstrated more directly by Frick and Scheid-Seydel (1958), and this has been confirmed subsequently (see Tourtellotte, 1970a). Tourtellotte et al. (1980) showed a close correlation between the IgG synthesis rate calculated by his empirical formula and the synthesis rate measured by radio-labeled IgG exchange between serum and CSF.

Not only is the elevation of IgG in CSF helpful in supporting the clinical diagnosis of MS, but IgG levels correlate with some clinical parameters. Olsson and Link (1973) found higher relative IgG levels in patients in relapse compared to the same patients in remission. Ewan and Lachmann (1979), using Tourtellotte's formula, found higher IgG synthesis rates in MS patients in relapse than in remission. Olsson et al. (1976) found a correlation between relative IgG level and disability, and levels were particularly high in those severely disabled after a short duration of the disease. An association between a benign course and a relatively low IgG index was found by Stendahl-Brodin and Link (1980). However, other investigators have not found correlations (Schmidt et al., 1977; Christensen et al., 1978). Correlations between the CSF IgG concentration and the CSF white cell count have also been found (see Tourtellotte, 1970a and b; Eickhoff et al., 1977).

ELECTROPHORESIS AND ISOELECTRIC FOCUSING PATTERNS

Oligoclonal bands of gamma-globulin in SSPE were first reported by Booij (1959) and Karcher et al. (1959), and this finding has since been documented by numerous investigators, using Agar, agarose, or cellulose acetate electrophoresis (Lowenthal et al., 1960; Laterre et al., 1970; Liano et al., 1971; Link et al., 1973; Peter et al., 1974; Siemes et al., 1977; Silva et al., 1981). In most series, 100% patients with SSPE have oligoclonal bands in their CSF, and this has also been our experience using polyacrylamide gel electrophoresis (see Table I). Recently, Mattson et al. (1981) reported that all 15 of their CSF specimens from SSPE patients showed oligoclonal bands by isoelectric focusing.

The presence of oligoclonal bands within the gamma region is one of the most commonly found abnormalities of the CSF in MS, and may be found when all other parameters are normal (Lowenthal et al., 1960; Link, 1967; Laterre et al., 1970; Schwartz et al., 1970; Link and Müller, 1971; Bader et al., 1973; Vandvik and Skrede, 1973; Olsson and Pettersson, 1976; Johnson et al., 1977; Thompson et al., 1979). These electrophoretic findings have been extended by isoelectric focusing (Kjellin and Vesterberg, 1974; Delmotte and Gonsette, 1977; Trotter et al., 1977; Laurenzi and Link, 1978; Poloni et al., 1979; Olsson and Nilsson, 1979; Hosein and Johnson, 1981; Mattson et al., 1981; Livrea et al., 1981). The precise percentage of MS patients showing oligoclonal bands varies in each series, but using modern techniques is around 90%.

Siemes et al. (1977) compared their agarose electrophoresis results in SSPE and MS, and noted differences between the two. Their patients with SSPE had more bands (6–7) than those with MS (1–5), and several of these bands were pronounced, with distinct "valleys" between the peaks on the densitometric scans. In the MS CSF specimens, the bands were less well demarcated from one another. Mattson et al. (1981) have made similar observations about the prominence of the bands in SSPE and MS displayed by isoelectric focusing. They found no difference in mean band number between MS and SSPE specimens, either by agarose gel electrophoresis or isoelectric focusing.

Lowenthal et al. (1960) observed that the abnormal gamma-globulins in CSF from both MS and SSPE patients migrated more cathodally than the CSF gamma-globulins from normal individuals. They stressed that the bulk of the gamma-globulin was of even slower relative mobility in SSPE than in MS. They also recorded an abnormal anodal gamma-globulin fraction in SSPE. Peter et al. (1974) noted that cathodal gamma-globulin fractions were more likely to be found in clinically progressive SSPE patients than in patients whose disease was static.

TABLE I

CLINICAL AND CSF LABORATORY DATA ON 14 PATIENTS WITH SSPE

The diagnosis in each case was made on: (i) clinical grounds; (ii) characteristic EEG abnormalities; (iii) high measles antibody titers in serum and CSF. The disease was progressive in every case. Clinical grading was as described by Jabbour et al. (1969). NA, not available.

Patient number	Age	Duration of illness (months)	Clinical stage	CSF cell count (μl^{-1})	CSF total protein concentration (mg/dl)	IgG % of total protein	Polyacrylamide gel electrophoresis	
							Blood–CSF barrier	Oligoclonal bands
1	5	1	2	4	30	23.3	Normal	2
2	5	6	2	< 1	20	NA	Normal	3
3	6	1	2	1	42	14.3	Normal	3
4	8	5	2	NA	38	NA	Normal	2
5	9	6	1	< 1	< 10	NA	Normal	3
6	11	11	2	NA	30	NA	Normal	3
7	11	11	2	1	58	40.5	Normal	3
8	13	10	2	1	44	44.3	Normal	3
9	13	2	2	12	68	15	Transudate	5
10	16	24	1	0	39	9.5	Normal	3
11	17	2	1	NA	100	NA	Transudate	2
12	17	7	2	0	25	22	Transudate	2
13	18	36	2	0	40	24.8	Normal	4
14	21	2	2	7	48	36.5	Normal	3

Abnormal anodal and cathodal gamma globulin fractions in SSPE CSF have also been demonstrated by immunoelectrophoresis (Dencker and Kolar, 1965; Liano et al., 1971). Many reports point out that the pathological gamma-globulin in MS migrates in the slow gamma region or focuses in the alkaline region by isoelectric focusing (Vandvik and Skrede, 1973; Delmotte and Gonsette, 1977; Laurenzi and Link, 1978; Olsson and Nilsson, 1979; Hosein and Johnson, 1981; Mattson et al., 1981). We compared the mean of the R_fs of the tallest band (measured by densitometry) of each of our SSPE CSF specimens to the mean of the R_fs of the tallest band of a series of patients with clinically definite MS, and found no significant difference. Link et al. (1973) were also not able to distinguish between MS and SSPE electrophoretic patterns using Agar gel electrophoresis.

CHANGES IN BANDS WITH TIME

A point stressed by a number of investigators is that the electrophoretic pattern of the gamma region is unique to each individual MS patient, but remains constant when CSF specimens obtained at different times are compared (Olsson and Link, 1973; Delmotte and Gonsette, 1977; Olsson and Nilsson, 1979). Recently anti-idiotype antibodies have been raised, to identify homogeneous IgG idiotypes in the CSF and serum of individual MS patients, and it has been shown that the idiotypes thus defined have been present in CSF specimens taken 5 or 6 years apart (Baird et al., 1980; Gerhard et al., 1981). However, others have noticed changes in oligoclonal patterns (Siden and Kjellin, 1978). Mattson et al. (1980) showed that there were differences in the oligoclonal patterns between IgG eluates from different plaques in the same

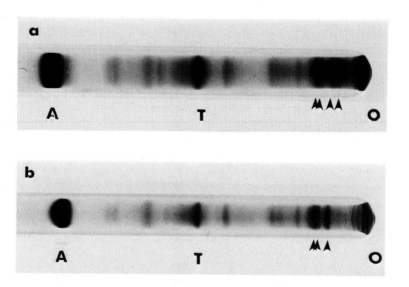

Fig. 1. Polyacrylamide rod gels, stained by Coomassie brilliant blue, after electrophoresis of unconcentrated cerebrospinal fluid from patient 13 (see Table I), at the time of initial investigation (a), and one month later (b), during which she had received isoprinosine, but during which her clinical condition had not changed significantly. A, albumin; T, transferrin; O, origin. The arrowheads show the 4 major oligoclonal bands in the gamma region in the first specimen (a), and there is loss of the most cathodal band in the second specimen (b).

patient, so one might expect that plaques developing during the disease would be reflected in alterations in the gamma-globulins in the CSF. Mattson et al. (1981) found alterations in the band patterns of CSF IgG from MS patients studied serially, and they also found a significant correlation between the number of bands demonstrated by isoelectric focusing and the duration of the disease. We also have data (unpublished observations) using polyacrylamide gel electrophoresis of unconcentrated CSF showing alterations of the oligoclonal band patterns in individual patients who have had more than one lumbar puncture.

By contrast there is universal agreement that the electrophoretic patterns change during the course of SSPE (Vandvik et al., 1973; Vandvik, 1977; Johnson and Nelson, 1977; Mattson et al., 1981). (See also Fig. 1). Vandvik et al. (1973) showed that, in one patient with SSPE, new bands appeared during an exacerbation of his illness, and these regressed when he remitted following the administration of transfer factor. Out of 5 SSPE patients whose CSF specimens were studied serially by Mattson et al. (1981), 3 showed an increase in band number in the second CSF specimen.

SUBCLASS RESTRICTION, KAPPA AND LAMBDA CHAINS, FREE LIGHT CHAINS AND IMMUNOGLOBULIN FRAGMENTS

Vandvik et al. (1976a) produced evidence that the oligoclonal IgG in CSF from both SSPE and MS patients was principally of the IgG_1 subclass. Eickhoff et al. (1979) and Kaschka et al. (1979) showed absolute increases in all IgG subclasses in MS CSF, but particularly IgG_1, so that the relative percentage of IgG_1 was elevated at the expense of the other subclasses. The predominance of one subclass in CSF in comparison to serum and normal CSF is further evidence of the restricted heterogeneity of the CSF IgG and of local synthesis of IgG (see Introduction). Keir et al. (1981) (submitted for publication) have shown that while the predominant subclass in MS CSF is IgG_1, oligoclonal bands of the other subclasses can also be demonstrated if the immunofixation technique used is sensitive enough.

There have been a number of reports concerning the kappa and lambda light chains of oligoclonal IgG in both SSPE and MS. Abnormal kappa:lambda light chain ratios were first reported in CSF from some, not all, MS patients by Link and Zetterval (1970). They found an increased kappa:lambda ratio in 6 out of 11 patients. In the other 5 it was normal. The ratio in the sera of all the patients was normal. The same authors (Zettervall and Link, 1970) subsequently showed that individual oligoclonal bands separated by Agar gel electrophoresis contained excesses of either kappa or lambda chains. These results were supported by similar findings by Vandvik (1977) using crossed immunoelectrophoresis for both MS and SSPE CSF specimens. Direct immunofixation is the highest resolution technique available for characterizing individual bands. It has been confirmed for MS that individual bands separated by agarose gel electrophoresis may contain only kappa or only lambda light chains, or may contain both (Link and Laurenzi, 1979), and even isoelectric focusing does not always resolve all the kappa chain immunoglobulins from the lambda chain immunoglobulins (Laurenzi et al., 1979). In general, IgG kappa bands predominate in number, but there are marked individual variations. These immunofixation studies presumably reflect the same phenomenon as measurements of kappa:lambda ratios, which are generally found to be raised in MS CSF, although some individuals have normal or low kappa:lambda ratios (Bollengier et al., 1975; Bollengier et al., 1976; Roberts-Thomson et al., 1976; Bollengier et al., 1978; Eickhoff et al., 1978; Link and Laurenzi, 1979).

Similarly disturbed kappa:lambda ratios have been found in the CSF of SSPE patients (Bollengier et al., 1975; Bollengier et al., 1978), and again there is wide individual variation.

The CSF of MS patients frequently contains free kappa and or lambda light chains (Bollengier et al., 1975; Bollengier et al., 1976; Vandvik, 1977; Bollengier et al., 1978; Link and Laurenzi, 1979; Laurenzi et al., 1979), and free kappa and lambda light chains were found in nearly all the cases of SSPE presented by Bollengier and co-workers (Bollengier et al., 1975; Bollengier et al., 1978). The pathological significance of free light chains is not clear. They may represent breakdown products of complete IgG molecules, or may represent defective synthesis of immunoglobulins in pathological conditions. Free light chains and other fragments of IgG molecules may underlie the double ring phenomenon seen when attempting to quantify kappa and lambda chains in MS and SSPE CSF by radial immunodiffusion (Iwashita et al., 1974; Bollengier et al., 1975; Bollengier et al., 1976; Bollengier et al., 1978), and also the doubling of immunoprecipitation arcs in immunoelectrophoresis, as described by a number of researchers (see Kolar et al., 1980). Bergmann et al. (1968) produced evidence for the presence of fragments of IgG molecules, similar to Fab fragments, in CSF from patients with SSPE. We have sometimes noticed gross discrepancies between the amount of IgG measured by electroimmunoassay and the amount of gamma-globulin stained by Coomassie brilliant blue after polyacrylamide gel electrophoresis, and it may be that the presence of fragments and free light chains interferes with quantification by immunological assays, a point to which Cutler et al. (1968) drew attention.

IDIOTYPES IN SSPE AND MS

One way to study the immunoglobulins produced by individual clones of B-cells is to raise anti-idiotype antibodies. This was achieved by Nordal et al. (1977) using measles virus-specific IgG from the serum of a patient with SSPE. They showed that the idiotype defined by their rabbit anti-idiotype antibody migrated in a cathodal band in both serum and CSF, and the serum:CSF ratio was 21, as opposed to 73 for IgG, suggesting strongly that the idiotype was synthesized intrathecally. They did not find cross-idiotypic specificity in 4 other SSPE patients. Strosberg et al. (1979), on the other hand, found cross-idiotypic specificity between 7/18 SSPE sera, with one anti-idiotype antibody against IgG from a patient with SSPE, and the same anti-idiotype also formed precipitin lines when set up against some MS sera, but never when control normal sera were used.

Ebers et al. (1979) defined a number of idiotypes in 2 SSPE patients and showed them to be present, either in both the serum and CSF of the patient in ratios suggesting systemic synthesis, or, in one case, in a serum:CSF ratio of 32 indicating intrathecal synthesis. Thus in SSPE there may be different clones synthesizing antibody inside and outside the central nervous system, although generally serum oligoclonal bands are found to have counterparts in CSF with the same electrophoretic mobility (Vandvik, 1977; Ebers et al., 1979). Ebers et al. (1979) found low titer cross-idiotypic specificity for 3 out of 14 SSPE patients only.

Idiotypes have also been looked at in MS. Baird et al. (1980) raised anti-idiotype antibodies using pooled concentrated CSF specimens from a single patient and found serum:CSF ratios which indicated intrathecal synthesis. Cross-idiotypic specificity was found in 1 out of 13 other MS patients. Nagelkerken et al. (1980) demonstrated intrathecal synthesis of homogeneous IgG in two patients, using anti-idiotype antibodies. No cross-idiotypic specificity was demonstrated between the two patients or with 13 other MS patients. The idiotype studied by Gerhard

(1981) from a patient with MS was consistently shown to be CNS derived, CSF:serum ratios being raised between 9 and 15 times those of total IgG. Their idiotype bound strongly to Theiler murine encephalomyelitis virus. Whether or not the patient's immunological system intended it to do so remains an open question. Ebers et al. (1979) also raised anti-idiotype antisera to intrathecally synthesized IgG idiotypes in 2 MS CSF specimens. They found no cross-idiotypic specificity.

VIRAL ANTIBODIES

Connolly et al. (1967) discovered the very high levels of measles virus antibodies in CSF and serum of SSPE patients, and these high titers are now a necessary diagnostic criterion (Bellman and Dick, 1980). In multiple sclerosis, measles virus antibody titers are frequently elevated in CSF, and serum:CSF ratios relative to other viral antibody titers indicate that there is local synthesis, but titers to viruses such as vaccinia, rubella and herpes simplex may also be elevated (reviewed by Norrby, 1978).

Vandvik and Norrby (1973) showed that oligoclonal bands in CSF of patients with SSPE represented antibodies to components of measles viruses. Subsequently Vandvik et al. (1976b) showed that the majority of the oligoclonal IgG in SSPE CSF could be absorbed out by measles virus antigen preparations. Some bands, however, were not absorbed out, although there was practically complete absorption by measles antigens of oligoclonal IgG eluted from SSPE brain. Mehta et al. (1977) confirmed the complete removal of oligoclonal IgG eluted from SSPE brain by absorption with measles antigens. Tourtellotte et al. (1981a) were unable to remove all the oligoclonal bands from CSF of two patients with SSPE by prior absorption of antibodies with a concentrated measles virus antigen preparation. Doing the same experiment on MS CSF, there was no electrophoretically demonstrable decrease of oligoclonal IgG after absorption with measles antigens (Vandvik et al., 1976b). The antibody subsequently retrieved from the measles antigen preparation was, however, shown to be electrophoretically homogeneous in those MS patients who showed evidence of local synthesis of measles antibodies as assessed by serum:CSF titers.

Nordal et al. (1978a) developed the technique of imprint electroimmunofixation (IEIF), in which antigen suspended or dissolved in a layer of agarose gel is layered on top of the agarose gel in which a CSF or serum sample has been electrophoresed. Specific antibody precipitates with antigen in the overlaid gel, and may be detected by ^{125}I-labeled anti-human IgG and autoradiography. Using this technique they demonstrated the measles virus specificity of oligoclonal IgG in CSF from a patient with SSPE. However there were discrepancies between the Coomassie-stained band patterns and the autoradiograph patterns. These were of two sorts. Firstly, not every Coomassie-stained band had its counterpart on the autoradiogram. Secondly, the band seen most intensely using autoradiography was not that most intensely stained by Coomassie. The explanation put forward was that the measles antigen preparation may have had some under-represented antigenic determinants. The technique was thought to work best for large or particulate antigens. Another explanation might be that the IgG present in greatest amount was not that with the highest association constant for its determinant. Panitch et al. (1979) have also found that IEIF does not identify all the oligoclonal bands in SSPE CSF specimens as anti-measles.

Nordal et al. (1978b) demonstrated intrathecal oligoclonal antibody responses to one or more of 4 viruses (measles, rubella, mumps and herpes simplex virus) in 9 out of 10 tested MS patients, but there was no association between the viral antibody bands displayed by autoradiography and the oligoclonal bands stained by Coomassie brilliant blue, indicating that the viral antibodies constituted only a small fraction of the locally produced IgG. This work was extended by Vartdal et al. (1980), who used IEIF to demonstrate the presence of oligoclonal locally synthesized antibodies to a variety of viruses (mainly neurotropic) in MS CSF specimens. Again there was a mismatch between the autoradiograph patterns and the Coomassie-stained patterns. They suggested that in MS there was non-specific activation of a variety of antibody-producing cell clones in the CNS. There is some evidence that in patients with CNS infections, including SSPE, there is synthesis within the CNS of small amounts of oligoclonal antibodies to unrelated viral antigens, as appears to be the case in MS (Vandvik and Norrby, 1980).

Schorr et al. (1981) have used the same IEIF technique after isoelectric focusing. They distinguished between oligoclonal and polyclonal zones of CSF IgG separated by isoelectric focusing, and found measles antibody activity in all of the oligoclonal zones and some of the polyclonal zones of all 3 SSPE CSF specimens tested. In MS CSF specimens they found measles antibody in some oligoclonal zones and some polyclonal zones. Their results differ slightly from those of Norrby and his co-workers in that they could match up autoradiograph bands with Coomassie bands in the MS specimens. However, in both diseases the relative intensities of autoradiograph bands and Coomassie bands were disparate. Roström et al. (1981) have extended these findings in MS CSF specimens, and have shown that there is intrathecal synthesis of antibody to other viral antigens (herpes simplex virus, mumps and rubella).

The absorption experiments provide good evidence that the majority, possibly all of the oligoclonal bands visible by agarose electrophoresis of concentrated CSF from SSPE patients consist of measles antibody, whereas the specificity of the bulk of the oligoclonal bands in MS remains unaccounted for. The immunoprint experiments are entirely qualitative and no assessment can be made of the binding affinity of the antibodies displayed by this technique. It has not been excluded that the antibodies detected are not cross-reacting, with primary specificities directed against other determinants. The experiment reported by Panitch et al. (1979) is relevant in this respect (see below).

Quantitative approaches to the problem of antibody specificity have been used in some centers. Mehta et al. (1977) calculated that the measles specific IgG in CSF from SSPE patients constituted 25–60% of the total IgG, in comparison with 10–20% of serum IgG. Of course, this does not tell one what percentage of intrathecally-synthesized IgG is measles virus-specific. They found that 40–75% of IgG eluted from SSPE brain was measles antibody.

Gorman et al. (1980) used Tourtellotte's formula and a solid-phase radioimmunoassay for measles antibodies to calculate the intracerebral synthesis rate of measles antibodies in SSPE and MS. They found values of 6.0 ± 2.3 mg/day in SSPE, more than 10 times higher than in MS, which was not different from other neurological diseases. Only 20% of intrathecally synthesized IgG was measles antibody. However, their radio-immunoassay did not assay antibodies to all the measles virus antigens, which may account for the differences between these results and those published recently by Tourtellotte et al. (1981a) who measured the amount of measles antibody by assaying IgG before and after absorption by a concentrated measles virus preparation. Measles antibody synthesis rates of 57 mg/day (59% of total IgG) and 145 mg/day (82% of total IgG) were found in two patients. By the same method, Tourtellotte et al. (1981c) found that 10–32% of IgG synthesized in MS was measles antibody in some patients, higher than predicted by the qualitative assessments using IEIF. Thus there are considerable discrepancies for both SSPE and MS between qualitative and quantitative assessments of the contribution of measles antibodies to the intrathecally synthesized IgG.

ANTIBODIES TO NON-VIRAL ANTIGENS

In broad terms, the etiology of SSPE is known, but further research into the specificities of antibodies synthesized during the disease may throw more light onto aspects of the pathogenesis of the disease, and may be of value in formulating ideas about the pathogenesis of related disorders whose etiology remains obscure, such as MS.

For instance, it is of interest that, while myelin basic protein antibodies are detected in MS CSF (Panitch et al., 1980) and the titers are higher in relapse than in remission, even higher levels are detected in SSPE. High levels of myelin basic protein antibodies in SSPE CSF have also been found by Frey et al. (1981). However, Panitch et al. (1979) showed that if measles antibodies were absorbed out of SSPE CSF, the myelin basic protein antibodies could then no longer be detected. One possible interpretation is that the myelin basic protein antibody detected represented cross-reacting measles virus antibody. Myelin basic protein antibodies were always found in oligoclonal bands which could be shown to contain measles antibodies. The possibility of cross-reaction applies to all the studies of antibody specificity mentioned. Specific anti-myelin basic protein antibodies have association constants of 10^8 M^{-1} or more, whereas non-specific interactions occur with association constants of the order of 10^4 M^{-1} (Varitek and Day, 1979).

Another problem is non-specific binding of IgG to putative antigens by the Fc component. Thus the oligodendrocyte antibody activity reported in MS sera by Abramsky et al. (1977) has been shown to be due to non-specific binding (Traugott et al., 1979; Ma et al., 1981).

Ryberg (1976, 1978) has reported the presence of anti-brain antibodies in CSF from a proportion of MS patients tested, and recently, Tourtellotte (1981b) has produced evidence which suggests binding of CSF IgG from MS patients to plaque and periplaque tissue, but not to normal-appearing white matter from MS brain.

CONCLUDING REMARKS

In spite of intensive research, the significance of CSF antibodies in MS remains totally unknown. So many antibody specificities have been demonstrated that it has been hypothesized that the intrathecally synthesized IgG represents "nonsense antibodies" (Mattson et al., 1980) whose existence is quite peripheral to the etiology and pathogenesis of the disease. Nevertheless, the antibody specificity of the bulk of the oligoclonal IgG remains undefined and may be as significant an indicator of the etiology of MS as measles antibodies are in SSPE, in which antibodies of other specificities have also been demonstrated.

Although measles antibodies have diagnostic importance in SSPE, their role in pathogenesis is not defined. T-cell-mediated immunological mechanisms are much more important in combatting measles infection (see Valdimarsson et al., 1979; ter Meulen and Siddell, 1981), but it may be that the presence of high titers of measles antibodies facilitate persistent infection by measles virus, possibly by mechanisms such as those documented by Oldstone and co-workers (Joseph and Oldstone, 1974; Oldstone and Tishon, 1978). Similarly, while variations in amounts of IgG synthesized intrathecally may occur in relapse and remission in MS, it may be that T-cell-changes in relation to relapse and remission are more closely bound up with the actual pathogenesis of demyelinating plaques.

REFERENCES

Abramsky, O., Lisak, R.P., Silberberg, D.H. and Pleasure, D.E. (1977) Antibodies to oligodendroglia in patients with multiple sclerosis. *New Engl. J. Med.*, 297: 1207–1211.

Bader, R., Rieder, H.P. and Kaesser, H.E. (1973) Die Bedeutung der diskontinuerlichen Zonierung des Immunglobulinbereiches für die Diagnose neurologischer Erkrankungen. *Z. Neurol.*, 206: 25–38.

Baird, L.G., Tachovsky, T.G., Sandberg-Wollheim, M., Koprowski, H. and Nisonoff, A. (1980) Identification of a unique idiotype in cerebrospinal fluid and serum of a patient with multiple sclerosis. *J. Immunol.*, 124: 2324–2328.

Bauer, H. (1956) Zur Frage der Identität der Liquorproteine mit den Eiweisskörpern des Blutserums. *Deutsch. Z. Nervenheilk.*, 175: 354–377.

Bellman, M.H. and Dick, G. (1980) Surveillance of subacute sclerosing panencephalitis. *Brit. Med. J.*, 281: 393–394.

Bergmann, L., Dencker, S.J. Johansson, B.G. and Svennerholm, L. (1968) Cerebrospinal fluid gamma globulins in subacute sclerosing leucoencephalitis. *J. Neurochem.*, 15: 781–785.

Bollengier, F., Lowenthal, A. and Henrotin, W. (1975) Bound and free light chains in subacute sclerosing panencephalitis and multiple sclerosis serum and cerebrospinal fluid. *Z. Klin. Chem. klin. Biochem.*, 13: 305–310.

Bollengier, F., Delmotte, P. and Lowenthal, A. (1976) Biochemical findings in multiple sclerosis. III. Immunoglobulins of restricted heterogeneity and light chain distribution in cerebrospinal fluid of patients with multiple sclerosis. *J. Neurol.*, 212: 151–158.

Bollengier, F., Rabinovitch, N. and Lowenthal, A. (1978) Oligoclonal immunoglobulins, light chain ratios and free light chains in cerebrospinal fluid and serum from patients affected with various neurological diseases. *J. clin. Chem. clin. Biochem.*, 16: 165–173.

Booij, J. (1958) The CSF aspects of leuko-encephalitis. *Folia psychiat. neerl.*, 61: 352–366.

Booij, J. (1959) Agar–agar electrophoresis as an aid in cerebrospinal fluid diagnostics. *Folia psychiat. neerl.*, 62: 247–253.

Bücher, Th., Matzelt, D. and Pette, D. (1952) Papier Electrophorese von Liquor cerebrospinalis. *Klin. Wschr.*, 30: 325–330.

Christensen, O., Clausen, J. and Fog, T. (1978) Relationships between abnormal IgG index, oligoclonal bands, acute phase reactants and some clinical data in multiple sclerosis. *J. Neurol.*, 218: 237–244.

Connolly, J.H., Allen, I.V., Hurwitz, L.J. and Millar, J.H.D. (1967) Measles virus antibody and antigen in subacute sclerosing panencephalitis. *Lancet*, i: 542–544.

Cutler, R.W.P., Merler, E. and Hammerstad, J.P. (1968) Production of antibody by the central nervous system in subacute sclerosing panencephalitis. *Neurology*, 18: 129–132.

Cutler, R.W.P., Watters, G.V. and Hammerstad, J.P. (1970) The origin and turnover rates of cerebrospinal fluid albumin and gamma-globulin in man. *J. neurol. Sci.*, 10: 259–268.

Delmotte, P. and Gonsette, R. (1977) Biochemical findings in multiple sclerosis. IV. Isoelectric focusing of the CSF gamma globulins in multiple sclerosis and other neurological diseases. *J. Neurol.*, 215: 27–37.

Dencker, S.J. and Kolar, O. (1965) The cerebrospinal fluid gamma-globulin profile in subacute sclerosing leuco-encephalitis. *Acta neurol. scand.*, 41, Suppl. 13, Part I: 135–140.

Ebers, G.C., Zabriskie, J.B. and Kunkel, H.G. (1979) Oligoclonal immunoglobulins in subacute sclerosing panencephalitis and multiple sclerosis: a study of idiotypic determinants. *Clin. exp. Immunol.*, 35: 67–75.

Eickhoff, K., Wikström, J., Poser, S. and Bauer, H. (1977) Protein profile of cerebrospinal fluid in multiple sclerosis with special reference to the function of the blood brain barrier. *J. Neurol.*, 214: 207–215.

Eickhoff, K., Heipertz, R. and Wikström, J. (1978) Determination of kappa/lambda immunoglobulin light chain ratios in CSF from patients with multiple sclerosis and other neurological diseases. *Acta neurol. scand.*, 57: 385–395.

Eickhoff, K., Kaschka, W., Skvaril, F., Theilkaes, L. and Heipertz, R. (1979) Determination of IgG subgroups in cerebrospinal fluid of multiple sclerosis patients and others. *Acta neurol. scand.*, 60: 277–282.

Ewan, P.W. and Lachmann, P.J. (1979) IgG synthesis within the brain in multiple sclerosis and subacute sclerosing panencephalitis. *Clin. exp. Immunol.*, 35: 227–235.

Frey, H., Ruutiainen, J. and Salmi, A. (1981) GFA-antibodies and myelin basic protein antibodies in MS, SSPE, brain tumours and other neurological diseases. In *Abstracts of the 12th World Congress of Neurology, International Congress Series 548*, Excerpta Medica, Amsterdam, no. 238.

Frick, E. and Scheid-Seydel, L. (1958) Untersuchungen mit J[131]-markiertem gamma-globulin zur Frage der Abstammung der Liquoreiweisskörper. *Klin. Wschr.*, 36: 857–863.

Gerhard, W., Taylor, A., Wroblewska, Z., Sandberg-Wollheim, M. and Koprowski, H. (1981) Analysis of a predominant immunoglobulin population in the cerebrospinal fluid of a multiple sclerosis patient by means of an anti-idiotypic hybridoma antibody. *Proc. nat. Acad. Sci. U.S.A.*, 78: 3225–3229.

Gorman, N.T., Habicht, J. and Lachmann, P.J. (1980) Intracerebral synthesis of antibodies to measles and distemper viruses in patients with subacute sclerosing panencephalitis and multiple sclerosis. *Clin. exp. Immunol.*, 39: 44–52.

Haber, E., Margolies, M.N. and Cannon, L.E. (1979) Insights gained from the study of homogeneous rabbit antibodies. In D. Karcher, A. Lowenthal and A.D. Strosberg (Eds.), *Humoral Immunity in Neurological Diseases, Nato Advanced Study Institute Series, Series A: Life Sciences, Vol. 24,* Plenum, New York, pp. 327–359.

Hershey, L.A. and Trotter, J.L. (1980) The use and abuse of the cerebrospinal fluid IgG profile in the adult: a practical evaluation. *Ann. Neurol.*, 8: 426–434.

Hosein, Z.Z. and Johnson, K.P. (1981) Isoelectric focusing of cerebrospinal fluid proteins in the diagnosis of multiple sclerosis. *Neurology*, 31: 70–76.

Iwashita, H., Grunwald, F. and Bauer, H. (1974) Double ring formation in single radial immunodiffusion for kappa chains in multiple sclerosis cerebrospinal fluid. *J. Neurol.*, 207: 45–52.

Jabbour, J.T., Garcia, J.H., Lemmi, H., Ragland, J., Duenas, D.A. and Sever, J.L. (1969) Subacute sclerosing panencephalitis: a multidisciplinary study of eight cases. *JAMA*, 207: 2248–2254.

Johnson, K.P. and Nelson, B.J. (1977) Multiple sclerosis: diagnostic usefulness of cerebrospinal fluid. *Ann. Neurol.*, 2: 425–431.

Johnson, K.P., Arrigo, S.C., Nelson, B.J. and Ginsberg, A. (1977) Agarose electrophoresis of cerebrospinal fluid in multiple sclerosis. *Neurology*, 27: 273–277.

Joseph, B.S. and Oldstone, M.B.A. (1974) Antibody-induced redistribution of measles virus antigen on the cell surface. *J. Immunol.*, 113: 1205–1209.

Karcher, D., van Sande, M. and Lowenthal, A. (1959) Micro-electrophoresis in agar gel of proteins of the cerebrospinal fluid and central nervous system. *J. Neurochem.*, 4: 135–140.

Kaschka, W., Theilkaes, L., Eickhoff, K. and Skvaril, F. (1979) Disproportional elevation of the immunoglobulin G1 concentration in cerebrospinal fluids of patients with multiple sclerosis. *Infect. Immun.*, 26: 933–941.

Kjellin, K.G. and Vesterberg, O. (1974) Isoelectric focusing of CSF proteins in neurological diseases. *J. neurol. Sci.*, 23: 199–213.

Kolar, O.J., Rice, P.H., Jones, F.H., Defalque, R.J. and Kincaid, J. (1980) Cerebrospinal fluid immunoelectrophoresis in multiple sclerosis. *J. neurol. Sci.*, 47: 221–230.

Laterre, E.C., Callewaert, A., Heremans, J.F. and Sfaello, Z. (1970) Electrophoretic morphology of gamma globulins in cerebrospinal fluid of multiple sclerosis and other diseases of the nervous system. *Neurology*, 20: 982–990.

Laurenzi, M.A. and Link, H. (1978) Comparison between agarose gel electrophoresis and isoelectric focusing of CSF for demonstration of oligoclonal immunoglobulin bands in neurological disorders. *Acta neurol. scand.*, 58, 148–156.

Laurenzi, M.A. Mavra, M., Kam-Hansen, S. and Link, H. (1979) Oligoclonal IgG and free light chains in multiple sclerosis demonstrated by thin-layer polyacrylamide gel isoelectric focusing and immunofixation. *Ann. Neurol.*, 8: 241–247.

Liano, H., Gimeno, A., Kreisler, M. and Ramirez, G. (1971) Cerebrospinal fluid proteins in subacute sclerosing panencephalitis. *Acta neurol. scand.*, 47: 579–593.

Link, H. (1967) Immunoglobulin G and low molecular weight proteins in human cerebrospinal fluid: chemical and immunological characterisation with special reference to multiple sclerosis. *Acta neurol. scand.*, 43, Suppl. 28: 1–136.

Link, H. (1973) Comparison of electrophoresis on agar gel and agarose gel in the evaluation of gamma-globulin abnormalities in cerebrospinal fluid and serum in multiple sclerosis. *Clin. Chim. Acta*, 46: 383–389.

Link, H. and Laurenzi, M.A. (1979) Immunoglobulin class and light chain type of oligoclonal bands in CSF in multiple sclerosis determined by agarose gel electrophoresis and immunofixation. *Ann. Neurol.*, 6: 107–110.

Link, H. and Müller, R. (1971) Immunoglobulins in multiple sclerosis and infections of the nervous system. *Arch. Neurol.*, 25: 326–344.

Link, H. and Tibbling, G. (1977) Principles of albumin and IgG analyses in neurological disorders. III. Evaluation of IgG synthesis within the central nervous system in multiple sclerosis. *Scand. J. Clin. lab. Invest.*, 37: 397–401.

Link, H. and Zettervall, O. (1970) Multiple sclerosis: disturbed kappa:lambda chain ratio of immunoglobulin G in cerebrospinal fluid. *Clin. exp. Immunol.*, 6: 435–438.

Link, H., Panelius, M. and Salmi, A.A. (1973) Immunoglobulins and measles antibodies in subacute sclerosing panencephalitis. *Arch. Neurol.*, 28: 23–30.

Livrea, P., Trojano, M., Simone, I.L., Zimatore G.B., Lamontanara, G. and Leante, R. (1981) Intrathecal IgG synthesis in multiple sclerosis: comparison between isoelectric focusing and quantitative estimation of cerebrospinal fluid IgG. *J. Neurol.,* 224: 159–169.

Lowenthal, A., van Sande, M. and Karcher, D. (1960) The differential diagnosis of neurological diseases by fractionating electrophoretically the CSF gamma globulins. *J. Neurochem.,* 6: 51–56.

Lowenthal, A., van Sande, M. and Karcher, D. (1971) Serum gamma globulins in 84 typical cases of subacute sclerosing panencephalitis. *Neurology,* 21: 277–280.

Ma, B.I., Joseph, B.S., Walsh, M.J., Potvin, A.R. and Tourtellotte, W.W. (1981) Multiple sclerosis serum and cerebrospinal fluid immunoglobulin binding to Fc receptors of oligodendrocytes. *Ann. Neurol.,* 9: 371–377.

Mattson, D.H., Roos, R.P. and Arnason, B.G.W. (1980) Isoelectric focusing of IgG eluted from multiple sclerosis and subacute sclerosing panencephalitis brains. *Nature (Lond.),* 287: 335–337.

Mattson, D.H., Roos, R.P. and Arnason, B.G.W. (1981) Comparison of agar gel electrophoresis and isoelectric focusing in multiple sclerosis and subacute sclerosing panencephalitis. *Ann. Neurol.,* 9: 34–41.

Mehta, P.D., Kane, A. and Thormar, H. (1977) Quantitation of measles virus-specific immunoglobulins in serum, CSF, and brain extract from patients with subacute sclerosing panencephalitis. *J. Immunol.,* 118: 2254–2261.

Nagelkerken, L., Aalberse, R.C., Van Walbeck, H.K. and Out, T.A. (1980) Preparation of antisera directed against the idiotype(s) of immunoglobulin G from the cerebrospinal fluid of patients with multiple sclerosis. *J. Immunol.,* 125: 384–389.

Nordal, H.J., Vandvik, B. and Natvig, J.B. (1977) Idiotyping of measles virus nucleocapsid-specific IgG kappa antibody in serum and cerebrospinal fluid in subacute sclerosing panencephalitis. *Scand. J. Immunol.,* 6: 1351–1356.

Nordal, H.J., Vandvik, B. and Norrby, E. (1978a) Demonstration of electrophoretically restricted virus-specific antibodies in serum and cerebrospinal fluid by immunoprint electroimmunofixation. *Scand. J. Immunol.,* 7: 381–388.

Nordal, H.J., Vandvik, B. and Norrby, E. (1978b) Multiple sclerosis: local synthesis of electrophoretically restricted measles, rubella, mumps and herpes simplex virus antibodies in the central nervous system. *Scand. J. Immunol.,* 7: 473–479.

Norrby, E. (1978) Viral antibodies in multiple sclerosis. *Progr. med. Virol.,* 24: 1–39.

Oldstone, M.B.A. and Tishon, A. (1978) Immunologic injury in measles virus infection. IV. Antigenic modulation and abrogation of lymphocyte lysis of virus-infected cells. *Clin. Immunol. Immunopathol.,* 9: 55–62.

Olsson, J.-E. and Link, H. (1973) Immunoglobulin abnormalities in multiple sclerosis. Relation to clinical parameters: exacerbations and remissions. *Arch. Neurol.,* 28: 392–399.

Olsson, J.-E. and Nilsson, K. (1979) Gamma globulins of CSF and serum in multiple sclerosis: isoelectric focusing on polyacrylamide gel and agar gel electrophoresis. *Neurology,* 29: 1383–1391.

Olsson, J.-E. and Pettersson, B. (1976) A comparison between agar gel electrophoresis and CSF serum quotients of IgG and albumin in neurological diseases. *Acta neurol. scand.,* 53: 308–322.

Olsson, J.-E., Link, H. and Müller, R. (1976) Immunoglobulin abnormalities in multiple sclerosis. Relation to clinical parameters: disability, duration and age of onset. *J. neurol. Sci.,* 27: 233–245.

Panitch, H.S., Swoveland, P. and Johnson, K.P. (1979) Antibodies to measles virus react with myelin basic protein. *Neurology,* 29: 548–549.

Panitch, H.S., Hooper, C.J. and Johnson, K.P. (1980) CSF antibody to myelin basic protein. *Arch. Neurol.,* 37: 206–209.

Peter, A. (1967) The plasma cells of the cerebrospinal fluid. *J. neurol. Sci.,* 4: 227–239.

Peter A., Lowenthal, A. and Juvancz, I. (1974) Changes of gamma globulins in serum and cerebrospinal fluid of patients with subacute sclerosing panencephalitis. *J. Neurol.,* 207: 85–92.

Poloni, M., Rocchelli, B., Scelsi, R. and Pinelli, P. (1979) Intrathecal IgG synthesis in multiple sclerosis and other neurological diseases: a comparative evaluation by IgG-index and isoelectric focusing. *J. Neurol.,* 221: 245–255.

Roberts-Thomson, P.J., Esiri, M.M., Young, A.C. and MacLennan, I.C.M. (1976) Cerebrospinal fluid immunoglobulin quotients, kappa/lambda ratios, and viral antibody titres in neurological disease. *J. clin. Pathol.,* 29: 1105–1115.

Roström, B., Link, H., Laurenzi, M.A., Kam-Hansen, S., Norrby, E. and Wahren, B. (1981) Viral antibody activity of oligoclonal and polyclonal immunoglobulins synthesized within the central nervous system in multiple sclerosis. *Ann. Neurol.,* 9: 569–574.

Ryberg, B. (1976) Complement-fixing antibrain antibodies in multiple sclerosis. *Acta neurol. scand.,* 54: 1–12.

Ryberg, B. (1978) Multiple specificities of antibrain antibodies in multiple sclerosis and chronic myelopathy. *J. neurol. Sci.,* 38: 357–382.

Schmidt, R., Rieder, H.P. and Wüthrich, R. (1977) The course of multiple sclerosis cases with extremely high gamma-globulin values in the cerebrospinal fluid. *Europ. Neurol.*, 15: 241–248.

Schorr, J., Roström, B. and Link, H. (1981) Antibodies to viral and non-viral antigens in subacute sclerosing panencephalitis and multiple sclerosis demonstrated by thin-layer polyacrylamide gel isoelectric focusing, antigen immunofixation and autoradiography. *J. neurol. Sci.*, 49: 99–108.

Schuller, E., Delasnerie, N., Deloche, G. and Loridan, M. (1973) Multiple sclerosis: a two-phase disease? *Acta neurol. scand.*, 49: 453–460.

Schwartz, S., Rieder, H.P. and Würthrich, R. (1970) The protein fractions in cerebrospinal fluid in the various states of multiple sclerosis. *Europ. Neurol.*, 4: 267–282.

Siden, A. and Kjellin, K.G. (1978) CSF protein examinations with thin-layer isoelectric focusing in multiple sclerosis. *J. neurol. Sci.*, 39: 131–146.

Siegelman, M. and Capra, J.D. (1979) Immunoglobulin structure and function: idiotyping and the oligoclonal response. In D. Karcher, A. Lowenthal and A.D. Strosberg (Eds.), *Humoral Immunity in Neurological Diseases, Nato Advanced Study Institute Series, Series A: Life Sciences, Vol. 24,* Plenum, New York, pp. 303–318.

Siemes, H., Siegert, M., Hanefeld, F., Kölmel, H.W. and Paul, F. (1977) Oligoclonal gamma-globulin banding of cerebrospinal fluid in patients with subacute sclerosing panencephalitis. *J. neurol. Sci.*, 32: 395–409.

Silva, C.A., Rio, M.E. and Cruz, C. (1981) Protein patterns of the cerebrospinal fluid of 30 patients with subacute sclerosing panencephalitis. *Acta neurol. scand.*, 63: 255–266.

Stendahl-Brodin, L. and Link, H. (1980) Relation between benign course of multiple sclerosis and low-grade humoral immune response in cerebrospinal fluid. *J. neurol. neurosurg. psychiat.*, 43: 102–105.

Strosberg, A.D., Marescau, B., Thielemans, K., Vray, B., Karcher, D. and Lowenthal, A. (1979) Cross-idiotypic specificity among immunoglobulins in subacute sclerosing panencephalitis and multiple sclerosis. In D. Karcher, A. Lowenthal and A.D. Strosberg (Eds.), *Humoral Immunity in Neurological Diseases, Nato Advanced Study Institute Series, Series A: Life Sciences, Vol. 24,* Plenum, New York, pp. 97–103.

Ter Meulen, V. and Siddell, S. (1981) Virus infections of the nervous system: molecular, biological and pathogenetic considerations. In A.N. Davison and R.H.S. Thompson (Eds.), *The Molecular Basis of Neuropathology,* Edward Arnold, London, pp. 150–187.

Thompson, E.J., Kaufman, P., Shortman, R.C., Rudge, P. and McDonald, W.I. (1979) Oligoclonal immunoglobulins and plasma cells in spinal fluid of patients with multiple sclerosis. *Brit. Med., J.,* i: 16–17.

Tibbling, G., Link, H. and Öhman, S. (1977) Principles of albumin and IgG analyses in neurological disorders. I. Establishment of reference values. *Scand. J. Clin. lab. Invest.*, 37: 385–390.

Tourtellotte, W.W. (1970a) Cerebrospinal fluid in multiple sclerosis. In P.J. Vinken and G.W. Bruyn (Eds.), *Handbook of Clinical Neurology, Vol. 9,* North-Holland, Amsterdam, pp. 324–382.

Tourtellotte, W.W. (1970b) On cerebrospinal fluid immunoglobulin-G quotients in multiple sclerosis and other diseases. A review and a new formula to estimate the amount of IgG synthesized per day by the central nervous system. *J. neurol. Sci.*, 10: 279–304.

Tourtellotte, W.W. and Ma, B.I. (1978) Multiple sclerosis: the blood-brain-barrier and the measurement of de novo central nervous system IgG synthesis. *Neurology,* 28: 76–83.

Tourtellotte, W.W. and Potvin, A.R. (1981) Cytomorphology of multiple sclerosis cerebrospinal fluid cells, clinical activity and de novo central nervous system IgG synthesis. In *Abstracts of the 12th World Congress of Neurology, International Congress Series 548,* Excerpta Medica, Amsterdam, no. 86.

Tourtellotte, W.W., Potvin, A.R., Fleming, J.O., Murthy, K.N., Levy, J., Syndulko, K. and Potvin, J.H. (1980) Multiple sclerosis: measurement and validation of central nervous system IgG synthesis rate. *Neurology,* 30: 240–244.

Tourtellotte, W.W., Ma, B.I., Brandes, D.B., Walsh, M.J. and Potvin, A.R. (1981a) Quantification of de novo central nervous system IgG measles antibody synthesis in SSPE. *Ann. Neurol.,* 9: 551–556.

Tourtellotte, W.W., Ma, B.I., Ingram, T.S., Cowan, T.M. and Potvin, A.R. (1981b) Quantitative absorption of multiple sclerosis and cerebrospinal fluid IgG by MS plaque and periplaque tissue. In *Abstracts of the 12th World Congress of Neurology, International Congress Series 548,* Excerpta Medica, Amsterdam, no. 394.

Tourtellotte, W.W., Ma, B.I. and Potvin, A.R. (1981c) Positive correlation between multiple sclerosis IgG measles antibody concentration and central nervous system IgG synthesis rate. In *Abstracts of the 12th World Congress of Neurology, International Congress Series 548,* Excerpta Medica, Amsterdam, no. 431.

Traugott, V., Snyder, D.S. and Raine, C.S. (1979) Oligodendrocyte staining by multiple sclerosis serum is non-specific. *Ann. Neurol.,* 6: 13–20.

Trotter, J.L., Banks, G. and Wang, P. (1977) Isoelectric focusing of gamma globulins in cerebrospinal fluid from patients with multiple sclerosis. *Clin. Chem.,* 23: 2213–2215.

Valdimarsson, H., Agnarsdottir, G. and Lachmann, P.J. (1979) Subacute sclerosing panencephalitis. In F.C. Rose (Ed.), *Clinical Neuroimmunology,* Blackwell Scientific Publications, Oxford, pp. 406–418.

Vandvik, B. (1976) Oligoclonal measles virus-specific IgG antibodies isolated from sera of patients with subacute sclerosing panencephalitis. *Scand. J. Immunol.,* 6: 641–649.

Vandvik, B. (1977) Oligoclonal IgG and free light chains in the cerebrospinal fluid of patients with multiple sclerosis and infectious diseases of the central nervous system. *Scand. J. Immunol.,* 6: 913–922.

Vandvik, B. and Norrby, E. (1973) Oligoclonal IgG antibody response in the central nervous system to different measles virus antigens in subacute sclerosing panencephalitis. *Proc. nat. Acad. Sci. U.S.A.,* 70: 1060–1063.

Vandvik, B. and Norrby, E. (1980) Viral antibody responses in the central nervous system of patients with multiple sclerosis. In H. Bauer, S. Poser and G. Ritter (Eds.), *Progress in Multiple Sclerosis Research,* Springer, Berlin, pp. 256–262.

Vandvik, B. and Skrede, S. (1973) Electrophoretic examination of cerebrospinal fluid proteins in multiple sclerosis and other neurological diseases. *Europ. Neurol.,* 9: 224–241.

Vandvik, B., Froland, S.S., Hoyeraal, H.M., Stien, R. and Degré, M. (1973) Immunological features in a case of subacute sclerosing panencephalitis treated with transfer factor. *Scand. J. Immunol.,* 2: 367–374.

Vandvik, B., Natvig, J.G. and Wiger, D. (1976a) IgG1 subclass restriction of oligoclonal IgG from cerebrospinal fluids and brain extracts in patients with multiple sclerosis and subacute encephalitides. *Scand. J. Immunol.,* 5: 427–436.

Vandvik, B., Norrby, E., Nordal, H.J. and Degré, M. (1976b) Oligoclonal measles virus-specific IgG antibodies isolated from cerebrospinal fluids, brain extracts, and sera from patients with subacute sclerosing panencephalitis and multiple sclerosis. *Scand. J. Immunol.,* 5: 979–992.

Varitek, V.A. and Day, E.D. (1979) Relative affinity of antisera for myelin basic protein and degree of affinity heterogeneity. *Molec. Immunol.,* 16: 163–172.

Vartdal, F., Vandvik, B. and Norrby, E. (1980) Viral and bacterial antibody responses in multiple sclerosis. *Ann. Neurol.,* 8: 248–255.

Zeman, W. (1978) Subacute sclerosing panencephalitis. In P.J. Vinken and G.W. Bruyn (Eds.), *Handbook of Clinical Neurology. Vol. 34,* North-Holland Amsterdam, pp. 343–368.

Zettervall, O. and Link, H. (1970) Electrophoretic distribution of kappa and lambda immunoglobulin light chain determinants in serum and cerebrospinal fluid in multiple sclerosis. *Clin. exp. Immunol.,* 7: 365–372.

Subject Index